Cutting Edge of Ophthalmic Su

Ulrich Spandau · Gabor B. Scharioth
Editors

Cutting Edge of Ophthalmic Surgery

From Childhood Myopia to Robotic Vitrectomy
From Childhood Myopia to Carlevale IOL

Second Edition

Springer

Editors
Ulrich Spandau
Department of Ophthalmology
Stockholm University Hospital
University of Stockholm
Stockholm, Sweden

Gabor B. Scharioth
Aurelios Augenzentrum
Recklinghausen, Nordrhein-Westfalen, Germany

University of Szeged
Szeged, Hungary

ISBN 978-3-031-84203-0 ISBN 978-3-031-84204-7 (eBook)
https://doi.org/10.1007/978-3-031-84204-7

This Springer imprint is published by the registered company Springer Nature Switzerland AG
The registered company address is: Gewerbestrasse 11, 6330 Cham, Switzerland

Preface

This is the second edition of *Cutting Edge of Ophthalmic Surgery*. We have added several new hot topics such as Trans-PRK, Carlevale IOL, Myopia treatment, and not last but least the implantation of amniotic membrane in vitreoretinal surgery.

This book contains the most innovative and modern ocular surgery of the complete eye: from the cornea to the retina. Only leading surgeons and pioneers in their field present their surgery with videos and detailed step-by-step instructions.

Progressive myopia in children is a topic that is currently experiencing a rapid increase in interest. The authors have an out-patient department for myopic patients. This chapter describes the examination and non-surgical treatment of myopic patients from a practical perspective.

Refractive corneal surgery can be made as a surface treatment (PRK) or a stromal treatment (LASIK). *TransPRK* is the most recent surface treatment and is a one-step ablation that combines a reverse aspheric PRK and a phototherapeutic keratectomy (PTK). Dr. Diego de Ortueta (Recklinghausen, Germany) describes this technique with the AMARIS laser platform.

SMILE stands for *small incision lenticule extraction* and is the most recent revolution in corneal refractive surgery. During the SMILE procedure, the femtosecond laser cuts a lenticule inside the corneal stroma which is removed by a side incision. A corneal flap with all the negative side effects is no longer necessary. This technique was developed by the company Zeiss together with Prof. Sekundo (Marburg, Germany), Prof. Blum (Erfurt, Germany), and Prof. Meyer (Cologne, Germany). The authors describe the development of this new technique and demonstrate the surgery step by step.

In 2015, the German glaucoma patient association declared *canaloplasty* as the new gold standard in glaucoma surgery, as this operation combines good results with a low risk profile. Prof. Körber from Cologne, Germany, is a pioneer in the surgery of canaloplasty. During this surgery, an illuminated microcatheter is introduced in Schlemm's canal and the canal is then widened through injection of viscoelastics. Prof. Scharioth from Gelsenkirchen, Germany, will demonstrate a novel technique for canaloplasty using a special suture from Onatec (Onalene, Germany).

Iris surgery has made a huge leap forward with the advent of a foldable iris prosthesis from Human Optics, Germany, and new iris instruments from Geuder, Germany. The iris prosthesis enables the treatment of aniridia with a 2.5 mm incision and the new instruments allow a simple surgery for traumatic mydriasis. Asst. Prof. Spandau will demonstrate the surgical techniques step by step and show several videos.

The most exciting development in *cataract surgery* is surely the advent of the laser. Prof. Nagy from Budapest, Hungary, is a developer of femtosecond cataract surgery. He will present his technique step by step and show the pros and cons of this exciting new surgery. Prof. Sauder from Stuttgart, Germany, will demonstrate a novel phaco handpiece which removes the nucleus with laser instead of ultrasound. And finally, Dr. Nyström from Gothenburg, Sweden, will demonstrate congenital cataract surgery and implantation of a Tassignon IOL.

The amount of implanted *special lenses* has augmented dramatically in recent years. In this book, we will present two special lenses, the macula lens for improved reading ability and the add-on IOL. Prof. Scharioth from Recklinghausen, Germany, designed a novel macula lens which is implanted as a piggyback IOL and allows near vision for patients with AMD. Prof. Sauder from Stuttgart, Germany, will present the use and implantation of add-on IOLs for spherical, astigmatic, and presbyopic correction in pseudophakic eyes.

Glued IOL and the intrascleral IOL are the most common techniques for *secondary* IOL implantations. Prof. Scharioth from Recklinghausen, Germany, will present his famous technique of intrascleral IOL fixation and the modified glued IOL technique. (WEG? UND MIT CARLEVALE IOL ERSETZEN? UNSICHER, das Kapitel ist hervorragend geschrieben).

The *Carlevale IOL* is the first foldable IOL specially designed to be used for scleral fixation. The Carlevale IOL is currently one of the most popular techniques for secondary IOL implantations. The inventor will describe the surgical technique step-by-step.

The *usage of amnion membranes* is a current hot topic in vitreoretinal surgery. The indications are a large macular hole, PVR perforations, optic disc pit and morning glory syndrome. Dr. Spandau from Stockholm, Sweden, will demonstrate a vitrectomy with usage amnion membrane in a patient with retinal detachment.

Will *robotic surgery* be the future in ocular surgery? Dr. Charles Mango from New York, USA, will report on the latest state of robotic technology for eye surgery.

Ophthalmology has always been an innovative field. With constant development of technical innovations and surgical techniques, the potential for the future is unlimited.

Stockholm, Sweden — Ulrich Spandau
Recklinghausen, Germany — Gabor B. Scharioth

Contents

List of Videos

Endoscopic Lacrimal Duct Surgery

Video 1.1 Microdrill dacryoplasty of a buttonhole stenosis of the lacrimal sac (Dr. Ungerechts)

Video 1.2 Microdrill dacryoplasty of a subtotal stenosis of the nasolacrimal duct (Dr. Ungerechts)

Video 1.3 Saccus stenosis: Microdrill dacryoplasty of dacryoliths and scars in the lacrimal sac (Dr. Ungerechts)

Video 1.4 Inflammation: Polyps and bleeding in the lacrimal sac due to chronic dacryocystitis (Dr. Ungerechts)

Cornea: ReLex-SMILE

Video 3.1 Capless SMILE (Dr. Meyer)

Video 3.2 Perfect SMILE (Dr. Meyer)

Video 3.3 Suction loss (Dr. Meyer)

Glaucoma: Canaloplasty

Video 4.1 Canaloplasty (Prof. Scharioth)

Video 4.2 Canaloplasty with Onalene (Prof. Scharioth)

Video 5.1 Canaloplasty (Prof. Körber)

Video 5.2 Descemet window (Prof. Körber)

Video 5.3 Descemet rupture (Prof. Körber)

You Tube Videos for Canaloplasty

Introduction: https://www.youtube.com/watch?v=dDp_6iqgsqo

https://www.youtube.com/watch?v=cyD64ScCvyo&list=PLu4WoZG_17A29Zy6gy73ogYyhM1Ys_4Go (German language)

Iris

Video 6.1 Foldable iris and IOL prosthesis (very short version) (Prof. Spandau)

Video 6.2 Combo IOL-iris prosthesis (long version) (Prof. Spandau)

Video 6.3 Combo IOL iris prosthesis in lens capsule (short) (Prof. Spandau)

You Tube Videos for Iris Surgery
https://www.youtube.com/watch?v=oC4O0mW3yLY

Cataract

You Tube Videos for Femto Cataract
Introduction: https://www.youtube.com/watch?v=qCS1P_7Oiao
https://www.youtube.com/watch?v=SMi5TqWqBaU
https://www.youtube.com/watch?v=Znwa109owbo
https://www.youtube.com/watch?v=r5kwgxdI-SE (German language)

Premium IOL

Secondary IOL Implantation with Scharioth Technique

Secondary IOL Implantation with Iris-Claw IOL

Retina
Pediatric Vitrectomy with 27G TDC Cutter

About the Authors

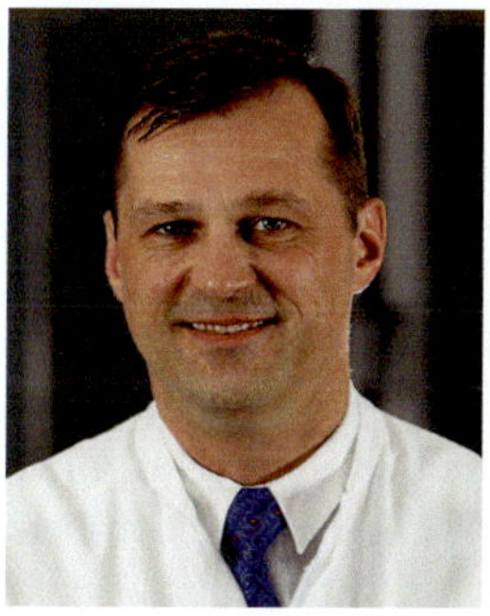

Marcus Blum, MD Marcus Blum is chairman of ophthalmology at the Helios Klinikum Erfurt GmbH, Germany. He graduated from Heidelberg University Medical School and was a resident at the Department of Ophthalmology in Heidelberg. From 1995 onwards, he was Fellow at the University of Jena and was appointed associate professor. In 2001, he became head of department in Erfurt. He was clinical investigator for several new technologies and published more than 100 papers. Together with Walter Sekundo, he was the first surgeon to perform FLEx and SMILE with a femtosecond laser.

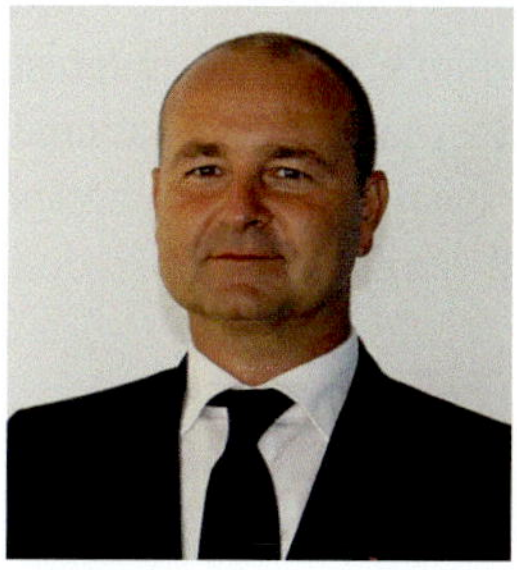

Carlo Carlevale, MD He graduated in Medicine and Surgery at "La Sapienza" Rome university, Majored in Ophthalmology at the Postgraduate School of Ophthalmology at "La Sapienza", University of Rome. He is Director of Ophthalmology Department at the "Karol Wojtyla Hospital" of Rome, and from 2001 till now he performs high volume surgeries mainly anterior segment. He is consultant surgeon at "Neuromed Hospital" in Pozzilli.

He developed the first flexible intraocular lens in the world with a sutureless scleral fixation system in 2011 and registered the relative trademark.

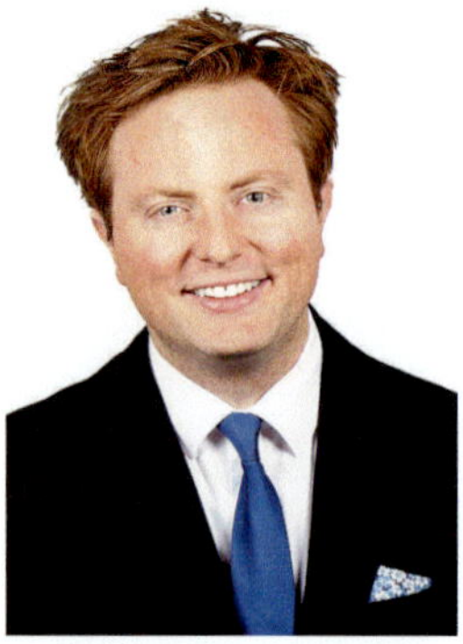

Dr. Gerhardt is a Clinician-Scientist and Head of the Clinical Study Center at the Department of Ophthalmology at Ludwig-Maximilians-University (LMU) Munich, Germany. His clinical focus is on diagnosing and treating vitreoretinal diseases, with a particular interest in inherited retinal diseases in children and gene therapy. The focus of his research is on developing minimal-invasive gene therapy approaches for age-related macular degeneration and inherited retinal dystrophies, along with the clinical characterization of retinopathies through deep phenotyping.

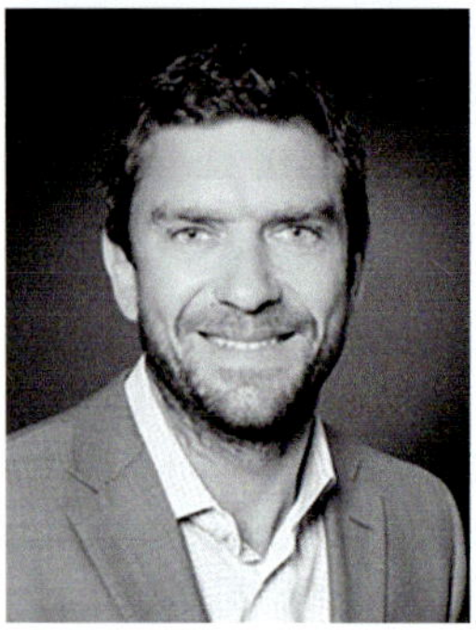

Jean-Pierre Hubschman, MD Jean-Pierre Hubschman is currently Associate Professor in Residence, Department of Ophthalmology, at the David Geffen School of Medicine—University of California Los Angeles (UCLA), Stein Eye Institute. Dr. Hubschman is also Chief of Retina at Olive View Medical Center at UCLA, and an Affiliate Faculty of the Bioengineering Department, Henry Samueli School of Engineering and Applied Science. Jean-Pierre Hubschman is the author of more than 100 peer-reviewed papers, numerous book chapters, and the principal investigator or co-investigator of several grants including the NIH and NEI institutes. Dr. Hubschman's research interest has focused, during the last 10 years on translational research in ophthalmology, specifically on robotics for ophthalmic surgery and surgical visualization improvement.

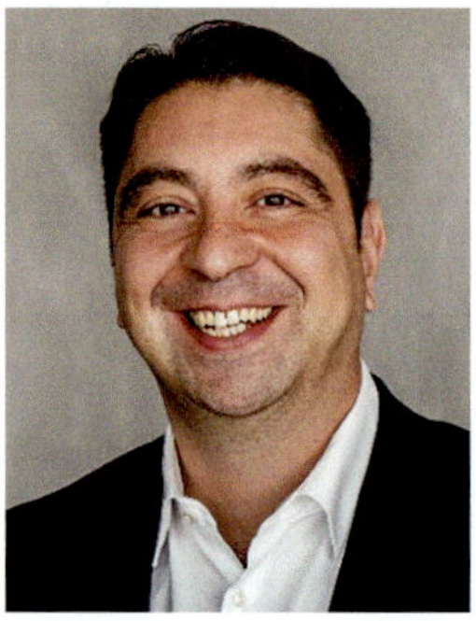

Hakan Kaymak, MD Prof. Hakan Kaymak, MD is a board-certified ophthalmologist & eye surgeon. He is head surgeon for the field of retina, macula and vitreous body at Breyer, Kaymak & Klabe Eye Surgery - one of the largest private ophthalmology practices in Germany.

He studied medicine at University of Tübingen and Heidelberg, and then specialized as Ophthalmologist and Ophthalmologic Surgeon.

Since 2017 he is head of the Macula and Retina Department of Breyer, Kaymak & Klabe in Düsseldorf, where he started in 2010 as partner and senior consultant ophthalmologist. Asides to his expertise in retinal diseases such as nAMD, he is also one of the leading experts for eye therapies including laser treatment, minimally invasive surgeries, and innovative therapies.

His personal interest lays in the field of myopia therapy. He already wrote his dissertation in 1999 on the effect of atropine on visual induced myopia in chicks and, starting in 2016, he was one of the first ophthalmologists in Germany to apply low-dose atropine therapy. Since late 2020 his new first-line choice for myopia therapy are the MiYOSMART lenses.

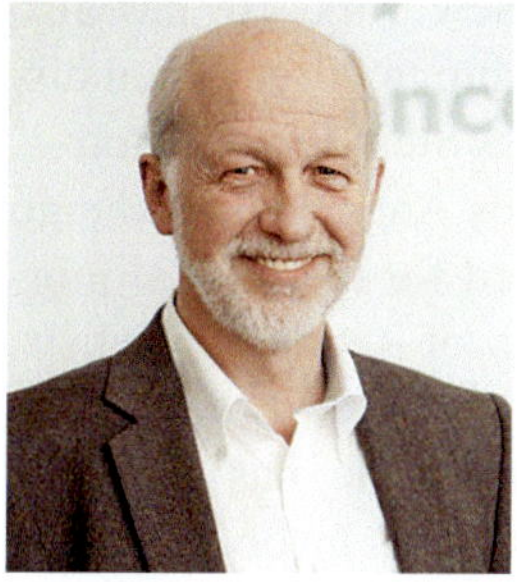

Norbert Körber, FEBO Norbert Körber is born in 1952 in Germany. He finished his medical studies (1972–1978) 1979 with a Ph.D. and 1984 he passed the exam as ophthalmologist. He is working in his own practice in Cologne since 1987; nowadays an ophthalmologic group practice with nine other colleagues. For > 25 years, he owned an ophthalmic outpatient surgery centre; a total of twelve surgeons are performing surgery in the centre (approximately 110000 intraocular cases per year). He specializes in cataract and glaucoma surgery.

He showed scientific activities in microcirculation and hemorheology and published about cataract surgery, refractive surgery, and glaucoma surgery.

(In total more than 150 publications and presentations.)

As guest professor, he has been teaching at the University Eye Hospital in Padova, Italy, since 2002 and is honorary member of the AISG (Italian Society on Studies of Glaucoma). Further memberships are at ESCRS, DGII, past chairman of the VOA North Rhine, and fellow of the European Board of Ophthalmologists.

His operative spectrum covers cataract, refractive IOLs, glaucoma surgery, vitrectomy, and oculoplastic surgery.

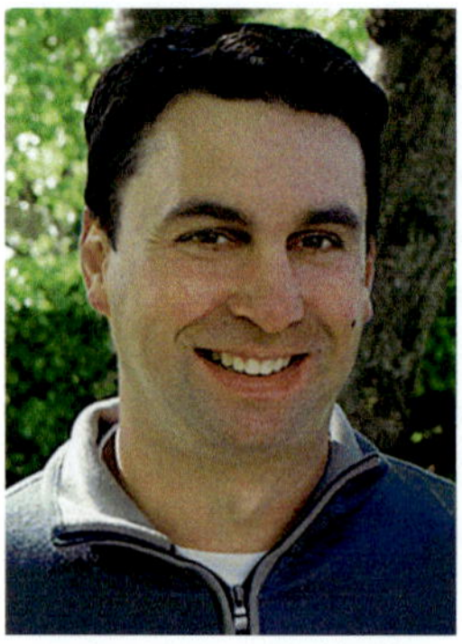

Charles W. Mango, MD Dr. Charles W. Mango is a Clinical Associate Professor of Ophthalmology at the Weill Cornell Medical College. He is a board-certified ophthalmologist whose clinical practice involves the medical and surgical management of vitreoretinal disorders. He is actively involved as a teaching professor in the vitreoretinal fellowship training program at New York Presbyterian Hospital. Dr. Mango completed a residency in Ophthalmology at the Weill Cornell Medical College—New York Presbyterian Hospital in New York. He has also completed a 2-year fellowship in vitreoretinal disease and surgery at the Jules Stein Eye Institute—University of California Los Angeles. Dr. Mango serves on the editorial board for the official journal of the American Society of Retina Specialists. He has published and contributes as a reviewer to the major scientific journals. He has authored multiple textbook chapters. He is involved in several scientific research projects, which include robotic ocular surgery, retinal imaging modalities, and evaluation of electronic advances in the field of retina. Dr. Mango has been a speaker and moderator at multiple national and international meetings. He has participated as a principal investigator and co-investigator in numerous clinical trials. Dr. Mango is a founder of the Vit-Buckle Society where he currently serves as an officer and executive board member. Will *robotic surgery* be the future in ocular surgery? Dr. Charles Mango from New York, USA, Jean-Pierre Hubschman from Los Angeles, USA, and Angelo Tsirbas from Sidney, Australia, will report on the latest state of robotic technology for eye surgery.

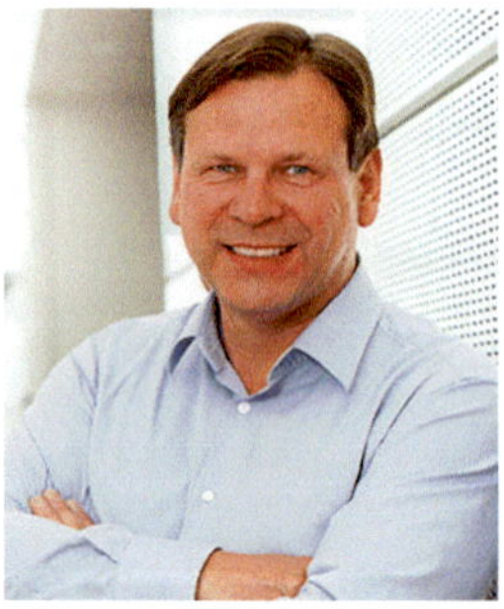

Bertram Meyer, MD Dr. Bertram Meyer is specialist in laser refractive surgery since 1992 and is performing SMILE procedures since 2010. He works in private clinics in Cologne and in Dubai. He gives continuous and regular lectures and updates during the annual meetings of DOG, DOC, DGII, and European Society of Cataract and Refractive Surgeons (ESCRS) about Femto-Lasik and ReLEx® SMILE. He is member of Advisory Board for Refractive Laser Surgery for Carl Zeiss Meditec for many years.

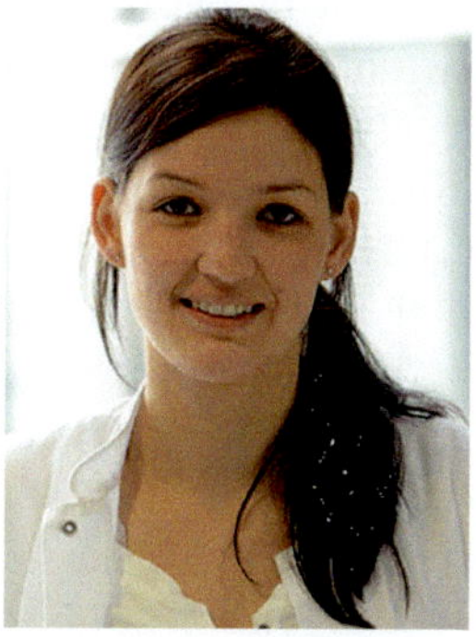

S. Mödl, MD Sarah Mödl is a senior registrar at the Eye Hospital Charlottenklinik in Stuttgart. She graduated from University of Ulm Medical School in 2010 and was afterwards a resident at Charlottenklinik. She performs cataract, oculoplastic and lacrimal surgery.

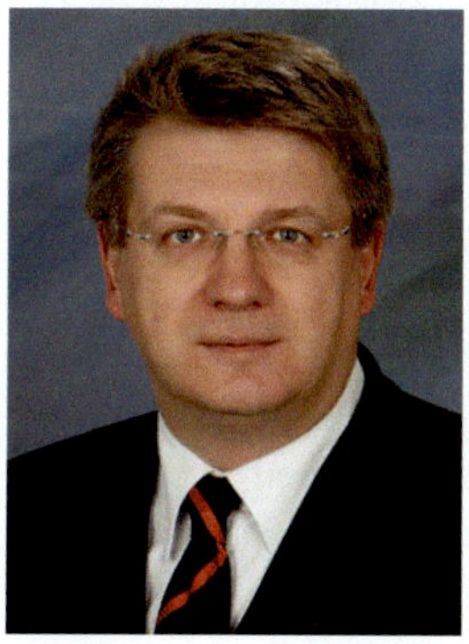

Zoltan Z Nagy, MD Zoltan Nagy has been working in ophthalmology since 1986. Currently he is the Head of the Department of Ophthalmology Semmelweis University, Budapest, Hungary, and serves as a Dean of the Faculty of Health Sciences. His main interest in ophthalmology is cataract and refractive surgery. He started refractive surgery first in Hungary in 1992, performed all kinds of refractive procedures: PRK, LASIK, epi-LASIK, LASEK, PTK, femto-LASIK, overall he operated more than 30,000 eyes with all kinds of refractive errors and more than 16,000 eyes with cataract. He discovered the role of harmful ultraviolet-B effect during corneal avascular wound healing, which has been published in Ophthalmology in 1997. He has published more than 139 articles in English and in Hungarian, contributed 5 books, and wrote 20 book chapters. Dr. Nagy was the first who performed femtolaser-assisted cataract surgery in the world in 2008. He has published more than 22 papers, 1 book, and 5 book chapters regarding the clinical results of femtolaser-assisted cataract surgeries in peer-reviewed ophthalmic journals since the first procedure. In 2010, he was awarded the Waring Medal for the best publication in Journal of Refractive Surgery. In 2012, he received the Casebeer Award from the International Society of Refractive Surgeons (ISRS) as a recognition of his pioneer role and scientific contribution in femtolaser-assisted cataract surgery. In 2014, he received the Presidential Award of the International Society of Refractive Surgeons. He is an invited speaker in many European and international congresses. He is a Board member of the Executive Board of the ISRS (International Society of Refractive

Surgeons) and a coopted member of the ESCRS Board (European Society of Cataract and Refractive Surgeons). Presently he serves as a President of the Hungarian Society of Cataract and Refractive Surgeons (SHIOL). He received an invitation to the Editorial Board of Journal of Cataract and Refractive Surgery in 2012 and also to the Journal of Refractive Surgery. The Semmelweis University awarded him with Jendrassik Prize in 2012, with Emil Grósz Prize in 2013, and he received the Batthyany-Strattmann Prize in 2014.

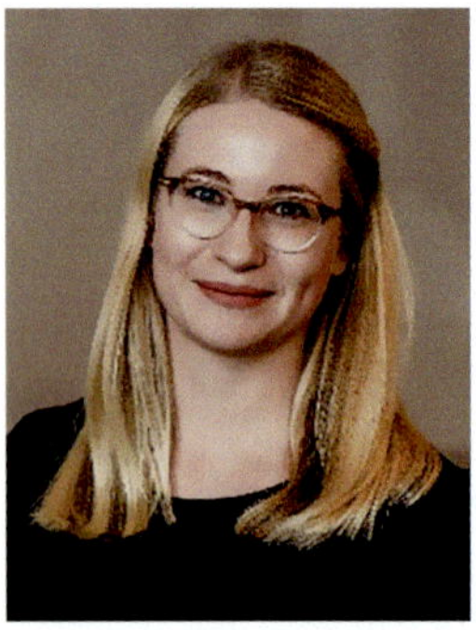

Birte Neller, Optometrist is a senior researcher at the private research lab Internationale Innovative Ophthalmochirurgie (I.I.O.) GbR at Breyer, Kaymak & Klabe Eye Surgery - one of the largest private ophthalmology practices in Germany.

2016 she finished her Bachelor's degree in Ophthalmic Optics & Optometry and in 2019 her Master's degree in Ophthalmic Optics & Psychophysics both at Aalen University, Germany.

Her research focuses on childhood myopia and treatments to inhibit myopia progression. In recent years, she has presented her work on this topic at several national and international conferences and thus built a reputation as a key opinion leader in myopia amongst well known researchers.

Alf Nyström, MD Dr. Alf Nyström works since 1992 as pediatric ophthalmologist at the University of Gothenburg, Sweden. He is responsible for congenital cataract and glaucoma. He operated approximately 2000 cases of congenital cataract (No photograph available).

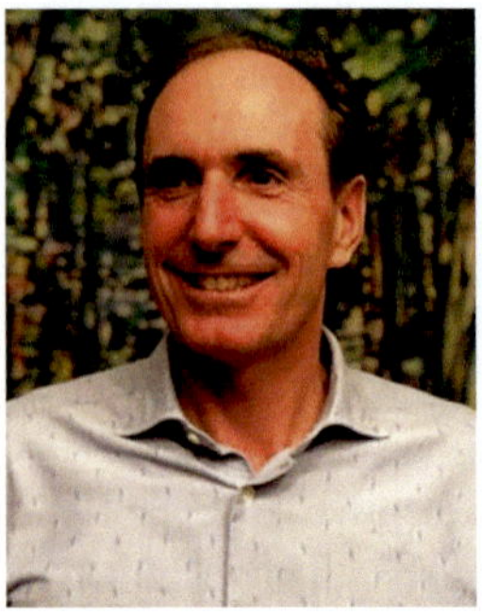

Diego de Ortueta, MD Diego de Ortueta is Consultant Chief Refractive department Aurelios Augenzentrum Recklinghausen since 2002 till now. He is born 1966 in Germany. He studied Medicine and wrote his PhD at the University of Navarra . He did his residency in Ophthalmology at the eye clinic Mülheim, University Düsseldorf. He is Fellow European Board Ophthalmology and Fellow World Refractive Surgeons. He published more than 50 articles about refractive surgery indexed in Pubmed or ORCID and is am reviewer of several ophthalmic indexed journals.

Dr. Diego de Ortueta is consultant and medical advisor for Schwind eye-tech solutions, Kleinostheim Germany

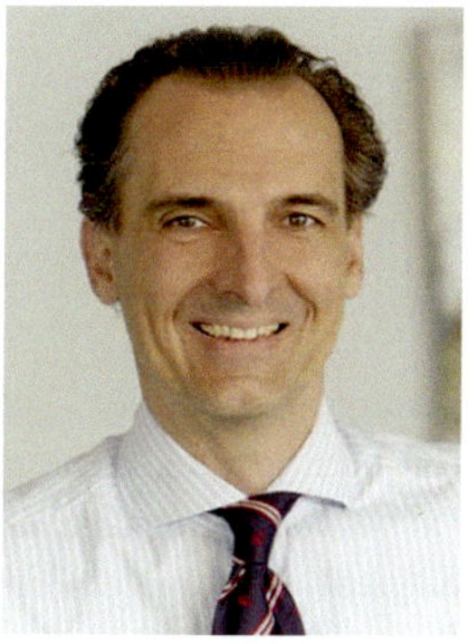

Gabor B. Scharioth, MD Gabor Scharioth graduated from Medical School in Humboldt University Berlin in 1993. During his residency program, he was trained in Augentagesklinik Groß-Pankow, Campus Virchow of University. Berlin, and Aravind Eye Hospitals, India. In 1998, he joined private practice in West Germany and founded Aurelios Eye Centers in 2004. His fields of expertise in ophthalmic surgery are cataract surgery, vitreoretinal surgery, reconstructive/trauma surgery, and modern glaucoma surgery. He has performed more than 30,000 surgeries during his career and trained many doctors around the world. He gave more than 250 scientific presentations at national and international conferences and performed more than 20 live surgeries at several international meetings around the world. Multiple scientific peer-reviewed publications are published and he was awarded several times at international meetings, including ASCRS, ESCRS, EVRS, and DOC. He is member of several ophthalmic organizations and scientific and advisory boards. During his professional career, he made several inventions like Scharioth Macula Lens for patients with advanced maculopathy, Glaucolight-assisted canaloplasty, microscope mounted angle viewing system, Light indentor for vitreoretinal surgery, and intrascleral haptic fixation of PCIOL in absence of capsular support. He was principal investigator and participated in multiple large prospective, multicenter studies. Since 2013, he is private professor at the University of Szeged in Hungary.

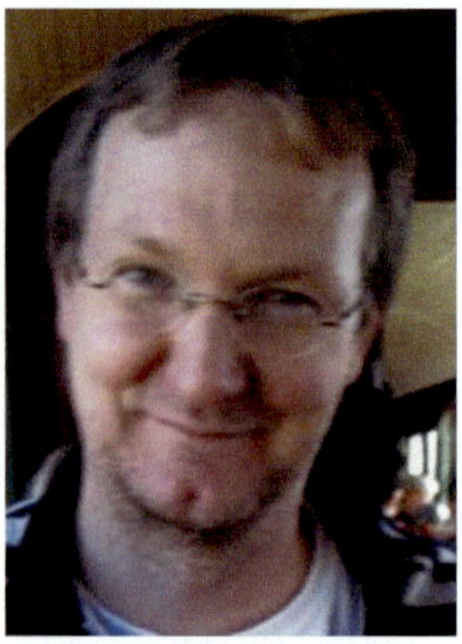

Lothar Schneider, MD Dr. Lothar Schneider works since 2011 at the University of Gothenburg, Sweden. He works with vitreoretinal and pediatric surgery.

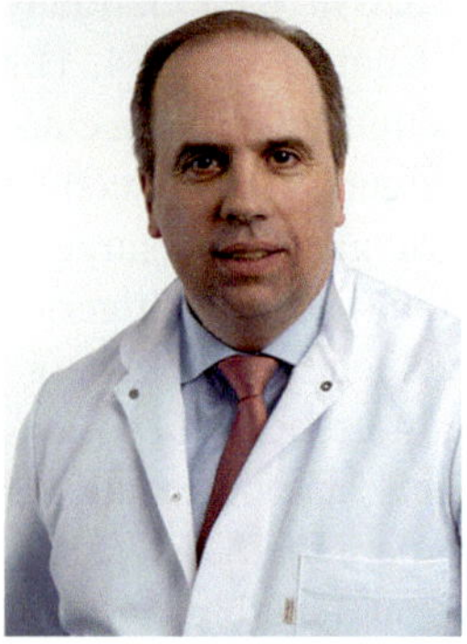

Gangolf Sauder, MD Gangolf Sauder is Director at the Eye Hospital Charlottenklinik in Stuttgart, Germany. He is a board-certified ophthalmologist, whose surgical management involves the complete ocular spectrum from oculoplastic surgery to vitreoretinal disorders.

Prof.Dr. Sauder studied medicine at the University of Bonn, Germany, from 1988 to 1994. He completed his residency in Ophthalmology at the Stiftsklinikum in Koblenz, Germany. He worked as Vice-Director at the University of Heidelberg-Mannheim from 2000 to 2006. Since 2006, he is Director at the Charlottenklinik in Stuttgart. A total of 6 surgeons are performing surgery at this hospital. Annually, the Charlottenklinik performs 8000 cataract surgeries, 600 glaucoma surgeries, and 1400 vitreoretinal surgeries.

Prof. Sauder operated more than 800 patients with Add-On IOL and performed more than 3000 cases of laser phaco.

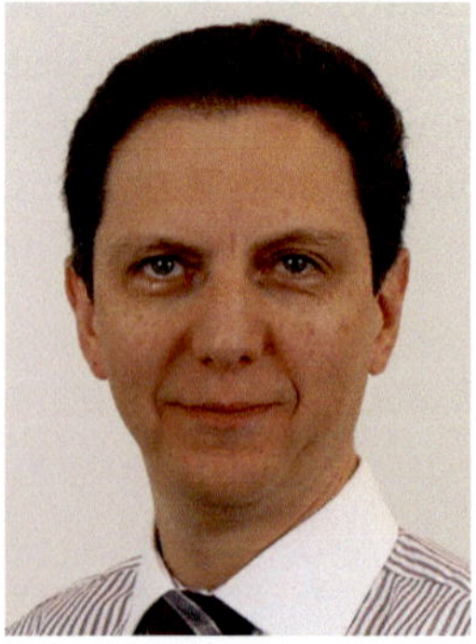

Walter Sekundo, MD Prof. Dr.med. Walter Sekundo is Professor and Chairman, Department of Ophthalmology, Philipps University of Marburg, Germany. He studied Medicine in Frankfurt (Germany), New Orleans and Durham (USA). He was a resident at the University of Bonn in Germany and a Fellow in Corneal and Refractive surgery at Moorfields Eyes Hospital (UK) and Ocular Pathology at the University of Glasgow, UK. He also has a degree of "Health

Care Manager". Prof. Sekundo has published over 100 original papers, 29 book chapters and is an editor of the newly appeared textbook on SMILE surgery. He gave over 300 presentations at national and international meetings. He is a reviewer for 21 Ophthalmic Journals and a Board Member of "Der Ophthalmologe". Prof. Sekundo performed over 20,000 surgical procedures in the entire field of ophthalmology and has been repeatedly named as one of the 30 top refractive and cataract surgeons in Germany. He was the first surgeon in the world who performed FLEx and SMILE.

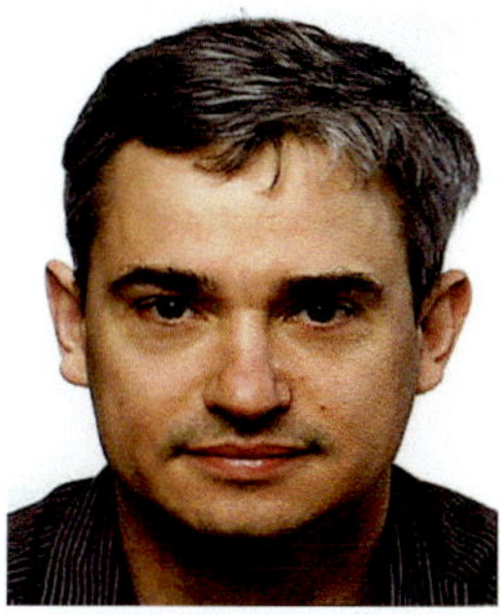

Ulrich Spandau, MD Ulrich Spandau is Assistant Professor at the University of Uppsala, Sweden. He is head of ocular surgery and works mainly as vitreoretinal surgeon. His special surgical interest is the diagnosis and treatment of vitreoretinal diseases of newborn.Dr. Spandau was born 1968 in Grahamstown, South Africa, and moved to Germany in 1978. He studied at the Medical School of the University of Wuerzburg, Germany. He completed his ophthalmological residency at the University of Heidelberg and his surgical education at the Stiftsklinikum in Koblenz and the University of Mannheim, Germany. In 2008, he moved to Uppsala, Sweden, to learn modern VR surgery. He works currently at the University clinic of Stockholm. Dr. Spandau is author of the textbooks Small Gauge Vitrectomy. A Practical Handbook, Complications During and After Cataract Surgery, Small Gauge Vitrectomy for Diabetic Retinopathy and 27G Vitrectomy and many more.

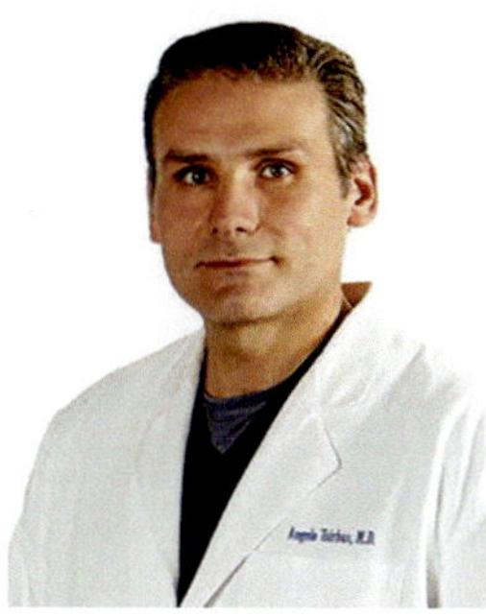

Angelo Tsirbas, MD Dr. Angelo Tsirbas is a world-renowned ophthalmic facial plastic and reconstructive surgeon with a distinguished background. He was trained in Australia and then worked in NYC and Los Angeles for many years. During his time as faculty professor at UCLA, he maintained a private aesthetic practice based in Beverly Hills. Dr. Tsirbas is sought after by patients from around the world for help in correcting some of the most challenging complicated cases with his innovative surgical techniques. Dr. Tsirbas popularized modern endoscopic lacrimal surgery in the ophthalmic and oculoplastic community. He developed surgical techniques in the 1990s that are still used all around the world today. His work now specializes in obtaining the finest and most natural results for blepharoplasty, brow-lift, and aging facial surgery. The demand for his expertise in functional, reconstruction, revision, and cosmetic surgery has also found him consulting all across Australia. Dr. Tsirbas is based in the heart of Sydney's beautiful Harbour district.

Part I
Myopia: Non-surgical Treatment of Myopia

Myopia and especially childhood myopia is a fast growing health hazard. Myopia is defined as SE < –0.5 D and high myopia as SE < –5 D. The worldwide prevalence of myopia is around 30%. A recent study from Korea, however, examined 19 y/o male conscripts and reports a 96% prevalence of myopia and 21% of high myopia [1]. In addition, a study from the UK reports that in children aged between 10 and 16 the proportion of myopes has more than doubled over the last 50 years [2]. The latter study indicates that urbanization and education rather than geographic variation may play more important roles in myopia etiology.

Birte Neller and Prof. Hakan Kaymak (Düsseldorf, Germany) have an out-patient department for myopic patients. This chapter describes the examination and non-surgical treatment of myopic patients from a hand-on perspective.

References

1. Jung SK, Lee JH, Kakizaki H, Jee D. Prevalence of myopia and its association with body stature and educational level in 19-year-old male conscripts in Seoul, South Korea. Invest Ophthalmol Vis Sci. 2012;53(9):5579.
2. McCullough SJ, O'Donoghue L, Saunders KJ. Six year refractive change among white children and young adults: evidence for significant increase in myopia among white UK children. PLoS One. 2016;11(1):e0146332.

Progressive Childhood Myopia: Treatment Options and Clinical Experience from a Specialist Myopia Clinic

1

Birte Neller and Hakan Kaymak

Abstract

Progressive myopia in children is a topic that is currently experiencing a rapid increase in interest. While research on this topic dates back to the nineteenth century, it has now reached the masses thanks to new treatment options. This chapter reviews different treatment options and evaluates their efficacy in terms of a universal target criterion: the age-matched physiological axial length growth. In addition to background knowledge, practitioners are provided with practical suggestions and helpful tools for implementing, performing and monitoring myopia treatment. By way of introduction, the authors would like to point out that this chapter deals with axial myopia, which develops in childhood or adolescence and progresses from then on. It must be differentiated from congenital syndromic myopia and also from refractive myopia, such as occurs with steep corneal radii.

Keywords

Progressive myopia · Low-dose atropine · Multifocal contact lenses · Spectacle lenses · Axial length · Biometry · Refraction · Physiological growth · Emmetropization

Findings on Myopia from the Nineteenth Century

As early as the nineteenth century, H. Cohn (1838–1906) had carried out and collected epidemiological studies on the prevalence and severity of myopia in various (type of) schools [1].

He found higher prevalence of myopia firstly in urban schools with higher levels of education and secondly in higher grades versus lower grades. Follow-up examinations revealed increasing level of myopia with increasing age and time spent on education. Correspondingly high prevalences of myopia were found at universities in degree programs attended by graduates of schools with higher levels of education, which also place intensive learning demands on

B. Neller · H. Kaymak (✉)
Internationale Innovative Ophthalmochirurgie, Breyer Kaymak Klabe Augenchirurgie, Düsseldorf, Germany
e-mail: dr.h.kaymak@gmail.com

B. Neller
Institute of Experimental Ophthalmology, Saarland University, Homburg, Germany

H. Kaymak
Gottfried O.H. Naumann-Institute of Epidemiology und Prevention of Myopia, Saarland University, Homburg, Germany

U. Spandau and G. B. Schariot (eds.), *Cutting Edge of Ophthalmic Surgery*,
https://doi.org/10.1007/978-3-031-84204-7_1

students, namely philosophy, theology, medicine, and law. Prevalence was significantly lower among craftsmen or farmers, who tend to carry out manual work, often outdoors. Cohn also notes that the earlier myopia begins, the greater the risk that it will eventually reach high levels.

Even then, H. Cohn named "reading and writing in poor lighting […] and excessive hours of consecutive reading and writing" as the main reason for the development and progression of myopia. He aptly described this myopia as "school myopia," a term that still describes the exact same aetiology of myopia today.

Why Should Progression Myopia Be Inhibited?

While in the past the main problem with myopia was that not all of those affected could be adequately fitted with visual aids and therefore suffered from low visual acuity, the structural consequences of (high) myopia were already recognized at that time: Already 1886 F. C. Donders (1818–1889) concluded that a myopic eye was a "diseased eye" [2]. He emphasized that "any progressive myopia was a concern for the future, because if it remained progressive, vision would soon deteriorate and not infrequently be irretrievably lost by the age of 50 or 60, if not much earlier, either by retinal detachment or hemorrhage, or eventually by atrophy and degeneration of the macula" [2]. By now, the increased risk of eye diseases in adulthood [3–5], such as i.e. glaucoma [6], earlier development of cataract [7], retinal detachment [8], myopic maculopathy [9, 10], choroidal neovascularization [11] and posterior staphyloma [12], in myopic eyes has been proven many times over.

Fortunately, modern therapeutic and surgical treatments can counteract or delay visual impairment, so Donders' statement needs to be put into perspective. Also the problem of undersupply with visual aids is no longer an issue today. However, for the sake of overall eye health, it would be beneficial to prevent these complications of pathological myopia from occurring by preventing myopia from becoming "too" high in the first place. It should be noted that there is no safe level of myopia and that also at low and moderate levels, the risk of eye diseases increases [3]. Early onset of myopia is associated with high myopia later in life [13, 14]. Therefore, myopia treatment should be started early to inhibit myopia progression and thus facilitate a higher quality of life in the long term. Eventually, every diopter saved reduces the risk of various myopia-related complications [15].

Consequently, to the epidemiological studies on myopia in schools, Cohn has also already given some thoughts to treatment options and defined the requirements for a healthy workplace: Together with various ergonomic aspects, he emphasizes the distance from the eye to the table top. He also points out that visual acuity drops in poor lighting conditions, resulting in a shorter reading distance, and therefore demands bright lighting. All of these points still apply to today's world to be, i.e. in [16–18].

Physiological Development Versus Myopic Development of the Eye During Childhood

After emmetropization, the physiological development of the eye, i.e. in eyes that remain emmetropic, is mainly characterized by the following changes [19–21]:

(1) thinning, flattening, and thus decreasing power of crystalline lens
(2) growth in axial length.

In doing so, the loss of lens power compensates for the physiological growth in axial length to maintain emmetropia [19–21]. This means that in emmetropic eyes, there is an age-dependent physiological growth in axial length (up to a certain age), while refraction does not change or hardly changes at all.

In children who become myopic, however, the lens stops thinning, flattening, and losing power within ± 1 year of myopia onset [19].

It has been hypothesized that development of myopia is caused by an inability to balance the refractive power (mainly by crystalline lens) and length of the eye to maintain emmetropia [22]. The axial length grows longer, the lens exhausts its compensatory capabilities, and this imbalance results in a myopic refractive error, which increases as the axial length continues to grow [20]. Unlike the physiological growth rate, which decreases over time and eventually stagnates near zero as the absolute axial length stabilizes, this appears to fail in myopic eyes, showing increased growth rate with little or no decrease [23].

By performing regular biometric measurements at an early stage, the development of myopia can be detected before it occurs in terms of refractive error [20, 24]. It is therefore useful to measure the biometry (in particular axial length) at any time, before the onset of myopia as well as after the onset.

Implementation of a Treatment

Which Examinations and Measurements Should Be Carried Out?

The pathophysiological mechanism for the development of myopia delivers two parameters that need to be measured and monitored: refraction and axial length, who are highly correlated. Both parameters have advantages and disadvantages but are indispensable for myopia management. A follow-up control visit should be carried out at least every 12 months, preferably every 6 months.

Refraction: When measuring refraction to quantify myopia, objective refraction is preferable to subjective refraction. However, a subjective fine adjustment should be made before prescribing spectacles. Objective refraction should be carried out under cycloplegia to avoid accommodation during the measurement and thus incorrect measurements. Refraction is a value that is usually known to parents, which makes communication easier.

However, refraction is merely a description of the optical (mis)conditions in the eye, i.e. the interaction of the refractive components and length of the eye. Therefore, refraction only provides limited information about the origin of myopia, i.e. whether axial myopia or refractive myopia is present.

Axial length: Firstly, axial length growth is the main determining factor of development of myopia and, ultimately, the goal of myopia treatment is to minimize the risk of pathological myopia. The cause of the anatomical changes in pathological myopia is excessive axial length growth, which is why this parameter is essential.

Axial length can be measured without cycloplegia, as this is largely unaffected by the accommodative state of the lens. With the development of modern optical biometers, such as those used for IOL calculation in cataract surgery, axial length can be measured easy, quickly, and contact-free. The devices currently available have satisfactory repeatability, even when measuring in children [25]. With their high repeatability, they are more sensitive to change than refraction [26]. However, it is important to ensure that the same device is always used, as the different devices sometimes give different values due to their different measurement methods [25]. Measurement of axial length by ultrasound is not recommended as they fail to achieve the required accuracy for myopia management.

In combination with refraction, axial length can be used to assess which components contribute to myopia and to what extent. It is important to know whether axial myopia is present, at least in part, when initiating treatment, as current treatment methods target to inhibit axial length growth. Refractive myopia, e.g. due to steep corneal radii, should be monitored otherwise (keratoconus screening).

Further useful examinations:

- To ensure that the child's eyes health, an orthoptic status should be obtained at least when initiating treatment.
- In addition, it makes sense to perform an OCT and a fundus photograph in children who are already highly myopic in order to detect and document pathological changes at an early stage.
- If treatment with atropine is an option, the pupil size and accommodative performance could also be monitored. In everyday clinical practice, however, it has been shown that these two examinations are of little value in determining whether a child can cope with the atropine eye drops or not.

How to Monitor the Progression of Myopia?

For precise evaluation of myopia progression, the axial length is more suitable than the refraction, as a change in axial length is not immediately reflected in the refraction (masked by compensatory refractive changes in the anterior segment of the eye, for example) [19].

The treatment goal for axial length growth should be based on age- and sex-specific physiological axial length growth, which is underlying the excessive myopic growth. The fact that physiological axial length growth is age-dependent means that a single threshold value (e.g. 0.2 mm per year) is not adequate for an accurate assessment of myopia progression [27].

A practical tool for assessing axial length growth based on physiological axial length growth is offered by Myopia Solutions (www.myopia-solutions.com), featuring the AMMC (Age-Matched Myopia Control) system. In addition to the familiar presentation of axial length measurements in percentile curves, this free, web-based online tool calculates the annual axial length growth rate from the axial length measurements entered and compares this with physiological growth. The implemented AMMC system is based on physiological axial growth rate, i.e. axial length growth as a function of age. Depending on how closely the observed annual axial length growth of a child's eyes approaches the physiological axial length growth rate, a conclusion can be made about the current treatment concept [27]. The color coding of the AMMC system provides the user with a classification of the axial length growth that has taken place at a glance (Fig. 1.1):

- The green zone describes an uncritical axial length growth rate, corresponding to physiological axial length growth (within a + 25% boundary to cover for variability in measurement). If the observed annual axial length growth rate is in the green zone, this means that there is no need for treatment at this time.
- The yellow zone describes a moderately excessive axial length growth rate in the range of + 25 to + 50% above the age-matched physiological AL growth rate, which means that a treatment is recommended.
- The red zone describes a highly excessive AL growth rate that is more than + 50% above the age-matched physiological AL growth rate. In the case of an annual axial length growth rate landing in red zone, a treatment is strongly recommended.

When Should Myopia Treatment Be Started and How Long Should It Last?

As there is no safe level of myopia, a treatment should be started as soon as a diagnosis of (at least partial) axial myopia has been made. Waiting to see if there is progression, or even severe progression, wastes valuable time and increases the risk of complications later in life. In fact, an axial myopic eye must have already undergone progression in the past, otherwise there would not be this imbalance between refractive power and axial length.

Due to the high prevalence of myopic children in Asia, the approach of treating even emmetropic children with low-dose atropine is being investigated to possibly delay or even prevent the onset of myopia [28, 29]. This is done

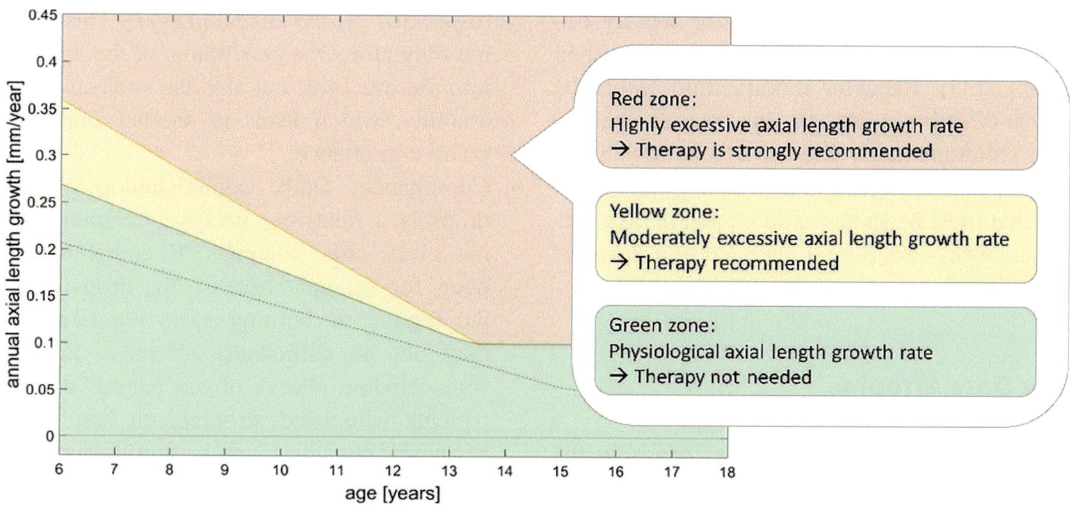

Fig. 1.1 The color-coded AMMC (age-matched myopia control) system: depending on the colour of the zone in which the observed annual axial length growth falls, a conclusion can be drawn about the effectiveness of the current treatment concept

under the assumption that most of them would become myopic anyway, which is why only a small proportion would be treated unnecessarily [30]. Therein the hyperopic reserve plays a crucial role in identifying those children who are at high risk of developing myopia [31].

> Key facts for implementation and monitoring of myopia treatment
>
> - Start upon diagnosis of (axial) myopia
> - Follow-up visit every 6 months, but at least every 12 months
> - Measurement of **refraction** and **axial length** at each visit
> - Treatment goal: age- and sex-matched physiological axial length growth (e.g. with www.myopia-solutions.com).

As most large clinical trials are ongoing and continue to provide more data, little is known about the optimal duration that treatment should be administered. What is known is that children with early myopia onset have a higher risk of further progression [20, 32, 33]. Stopping treatment too "early" can again lead to myopia progression and increased axial length growth [34]. To be on the safe side, any myopia treatment should be continued until stable physiological axial length growth has been achieved. Due to the critical phase of higher axial length growth up to around 15 years of age, treatment should be carried out until the late teenage years.

Treatment Options

While ideally the onset of myopia would be prevented or delayed, current treatment methods focus mainly on slowing the progression of myopia. The following describes various treatment approaches currently in use:

Behavior Modification

As lot of near work (reading, tablet use etc.) and time spent indoor is associated with high prevalence rates of myopia, encouraging outdoor activities, limiting time and implementing regular breaks of near work could delay the onset the myopia and thus its final level [35]. It is uncertain whether more outdoor activity can also inhibit progression of already established myopia [35]. Behavior modification would be a cost-effective approach, but not compatible with children's daily life on a voluntary basis. Government-mandated breaks during the school day that must be spent outdoors and breaks during the near-work period have led to a decrease in the prevalence of myopia in Taiwan [36].

Low-Dose Atropine

Low-dose atropine eye drops are probably the oldest myopia treatment [1] and are widely used to slow myopia progression. There are several possible approaches to the mechanism by which atropine inhibits axial growth, but the actual mechanism of action remains unclear [37, 38]. Atropine drops are applied once in the evening (1 drop per eye). The advantage of this is that disturbing ocular side effects such as dilated pupil or reduced accommodation mainly occur when the eye is closed because the child is asleep. It is known that the higher the dose, the better the inhibition of myopia progression [39, 40]. However, high-dose atropine showed a strong rebound effect after discontinuation [41] and the higher the dose, the more likely children are to notice disturbing ocular side effects. Because of the favorable side effect profile [42] and consistent beneficial effect [40], 0.01% atropine eye drops are commonly used. However, some publications question the efficacy of this dosage [39, 43]. A higher dosage, e.g. 0.025%, has shown a better effect in terms of myopia inhibition with questionably disturbing ocular side effects [39, 44].

In addition, there are a few other critical points to consider with atropine treatment:

- Formulation: To date, there is no approved atropine solution on the market in Europe and therefore the atropine solutions used come from different compounding pharmacies. The lack of a standardized solution leads to variation between the formulations, e.g. with regard to pH-value, osmolarity, ingredients (especially preservatives) [45–47]. This could not only affect the penetration of the atropine into the eye [48], but also the subjective tolerability, which leads to another important point: compliance.
- Compliance: Daily administration of eye drops is a relatively invasive treatment that not every child tolerates. If compliance is poor, for example because the drops create the feeling of burning eyes, the treatment may not be sufficiently effective. In fact, some random checks of the records of own patients who used atropine, on how much atropine was left in their supply and how often new prescriptions were picked up, led to the suspicion that atropine use was not as regular as claimed [49].
- Administration: Along with the lack of standardized formulation of atropine drops, the available products of compounding pharmacies also vary in their dosage form and therefore also in drop size. The statement "put one drop in each eye daily in the evening" is therefore inadequate. It is understandable that a smaller drop brings less active ingredient into the eye, but a drop that is too large may not be absorbed by the child's eye and the active ingredient is more likely to be washed out than to penetrate the eye.

> Key facts for low-dose atropine treatment:
>
> - application of 1 drop in each eye in the evening
> - invasive treatment
> - the higher the dose, the greater the effect but also the side effects
> - high variability in available compounded solutions.

Figure 1.2 shows the results of two different studies of low-dose atropine using the AMMC system. The plotted values describe the mean age after one year of treatment and the axial length growth measured during this time for each study arm.

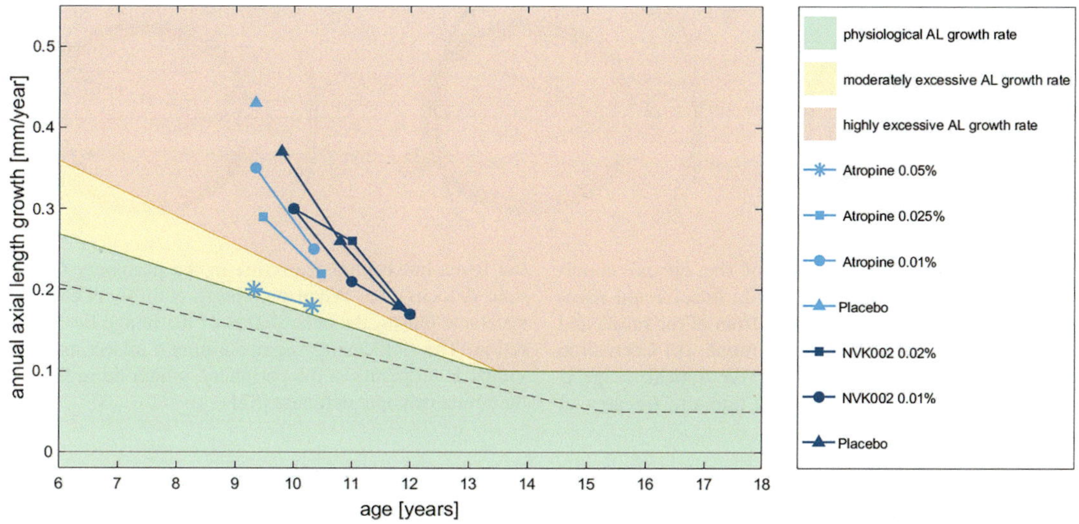

Fig. 1.2 Results of two different studies of low-dose atropine: LAMP study [44] and NVK002 by Vyluma [50]

1. 2-year results of LAMP Study by Yam et al. [44] testing atropine 0.05%, atropine 0.025%, atropine 0.01% versus placebo (only data available for one year, because placebo switched to atropine 0.05% in the second year).
2. 3-year results of NVK002 (Vyluma) 0.01 and 0.02% atropine versus placebo by Zadnik et al. [50].

The results of the LAMP study [44] clearly show the dose dependent effect of atropine: The higher the dose, the closer the average annual growth to the green zone. Puzzlingly, contrary to the well-established finding of this dose-dependency, this effect was not seen in the study with NVK002 [50], where 0.01% and 0.02% showed similar efficacy. Common to both studies is that 0.01% and 0.02%/0.025% did not achieve the treatment goal of physiological growth in axial length. Only 0.05% atropine gave acceptable results regarding this treatment goal.

Optical Treatment Options

Please note that the list of products is not exhaustive and not all products are available in all countries.

Most optical treatment options currently available are based on the approach of imposing myopic defocus on peripheral retina: From animal studies it is known that myopic defocus on the retina (focus in front of the retina) induced by positive lenses inhibits axial length growth, whereas hyperopic defocus (focus behind the retina) induced by negative lenses promotes growth [51]. Depending on the optical design, a second image is created in front of the peripheral retina, or the image is "bent" so that it lies in front of the peripheral retina (Fig. 1.3).

All optical treatments have the advantage that an optical correction of the myopic refractive error is required anyway. This means that children receive myopia correction and treatment in one.

Orthokeratology lenses

This non-surgical approach involves wearing specially designed gas permeable contact lenses overnight to temporarily modulate the elastic cornea to correct refractive error. This is done by flattening the central cornea for distance correction. Doing so, a bulge of tissue around the central zone is created, in which the cornea is

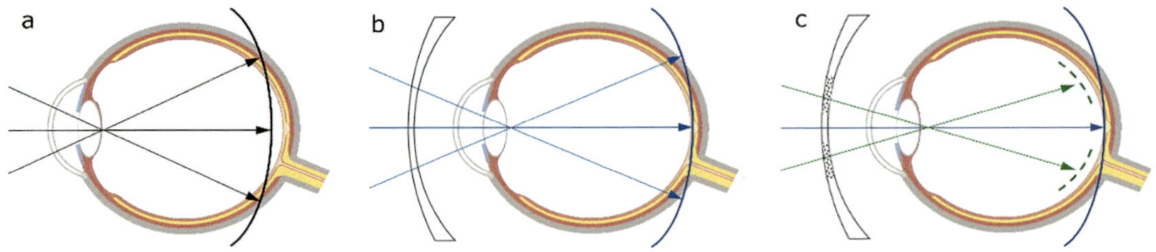

Fig. 1.3 Schematic presentation of the optical conditions in the eye (not to scale): (a) In uncorrected myopia the image shell lies centrally in front of the retina and in the periphery partly behind the retina. (b) Correction with a conventional spectacle lens, the optical image is shifted so that it is centered on the retina in the area of the fovea but behind the retina in the periphery (hyperopic defocus). (c) When correcting with MiYOSMART spectacle lenses, the central area of the image lies on the retina. The defocusing segments create additional individual focal points in the periphery, which lie in front of the retina (myopic defocus) [52]

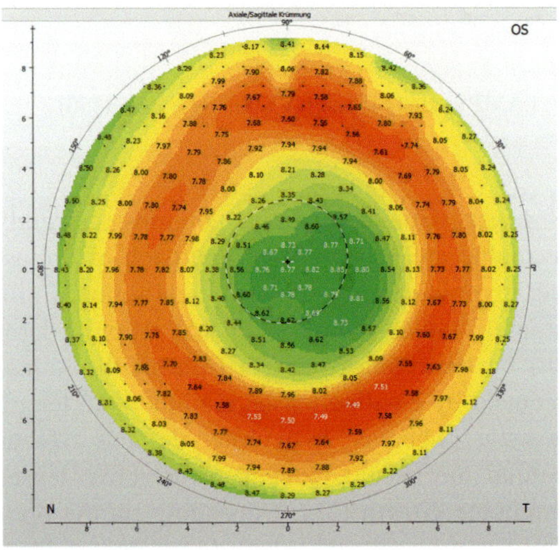

Fig. 1.4 Topographic map of cornea modulated after use of Orthokeratology lenses

thicker and more steeply curved (Fig. 1.4). This refracts the light more strongly and the image is "bent" in front of the retina in the corresponding peripheral area. Examples of orthokeratology lenses that are used in myopia control are (*with CE approval for myopia management in Europe; $^{+}$with U.S. FDA approval for myopia management): DreamLite MC (CooperVision)*, Bloom Night (Menicon)*, Abiliti Overnight Therapeutic Lenses (Johnson & Johnson)$^{+}$, Paragon CRT (CooperVision)$^{+}$, FOK MC (Falco), Luna (Galifa), myLIFE seefree (Hecht), NightFlex (SwissLens), Sleeplens (Techlens), Oke (Wöhlk).The ability of orthokeratology lenses to inhibit myopia progression has been known for a long time. Accordingly, there are numerous (long term) studies on efficacy and safety [53–55].

Caution:

To wear these contact lenses successfully in the long term and benefit from the myopia control effect, all types of contact lenses require a high level of handling and hygiene. Parents and children should be informed about the risks and symptoms of contact lens-related diseases during or before fitting.

Contact lenses

In soft and rigid contact lenses there are different variations of how an additional image is created in front of the retina, which are very similar to the designs of multifocal lenses for the correction of presbyopia (Fig. 1.5). Thus, there are lenses that implement the additional defocus via concentric rings that surround a clear zone (i.e. MiSight (CooperVision), Acuvue Abiliti 1-Day (Johnson & Johnson), proASSIST (Appenzeller), myLIFE (Hecht)), while other lenses utilise the "Extended Depth Of Focus (EDOF)"-Technology i.e. Mylo (Markennovy), Bloom Day (Menicon), or use a progressive design (i.e. Scalia2 (Galifa)). In fact, there are also approaches to use common multifocal lenses, originally intended for presbyopia correction [56].

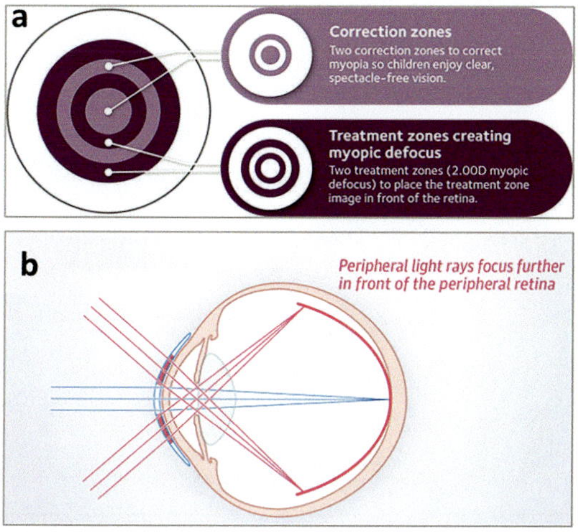

Fig. 1.5 Myopia control soft contact lenses (a) MiSight (CooperVision) [57], (b) Biofinity multifocal high add (CooperVision) [56]

Key facts for contact lens treatment:

- optical correction of myopia needed anyway
- available in soft, rigid and orthokeratology contact lenses
- high demands on hygiene and handling
- invasive treatment
- should be worn every waking hour for best effect.

Spectacle lenses

Spectacle lenses are the latest development in optical treatment options. Due to its simplicity, this treatment option is probably the most widely used of the optical treatment options currently available. There are two ways to induce peripheral myopic defocus in spectacle lenses: either (1) as an additional power circularly around a defocus free zone with distance correction, or (2) as a progressive design with increasing power towards the periphery of the lens.

(1) These myopia control spectacle lenses correct the refractive error over the entire lens surface and at the same time provide targeted defocusing in the retinal periphery with additional multiple lens segments, i.e. MiYOSMART (Hoya), Stellest (Essilor) and MyoCare (Zeiss). However, the lenses differ in the design, arrangement, and power of the defocusing segments (Fig. 1.6a–c).

(2) As with progressive designs for presbyopes, these lenses only correct the refractive error in the central area. Outward the power progressively increases to create a curved image in front of the according retinal areas. Here, too, the design of the outward power increase varies: e.g., power increase only in the horizontal plane (these progressive designs are not intended to support accommodation), or not uniform power increase, i.e. MyCon (Rodenstock, Fig. 1.6d), MyoSlow DF (Visall).

Key facts for spectacle lenses treatment:

- optical correction of myopia needed anyway
- not-invasive treatment
- easy in handling
- should be worn every waking hour for best effect.

Effectiveness of optical treatment methods

For the above-mentioned optical treatment one can also observe a kind of "dose"-dependent effect, because the more, stronger, and longer the myopic defocus works in the eye, the better the effectiveness:

- For multifocal contact lenses, higher addition was observed to be more effective than medium addition in both refractive myopia progression and axial length growth [56]; *see* Fig. 1.7*: High Add vs. Medium Add.* Similar was found for spectacle lenses, with a better effect from the highly aspherical lenslets (HAL) than the slightly aspherical lenslets (SAL), which are embedded in the lens around a free central zone [62]; *see* Fig. 1.8*: HAL vs. SAL.* With orthokeratology

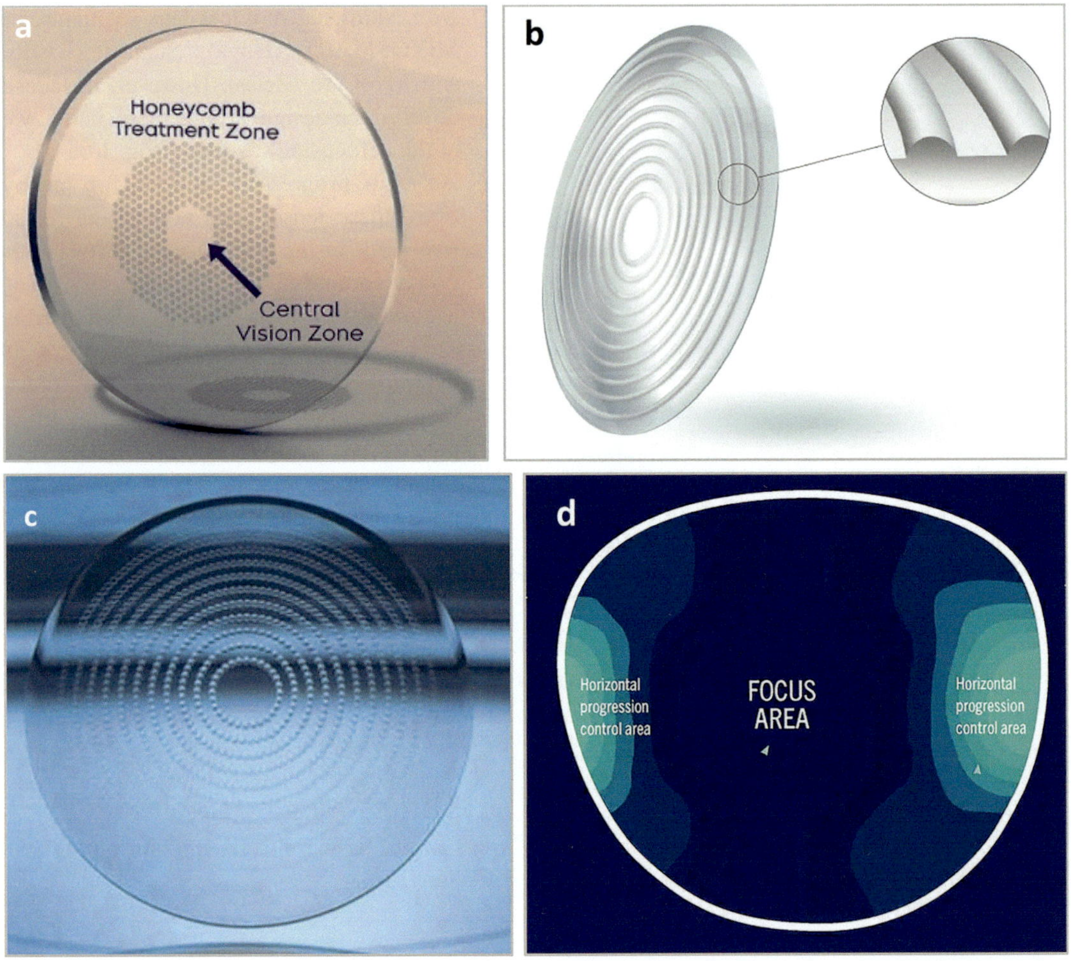

Fig. 1.6 Different designs of myopia control spectacle lenses based on the approach of imposing myopic defocus on the peripheral retina (a) MiYOSMART (Hoya) [58], (b) MyoCare (Zeiss) [59], (c) Stellest (Essilor) [60], (d) MyCon (Rodenstock) [61]

lenses it was found that the size of the optical zone has an influence on the effectiveness: the smaller the optical zone, meaning more peripheral plus power, the less axial length growth was observed [63].

- A duration-dependent effect was also observed, as the longer the daily wearing time of such peripheral defocusing optics, the greater the inhibitory effect with regard to myopia progression and axial length growth [62, 64]. Therefore, myopia contact and spectacle lenses should be worn every waking hour.

In general, the optical treatment methods, especially spectacle lenses, are very well tolerated after getting used to them [65, 66] and show no relevant restrictions in visual functions [67–69].

The effectiveness of the various treatment methods is clearly presented in current reviews, for example by Logan and Bullimore [70]. No or less rebound effect was observed for optical treatment methods compared to other treatment approaches [71–73]. In addition, the optical treatments can be combined with low-dose

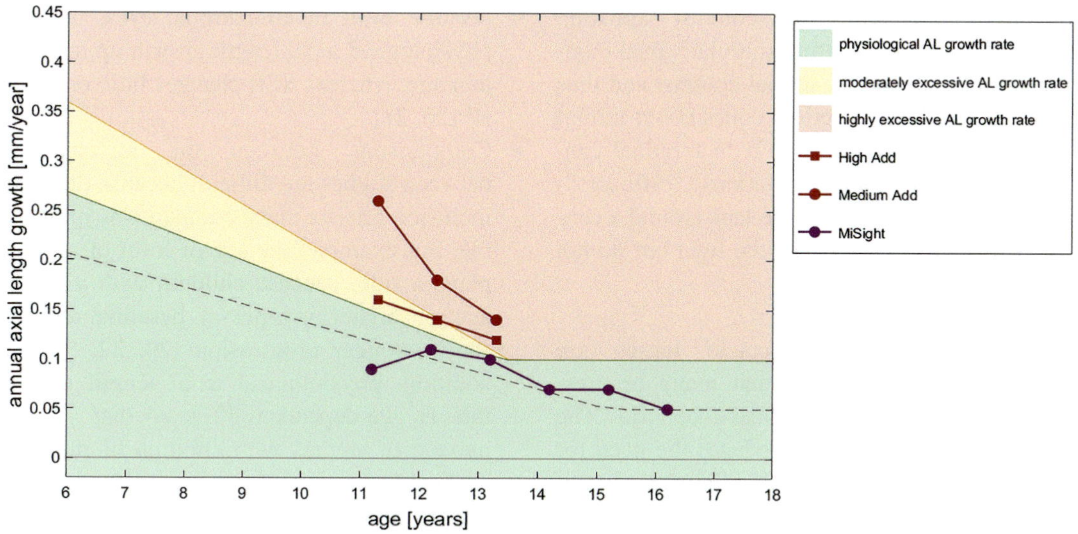

Fig. 1.7 Results of three different soft contact lenses: multifocal contact lenses (high and medium addition) by CooperVision [56] and MiSight contact lens by CooperVision [80]

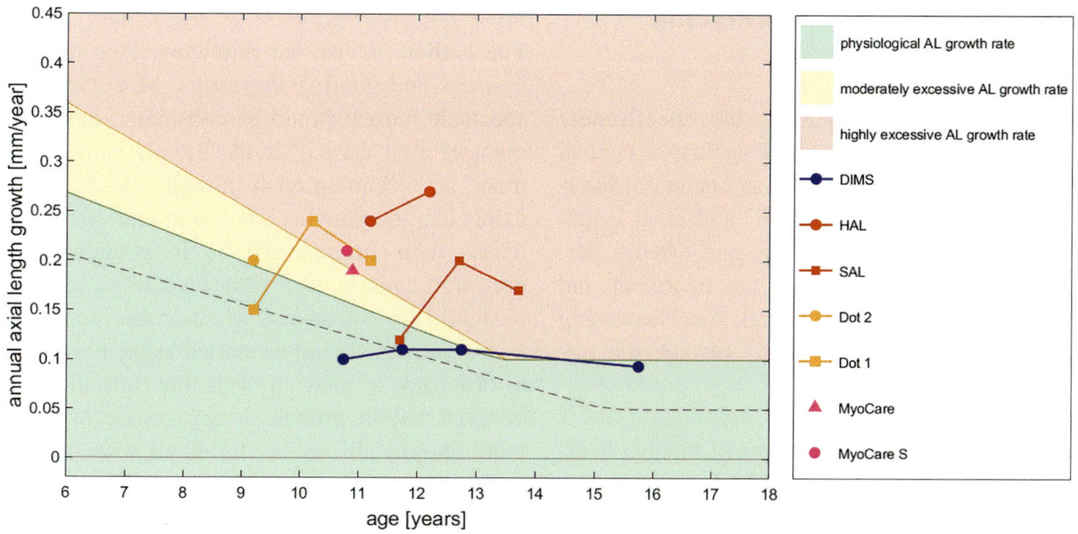

Fig. 1.8 Results of different myopia control spectacle lenses: MiYOSMART (DIMS = defocus incorporated multiple segments) by Hoya [71]; Stellest (HAL = highly aspherical lenslets) and SAL (= sligthly aspherical lenslets) by Essilor [81]; DOT (diffusion optics technology) lenses by SightGlass [82, 83]; MyoCare and MyoCare S by Zeiss [84]

atropine treatment to increase the effectiveness of the treatment [74–78]. A reduced tolerance of the myopia control optics due to the additional administration of atropine is not to be expected [79].

Other approaches of optical treatments

Reduction of retinal image contrast: SightGlass Vision's DOT (Diffusion Optics Technology) spectacle lenses take a different approach: Based on the finding, that high contrast signaling between cones in the retina stimulate axial elongation, in turn lowering retinal contrast and thus reducing signaling of retinal cones could inhibit myopia progression [82]. To reduce retinal contrast, numerous small indentations ("diffusors") are lasered on the front of the lens around a central free zone, which scatter the light but do not defocus it.

Near-addition: These spectacle lenses are based on the observation, that many progressive myopes also exhibit near-esophoria. The implemented near addition reduces the need for accommodation and thus accommodative convergence and reduces or eliminates esophoria at near, i.e. Myoslow Eso (Visall).

Comparison of Study Results on the Effectiveness of Various Myopia Treatments

As usual in clinical studies, the effectiveness of the treatment is assessed against a control group. In particular, the two parameters of interest, spherical equivalent (SER) and axial length (AL), are observed over time and often a percentage difference between the treatment and control group is then calculated. When assessing and comparing different study results, the following should be noted:

- The percentage effectiveness of myopia treatment depends significantly on the outcome of the control group. In this context, the control intervention also plays a role: myopia control spectacle lenses are usually tested against single vision (SV) spectacle lenses, but with myopia control contact lenses the control intervention could be both SV spectacle lenses or SV contact lenses, which might already have a different influence on myopia progression due to their different optical mode of action [85].
- While it is clear, that the treatment goal concerning SER is no or only minor increase, this does not apply to axial length. This is because even in emmetropic eyes, there is physiological axial length growth up to a certain age, whereas SER changes little or not at all [20, 21].
- Comparisons between the effectiveness between studies are difficult because different inclusion criteria make comparisons impossible. For example, the age or level of myopia plays a role, because children with younger age or higher myopia at baseline tend to show stronger progression [20, 32, 33]. In addition, physiological axial length growth rate is age-dependent [21], so that a comparison of studies with children of different ages with regard to the observed axial length growth is inadmissible.

Treatment Recommendation of the Authors

The authors advise the following: Due to their easiness and good study results, MiYOSMART spectacle lenses should be considered the treatment of first choice. If the biometry measurement at follow-up visit reveals an excessive axial length growth rate, combine spectacle lenses with atropine 0.05%. In younger children and eyes with already high axial lengths, it should be considered whether this combination treatment should be started at the beginning in order not to miss any valuable time in terms of axial length growth. Every choice of treatment should always be discussed with parents and patients. For example, if a child generally refuses to wear spectacle lenses, contact lenses or orthokeratology contact lenses should be considered.

Outlook

Since early onset of myopia is considered risky for the development of high myopia, future steps of myopia control activities should aim to delay or even prevent the onset of myopia. This requires early screening with cycloplegic objective refraction and axial length measurements.

However, neither the parents, who are responsible to take their children to the doctor, nor the pediatricians and ophthalmologists, who could inform them to do so, nor the health insurances or governments, who are in charge to create the conditions for these examinations to become standard, are aware of this. In Germany, for example, mandatory examinations of children include eye screening up to the age of 5 (i.e. before starting school). This involves testing for refractive error, strabismus and amblyopia. Once the risk of these developmental anomalies has been averted, the eye appears to be considered organically mature and no further screenings are carried out, although this does not mean that the eye will not continue to develop (and may develop school myopia in case of excessive growth).

Diligent education about myopia stays relevant even in adulthood: An own survey [86] showed that only 32% of (myopic) patients who underwent refractive surgery were aware that the risk for secondary eye diseases, such as retinal detachment, increases with higher levels of myopia. Moreover, 27% of these patients thought that these risks would decrease after refractive surgery. Most patients (55%) would wait about a week to see an ophthalmologist if they experienced symptoms such as floaters, dark spots, flashes of light or a shadow, rather than going straight away. To facilitate patient education, a distinction between optical and anatomical myopia may be useful.

Clinical Case 1: Low-dose Atropin (Fig. 1.9)

- Baseline Visit on 20-SEP-2022
  - female patient, 8.25 yrs old
  - mother highly myopic and thus seeking for treatment for her daughter
  - Spherical Equivalent: OD − 1.63 D / OS − 1.38 D
  - Axial Length: OD 23.49 mm / OS 23.27 mm

  → axial myopia is present
  - Treatment: The physician's recommendation was to start with atropine 0.025%, but the mother had only read about **atropine 0.01%** and wanted to start with that first because she was worried about the side effects. Treatment with atropine 0.01% was therefore started. A follow-up visit in 6 months was recommended.
- Follow-up on 07-MAR-2023
  - Spherical Equivalent: OD − 2.13 D / OS − 1.75 D
  - Axial Length: OD 23.75 mm / OS 23.44 mm
  - Treatment: Due to high axial length growth compared to physiological axial length growth, the atropine dose was **increased to atropine 0.025%** in agreement with the mother. A follow-up visit in 6 months was recommended.
- Follow-up on 19-SEP-2023
  - Spherical Equivalent: OD − 2.50 D / OS − 1.88 D
  - Axial Length: OD 23.88 mm / OS 23.54 mm
  - Treatment: As the axial growth has now approached physiological growth and the child did not report any disturbing side effects, a **continuation of the 0.025% atropine** treatment was agreed. Due to the now noticeable increase in myopic refraction and scratched lenses, new lenses were prescribed. A follow-up visit in 6 months was recommended.
- Follow-up on 02-MAY-2024
  - Spherical Equivalent: OD − 2.63 D / OS − 2.00 D
  - Axial Length: OD 24.00 mm / OS 23.63 mm
  - Treatment: The growth in axial length with this treatment is within the range of physiological axial length growth, so a **continuation**

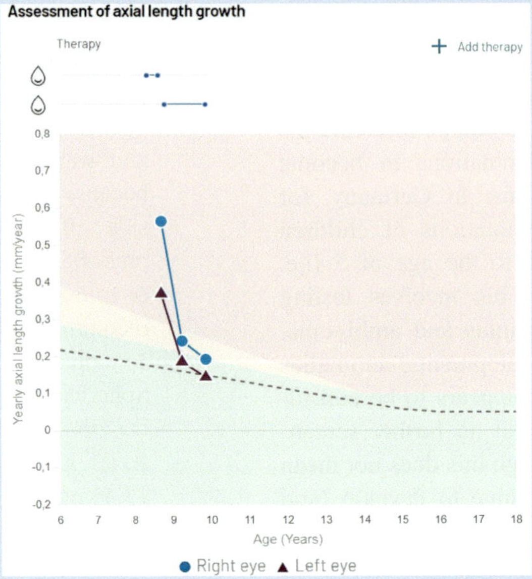

Fig. 1.9 **First data point**: in the first time interval (SEP 2022 to MAR 2023), an axial length growth of 0.26 mm (OD) and 0.17 mm (OS) was observed under atropine 0.01%, resulting in a calculated annual growth in the red zone, which was why the atropine dose was increased. **Second data point**: in the second time interval (MAR 2023 to SEP 2023), a growth of 0.13mm (OD) and 0.10mm (OS) was observed under 0.025% atropine, resulting in a calculated annual growth in the yellow (OD) and green (OS) zone, respectively. Due to the favorable development, this atropine treatment was continued. **Third data point**: in the third time interval from SEP 2023 to MAY 2024, the calculated annual growth under 0.025% atropine was in the green zone for both eyes, so this treatment was continued to maintain the good status (screenshot Myopia-Solutions.com)

of atropine 0.025% was agreed. A follow-up visit in 6 months was recommended. Myopia treatment is planned to continue until patient is at least 15 years old.

Clinical Case 2: Myopia Control Spectacle Lenses (MiYOSMART) (Fig. 1.10)

- Baseline Visit on 14-APR-2022
  - male patient, 13.75 yrs old
  - tried already low-dose atropine and contact lenses but did not tolerate either
  - Spherical Equivalent: OD – 5.00 D / OS – 5.75 D
  - Axial Length: OD 26.07 mm / OS 26.53 mm

  → axial myopia is present
  - Treatment: As treatment with low-dose atropine and contact lenses was not tolerated, **MiYOSMART** spectacle lenses were chosen as the future treatment.
- Follow-up on 27-OCT-2022
  - Spherical Equivalent: OD – 5.13 D / OS – 5.88 D
  - Axial Length: OD 26.10 mm / OS 26.58 mm

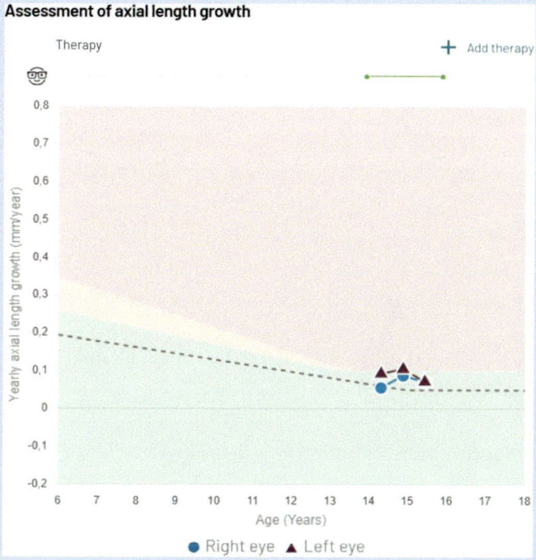

Fig. 1.10 **First data point**: in the first time interval (APR 2022 to OCT 2022), an axial length growth of 0.03 mm (OD) and 0.05 mm (OS) was observed under treatment with MiYOSMART spectacle lenses, resulting in a calculated annual growth in the green zone. Due to the favorable result, this treatment was continued. **Second data point**: in the second time interval (OCT 2022 to MAY 2023), a growth of 0.05mm (OD) and 0.06 mm (OS) was observed under treatment with MiYOSMART spectacle lenses, resulting in a calculated annual growth in the green zone for OD, but in red zone for OS. Nevertheless, as the growth appeared stable, and only one eye showed excessive growth, the treatment was continued. **Third data point**: in the third time interval from MAY 2023 to DEC 2023, a stable growth of 0.04mm (OD) and 0.04 mm (OS) was observed under treatment with MiYOSMART spectacle lenses, resulting in a calculated annual growth in the green zone for both eyes. Treatment with MiYOSMART was continued (screenshot Myopia-Solutions.com)

  - Treatment: As the axial length remained stable, it was agreed to continue wearing the **MiYOSMART** spectacle lenses. Patient reported to have tolerated the glasses well from the beginning.
- Follow-up on 24-MAY-2023
  - Spherical Equivalent: OD − 5.38 D / OS − 6.00 D
  - Axial Length: OD 26.15 mm / OS 26.64 mm
  - Treatment: The patient did not (yet) notice in everyday life that refraction has changed, and that visual acuity has reduced a little. The parents therefore wanted to wait for the next follow-up and the patient continued with the **MiYOSMART** spectacle lenses.
- Follow-up on 13-DEC-2023
  - Spherical Equivalent: OD − 5.38 D / OS − 6.25 D
  - Axial Length: OD 26.19 mm / OS 26.68 mm
  - Treatment: As the increase in refraction has now been confirmed, it was again recommended to adjust the **MiYOSMART** spectacle lenses. The parents agree, as the patient would also like a new spectacle frame.

Clinical Case 3: Combination Treatment (Fig. 1.11)

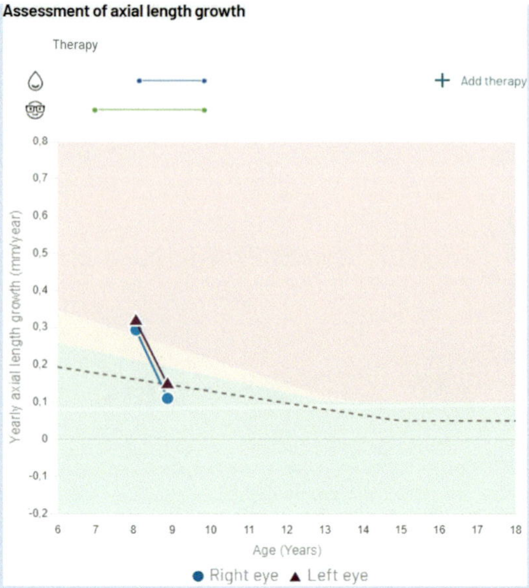

Fig. 1.11 **First data point**: in the first time interval (OCT 2021 to AUG 2022), an axial length growth of 0.25 mm (OD) and 0.27 mm (OS) was observed under treatment with MiYOSMART spectacle lenses, resulting in a calculated annual growth in the red zone. Therefore 0.05% atropine was added to treatment with MiYOSMART. **Second data point**: in the second time interval (AUG 2022 to JUN 2023), a growth of 0.09mm (OD) and 0.12 mm (OS) was observed under combination treatment with MiYOSMART spectacle lenses + 0.05% atropine, resulting in a calculated annual growth in the green zone for both eyes. Therefore, this treatment was continued (screenshot Myopia-Solutions.com)

- Baseline Visit on 13-OCT-2021
  - male patient, 7.2 yrs old
  - due to high myopia child already started with MiYOSMART spectacle lenses, given to the child by an optometrist early 2021, who told parents to also see an ophthalmologist
  - Spherical Equivalent: OD − 3.75 D / OS − 3.38 D
  - Axial Length: OD 24.30 mm / OS 24.14 mm

  → axial myopia is present
  - Treatment: As the child already received **MiYOSMART lenses**, no further treatment was initiated.
- Follow-up on 18-AUG-2022
  - Spherical Equivalent: OD − 4.00 D / OS − 3.63 D
  - Axial Length: OD 24.55 mm / OS 24.41 mm
  - Treatment: As a high axial length growth was observed, **combination treatment** was initiated by adding **0.05% atropine to MiYOSMART**.
- Follow-up on 13-JUN-2023
  - Spherical Equivalent: OD − 4.00 D / OS − 3.88 D
  - Axial Length: OD 24.64 mm / OS 24.53 mm
  - Treatment: Due to the increase in refraction new MiYOSMART lenses were prescribed. As the axial length growth decreased the **combination treatment** was maintained.

References

1. Cohn H. Lehrbuch der Hygiene des Auges. Wien und Leipzig: Urban & Schwarzenberg; 1892.
2. Donders FC. Die Anomalien der Refraction und Accomodation des Auges. Wien: Wilhelm Braumüller; 1866.

3. Haarman AEG, Enthoven CA, Tideman JWL, Tedja MS, Verhoeven VJM, Klaver CCW. The complications of myopia: a review and meta-analysis. Invest Ophthalmol Vis Sci. 2020;61:49. https://doi.org/10.1167/iovs.61.4.49.
4. Saw S-M, Gazzard G, Shih-Yen EC, Chua W-H. Myopia and associated pathological complications. Ophthalmic Physiol Opt. 2005;25:381–91. https://doi.org/10.1111/j.1475-1313.2005.00298.x.
5. Flitcroft DI. The complex interactions of retinal, optical and environmental factors in myopia aetiology. Prog Retin Eye Res. 2012;31:622–60. https://doi.org/10.1016/j.preteyeres.2012.06.004.
6. Marcus MW, de Vries MM, Junoy Montolio FG, Jansonius NM. Myopia as a risk factor for open-angle glaucoma: a systematic review and meta-analysis. Ophthalmology. 2011;118:1989–1994.e2. https://doi.org/10.1016/j.ophtha.2011.03.012.
7. Chang MA, Congdon NG, Bykhovskaya I, Munoz B, West SK. The association between myopia and various subtypes of lens opacity: SEE (Salisbury Eye Evaluation) project. Ophthalmology. 2005;112:1395–401. https://doi.org/10.1016/j.ophtha.2005.02.017.
8. van Leeuwen R, Haarman AEG, van de Put MAJ, Klaver CCW, Los LI. Association of rhegmatogenous retinal detachment incidence with myopia prevalence in the Netherlands. JAMA Ophthalmol. 2021;139:85–92. https://doi.org/10.1001/jamaophthalmol.2020.5114.
9. Vongphanit J, Mitchell P, Wang JJ. Prevalence and progression of myopic retinopathy in an older population. Ophthalmology. 2002;109:704–11. https://doi.org/10.1016/s0161-6420(01)01024-7.
10. Liu HH, Xu L, Wang YX, Wang S, You QS, Jonas JB. Prevalence and progression of myopic retinopathy in Chinese adults: the Beijing Eye Study. Ophthalmology. 2010;117:1763–8. https://doi.org/10.1016/j.ophtha.2010.01.020.
11. Wong TY, Ferreira A, Hughes R, Carter G, Mitchell P. Epidemiology and disease burden of pathologic myopia and myopic choroidal neovascularization: an evidence-based systematic review. Am J Ophthalmol. 2014;157:9-25.e12. https://doi.org/10.1016/j.ajo.2013.08.010.
12. Ohno-Matsui K, Wu P-C, Yamashiro K, Vutipongsatorn K, Fang Y, Cheung CMG, et al. IMI pathologic myopia. Invest Ophthalmol Vis Sci. 2021;62:5. https://doi.org/10.1167/iovs.62.5.5.
13. Chua SYL, Sabanayagam C, Cheung Y-B, Chia A, Valenzuela RK, Tan D, et al. Age of onset of myopia predicts risk of high myopia in later childhood in myopic Singapore children. Ophthalmic Physiol Opt. 2016;36:388–94. https://doi.org/10.1111/opo.12305.
14. Pärssinen O, Kauppinen M. Risk factors for high myopia: a 22-year follow-up study from childhood to adulthood. Acta Ophthalmol. 2019;97:510–8. https://doi.org/10.1111/aos.13964.
15. Bullimore MA, Brennan NA. Myopia control: why each diopter matters. Optom Vis Sci. 2019;96:463–5. https://doi.org/10.1097/OPX.0000000000001367.
16. Hsu C-C, Huang N, Lin P-Y, Fang S-Y, Tsai D-C, Chen S-Y, et al. Risk factors for myopia progression in second-grade primary school children in Taipei: a population-based cohort study. Br J Ophthalmol. 2017;101:1611–7. https://doi.org/10.1136/bjophthalmol-2016-309299.
17. Pärssinen O, Kauppinen M. Associations of reading posture, gaze angle and reading distance with myopia and myopic progression. Acta Ophthalmol. 2016;94:775–9. https://doi.org/10.1111/aos.13148.
18. Li S-M, Li S-Y, Kang M-T, Zhou Y, Liu L-R, Li H, et al. Near work related parameters and myopia in Chinese children: the Anyang childhood eye study. PLoS One. 2015;10: e0134514. https://doi.org/10.1371/journal.pone.0134514.
19. Mutti DO, Mitchell GL, Sinnott LT, Jones-Jordan LA, Moeschberger ML, Cotter SA, et al. Corneal and crystalline lens dimensions before and after myopia onset. Optom Vis Sci. 2012;89:251–62. https://doi.org/10.1097/OPX.0b013e3182418213.
20. Rozema J, Dankert S, Iribarren R, Lanca C, Saw S-M. Axial growth and lens power loss at myopia onset in Singaporean children. Invest Ophthalmol Vis Sci. 2019;60:3091–9. https://doi.org/10.1167/iovs.18-26247.
21. Rozema JJ. Refractive development I: biometric changes during emmetropisation. Ophthalmic Physiol Opt. 2023;43:347–67. https://doi.org/10.1111/opo.13094.
22. Flitcroft DI. Is myopia a failure of homeostasis? Exp Eye Res. 2013;114:16–24. https://doi.org/10.1016/j.exer.2013.02.008.
23. Jones LA, Mitchell GL, Mutti DO, Hayes JR, Moeschberger ML, Zadnik K. Comparison of ocular component growth curves among refractive error groups in children. Invest Ophthalmol Vis Sci. 2005;46:2317–27. https://doi.org/10.1167/iovs.04-0945.
24. Mutti DO, Hayes JR, Mitchell GL, Jones LA, Moeschberger ML, Cotter SA, et al. Refractive error, axial length, and relative peripheral refractive error before and after the onset of myopia. Invest Ophthalmol Vis Sci. 2007;48:2510–9. https://doi.org/10.1167/iovs.06-0562.
25. Mattern A-I, Neller K, Devenijn M, Schwahn H, Langenbucher A, Seitz B, Kaymak H. A comparison of optical biometers used in children for myopia control. Klin Monbl Augenheilkd. 2023;240:1306–13. https://doi.org/10.1055/a-2117-9335.
26. Bullimore MA, Brennan NA. Juvenile-onset myopia-who to treat and how to evaluate success. Eye (Lond). 2024;38:450–4. https://doi.org/10.1038/s41433-023-02722-6.
27. Graff B, Lam CSY, Vlasak N, Kaymak H. Age-matched analysis of axial length growth in myopic children wearing defocus incorporated multiple segments spectacle lenses. Br J Ophthalmol. 2023. https://doi.org/10.1136/bjo-2023-324508.
28. Lee S-H, Tseng B-Y, Wang J-H, Chiu C-J. Efficacy and safety of low-dose atropine on myopia prevention in premyopic children: systematic review

and meta-analysis. J Clin Med. 2024. https://doi.org/10.3390/jcm13051506.
29. Yam JC, Zhang XJ, Zhang Y, Yip BHK, Tang F, Wong ES, et al. Effect of low-concentration atropine eyedrops vs placebo on myopia incidence in children: the LAMP2 randomized clinical trial. JAMA. 2023;329:472–81. https://doi.org/10.1001/jama.2022.24162.
30. Schaeffel F. Prävention der Myopie [Prevention of myopia]. Ophthalmologe. 2019;116:509–17. https://doi.org/10.1007/s00347-019-0892-4.
31. Zhang XJ, Zhang Y, Kam KW, Tham CC, Chen LJ, Pang CC, Yam JC. Hyperopic reserve as a treatment indicator for low-concentration atropine to delay myopia onset in children (LAMP 2 Study). IOVS. 2024;65:ARVO E-Abstract 425.
32. Fu A, Stapleton F, Wei L, Wang W, Zhao B, Watt K, et al. Risk factors for rapid axial length elongation with low concentration atropine for myopia control. Sci Rep. 2021;11:11729. https://doi.org/10.1038/s41598-021-88719-1.
33. Polling JR, Tan E, Driessen S, Loudon SE, Wong H-L, van der Schans A, et al. A 3-year follow-up study of atropine treatment for progressive myopia in Europeans. Eye (Lond). 2020;34:2020–8. https://doi.org/10.1038/s41433-020-1122-7.
34. Zhang XJ, Zhang Y, Yip BHK, Kam KW, Tang F, Ling X, et al. Five-year clinical trial of the low-concentration atropine for myopia progression (LAMP) study: phase 4 report. Ophthalmology. 2024. https://doi.org/10.1016/j.ophtha.2024.03.013.
35. Xiong S, Sankaridurg P, Naduvilath T, Zang J, Zou H, Zhu J, et al. Time spent in outdoor activities in relation to myopia prevention and control: a meta-analysis and systematic review. Acta Ophthalmol. 2017;95:551–66. https://doi.org/10.1111/aos.13403.
36. Wu P-C, Chang L-C, Niu Y-Z, Chen M-L, Liao L-L, Chen C-T. Myopia prevention in Taiwan. Ann Eye Sci. 2018;3:12. https://doi.org/10.21037/aes.2018.01.05.
37. Mathis U, Feldkaemper M, Wang M, Schaeffel F. Studies on retinal mechanisms possibly related to myopia inhibition by atropine in the chicken. Graef Arch Clin Exp. 2020;258:319–33. https://doi.org/10.1007/s00417-019-04573-y.
38. Upadhyay A, Beuerman RW. Biological mechanisms of atropine control of myopia. Eye Contact Lens. 2020;46:129–35. https://doi.org/10.1097/ICL.0000000000000677.
39. Yam JC, Jiang Y, Tang SM, Law AKP, Chan JJ, Wong E, et al. Low-concentration atropine for myopia progression (LAMP) study: a randomized, double-blinded, placebo-controlled trial of 0.05%, 0.025%, and 0.01% atropine eye drops in myopia control. Ophthalmology. 2019;126:113–24. https://doi.org/10.1016/j.ophtha.2018.05.029.
40. Chia A, Lu Q-S, Tan D. Five-year clinical trial on atropine for the treatment of myopia 2: myopia control with atropine 0.01% eyedrops. Ophthalmology. 2016;123:391–9. https://doi.org/10.1016/j.ophtha.2015.07.004.
41. Tong L, Huang XL, Koh ALT, Zhang X, Tan DTH, Chua W-H. Atropine for the treatment of childhood myopia: effect on myopia progression after cessation of atropine. Ophthalmology. 2009;116:572–9. https://doi.org/10.1016/j.ophtha.2008.10.020.
42. Joachimsen L, Farassat N, Bleul T, Böhringer D, Lagrèze WA, Reich M. Side effects of topical atropine 0.05% compared to 0.01% for myopia control in German school children: a pilot study. Int Ophthalmol. 2021;41:2001–8. https://doi.org/10.1007/s10792-021-01755-8.
43. Repka MX, Weise KK, Chandler DL, Wu R, Melia BM, Manny RE, et al. Low-dose 0.01% atropine eye drops vs placebo for myopia control: a randomized clinical trial. JAMA Ophthalmol. 2023. https://doi.org/10.1001/jamaophthalmol.2023.2855.
44. Yam JC, Li FF, Zhang X, Tang SM, Yip BHK, Kam KW, et al. Two-year clinical trial of the low-concentration atropine for myopia progression (LAMP) study: phase 2 report. Ophthalmology. 2020;127:910–9. https://doi.org/10.1016/j.ophtha.2019.12.011.
45. Richdale K, Skidmore KV, Tomiyama ES, Bullimore MA. Compounded 0.01% atropine-what's in the bottle? Eye Contact Lens. 2023;49:219–23. https://doi.org/10.1097/ICL.0000000000000990.
46. Richdale K, Tomiyama ES, Novack GD, Bullimore MA. Compounding of low-concentration atropine for myopia control. Eye Contact Lens. 2022;48:489–92. https://doi.org/10.1097/ICL.0000000000000932.
47. Hoerst A, Schwahn H, Graff B, Neller K, Kaymak H. Personalisierte Atropintherapie für ein optimiertes Myopiemanagement (252) - Abstractband DOG 2020. Ophthalmologe. 2020;117:43–190. https://doi.org/10.1007/s00347-020-01197-0.
48. Austermann H, Schaeffel F, Mathis U, Hund V, Mußhoff F, Ziemssen F, Schnichels S. Corneal penetration of low-dose atropine eye drops. J Clin Med. 2021. https://doi.org/10.3390/jcm10040588.
49. Kaymak H, Graff B, Nienhaus S, Schwahn H. Atropintherapie in der klinischen Routine – eine mehrjährige Beobachtung (395) - Abstractband DOG 2020. Ophthalmologe. 2020;117:43–190. https://doi.org/10.1007/s00347-020-01197-0.
50. Zadnik K, Schulman E, Flitcroft I, Fogt JS, Blumenfeld LC, Fong TM, et al. Efficacy and safety of 0.01% and 0.02% atropine for the treatment of pediatric myopia progression over 3 years: a randomized clinical trial. JAMA Ophthalmol. 2023;141:990–9. https://doi.org/10.1001/jamaophthalmol.2023.2097.
51. Wallman J, Winawer J. Homeostasis of eye growth and the question of myopia. Neuron. 2004;43:447–68. https://doi.org/10.1016/j.neuron.2004.08.008.
52. Kaymak H, Graff B, Neller K, Langenbucher A, Seitz B, Schwahn H. Myopietherapie und Prophylaxe mit „Defocus Incorporated Multiple

Segments"-Brillengläsern [Myopia treatment and prophylaxis with defocus incorporated multiple segments spectacle lenses]. Ophthalmologe. 2021;118: 1280–6. https://doi.org/10.1007/s00347-021-01452-y.
53. Hiraoka T. Myopia control with orthokeratology: a review. Eye Contact Lens. 2022;48:100–4. https://doi.org/10.1097/ICL.0000000000000867.
54. Li X, Xu M, San S, Bian L, Li H. Orthokeratology in controlling myopia of children: a meta-analysis of randomized controlled trials. BMC Ophthalmol. 2023;23:441. https://doi.org/10.1186/s12886-023-03175-x.
55. Bullimore MA, Johnson LA. Overnight orthokeratology. Cont Lens Anterior Eye. 2020;43:322–32. https://doi.org/10.1016/j.clae.2020.03.018.
56. Walline JJ, Walker MK, Mutti DO, Jones-Jordan LA, Sinnott LT, Giannoni AG, et al. Effect of high add power, medium add power, or single-vision contact lenses on myopia progression in children. JAMA. 2020;324:571. https://doi.org/10.1001/jama.2020.10834.
57. VisionExpress. MiSight 1 day & children's myopia. https://www.eye-deology.com/eyewear/hoya-miyosmart-myopia-control-eyeglass-lenses. Accessed 24 May 2024.
58. eye-deology Vision Care. MiYOSMART myopia control eyeglass lenses. https://www.eye-deology.com/eyewear/hoya-miyosmart-myopia-control-eyeglass-lenses. Accessed 24 May 2024.
59. Zeiss, editor. MyoCare clinical insights paper; 2023.
60. Eyefox. Essilor Stellest Brillengläser. 2023. https://www.eyefox.com/videos/413/essilor-stellest-brillenglaeser.html. Accessed 24 May 2024.
61. mivision - THE OPHTHALMIC JOURNAL. Rodenstock Launches MyCon Myopia Lens. 2023. https://mivision.com.au/2023/05/rodenstock-launches-mycon-myopia-lens/. Accessed 24 May 2024.
62. Bao J, Huang Y, Li X, Yang A, Zhou F, Wu J, et al. Spectacle lenses with aspherical lenslets for myopia control vs single-vision spectacle lenses: a randomized clinical trial. JAMA Ophthalmol. 2022;140:472–8. https://doi.org/10.1001/jamaophthalmol.2022.0401.
63. Pauné J, Fonts S, Rodríguez L, Queirós A. The role of back optic zone diameter in myopia control with orthokeratology lenses. J Clin Med. 2021. https://doi.org/10.3390/jcm10020336.
64. Lam CSY, Tang WC, Tse DY-Y, Tang YY, To CH. Defocus Incorporated Soft Contact (DISC) lens slows myopia progression in Hong Kong Chinese schoolchildren: a 2-year randomised clinical trial. Br J Ophthalmol. 2014;98:40–5. https://doi.org/10.1136/bjophthalmol-2013-303914.
65. Lu Y, Lin Z, Wen L, Gao W, Pan L, Li X, et al. The adaptation and acceptance of defocus incorporated multiple segment lens for Chinese children. Am J Ophthalmol. 2020;211:207–16. https://doi.org/10.1016/j.ajo.2019.12.002.
66. Bao J, Yang A, Huang Y, Li X, Pan Y, Ding C, et al. One-year myopia control efficacy of spectacle lenses with aspherical lenslets. Br J Ophthalmol. 2022;106:1171–6. https://doi.org/10.1136/bjophthalmol-2020-318367.
67. Lam CSY, Tang WC, Qi H, Radhakrishnan H, Hasegawa K, To CH, Charman WN. Effect of defocus incorporated multiple segments spectacle lens wear on visual function in myopic Chinese children. Transl Vis Sci Technol. 2020;9:11. https://doi.org/10.1167/tvst.9.9.11.
68. Gao Y, Lim EW, Yang A, Drobe B, Bullimore MA. The impact of spectacle lenses for myopia control on visual functions. Ophthalmic Physiol Opt. 2021;41:1320–31. https://doi.org/10.1111/opo.12878.
69. García-Marqués JV, Macedo-De-Araújo RJ, Cerviño A, García-Lázaro S, McAlinden C, González-Méijome JM. Comparison of short-term light disturbance, optical and visual performance outcomes between a myopia control contact lens and a single-vision contact lens. Ophthalmic Physiol Opt. 2020;40:718–27. https://doi.org/10.1111/opo.12729.
70. Logan NS, Bullimore MA. Optical interventions for myopia control. Eye (Lond). 2024;38:455–63. https://doi.org/10.1038/s41433-023-02723-5.
71. Lam CSY, Tang WC, Zhang HY, Lee PH, Tse DYY, Qi H, et al. Long-term myopia control effect and safety in children wearing DIMS spectacle lenses for 6 years. Sci Rep. 2023;13:5475. https://doi.org/10.1038/s41598-023-32700-7.
72. Sánchez-Tena MÁ, Ballesteros-Sánchez A, Martinez-Perez C, Alvarez-Peregrina C, De-Hita-Cantalejo C, Sánchez-González MC, Sánchez-González J-M. Assessing the rebound phenomenon in different myopia control treatments: a systematic review. Ophthalmic Physiol Opt. 2024;44:270–9. https://doi.org/10.1111/opo.13277.
73. Ruiz-Pomeda A, Prieto-Garrido FL, Hernández Verdejo JL, Villa-Collar C. Rebound effect in the misight assessment study Spain (Mass). Curr Eye Res. 2021;46:1223–6. https://doi.org/10.1080/02713683.2021.1878227.
74. Xu S, Li Z, Zhao W, Zheng B, Jiang J, Ye G, et al. Effect of atropine, orthokeratology and combined treatments for myopia control: a 2-year stratified randomised clinical trial. Br J Ophthalmol. 2023;107:1812–7. https://doi.org/10.1136/bjo-2022-321272.
75. Kinoshita N, Konno Y, Hamada N, Kanda Y, Shimmura-Tomita M, Kakehashi A. Additive effects of orthokeratology and atropine 0.01% ophthalmic solution in slowing axial elongation in children with myopia: first year results. Jpn J Ophthalmol. 2018;62:544–53. https://doi.org/10.1007/s10384-018-0608-3.
76. Erdinest N, London N, Lavy I, Levinger N, Pras E, Morad Y. Myopia control utilizing low-dose atropine as an isolated therapy or in combination with other optical measures: a retrospective cohort study.

Taiwan J Ophthalmol. 2023;13:231–7. https://doi.org/10.4103/tjo.tjo_31_22.
77. Tsai H-R, Wang J-H, Huang H-K, Chen T-L, Chen P-W, Chiu C-J. Efficacy of atropine, orthokeratology, and combined atropine with orthokeratology for childhood myopia: a systematic review and network meta-analysis. J Formos Med Assoc. 2022;121:2490–500. https://doi.org/10.1016/j.jfma.2022.05.005.
78. Vagge A, Frattolillo A, Nucci P, Samassa F, Barosco G, Rapizzi E, et al. Highly Aspherical Lenslet Target (HALT) technology in combination with low-dose atropine to control myopia progression. IOVS. 2024;65:ARVO E-Abstract 425.
79. Kaymak H, Mattern A-I, Graff B, Neller K, Langenbucher A, Seitz B, Schwahn H. Sicherheit von Brillengläsern mit DIMS-Technologie und Atropin in der Kombinationstherapie der Myopieprogression [Safety of DIMS Spectacle Lenses and Atropine as Combination Therapy for Myopia Progression]. Klin Monbl Augenheilkd. 2022;239:1197–205. https://doi.org/10.1055/a-1930-7116.
80. Chamberlain P, Bradley A, Arumugam B, Hammond D, McNally J, Logan NS, et al. Long-term effect of dual-focus contact lenses on myopia progression in children: a 6-year multicenter clinical trial. Optom Vis Sci. 2022;99:204–12. https://doi.org/10.1097/OPX.0000000000001873.
81. Li X, Huang Y, Yin Z, Liu C, Zhang S, Yang A, et al. Myopia control efficacy of spectacle lenses with aspherical lenslets: results of a 3-year follow-up study. Am J Ophthalmol. 2023;253:160–8. https://doi.org/10.1016/j.ajo.2023.03.030.
82. Rappon J, Chung C, Young G, Hunt C, Neitz J, Neitz M, Chalberg T. Control of myopia using diffusion optics spectacle lenses: 12-month results of a randomised controlled, efficacy and safety study (CYPRESS). Br J Ophthalmol. 2023;107:1709–15. https://doi.org/10.1136/bjo-2021-321005.
83. Chalberg T, Laughton D, Hill J, Tasso V, Young G, Hunt C, et al. Control of myopia using diffusion optics spectacle lenses: efficacy and safety study (CYPRESS) 42-month results. Invest Ophthalmol Vis Sci. 2023;64.
84. Chen X, Wu M, Yu C, Ohlendorf A, Padmaja S, Rifai K, et al. Slowing myopia progression with cylindrical annular refractive elements (CARE)—12-month interim results from a 2-year prospective multi-center trial. IOVS. 2024;65:ARVO E-Abstract 425.
85. Malinowski A, Mrugacz M, Stopa M, Filipek E, Moniuszko-Malinowska A, Czupryna P. A clinical study of the impact of soft contact lenses on the progression of myopia in young patients. Clin Ophthalmol. 2022;16:51–62. https://doi.org/10.2147/OPTH.S338199.
86. Kaymak H, Devenijn M, Neller K, Langenbucher A, Seitz B, Schwahn H. Post-SMILE – Was Myope über ihre emmetropen Augen wissen! - Abstractband DOG 2022 [Not Available]. Ophthalmologie. 2022;119:157–344. https://doi.org/10.1007/s00347-022-01723-2

Part II
Cornea

Refractive corneal surgery can be made as a surface treatment (PRK) or a stromal treatment (LASIK, SMILE). TransPRK is the most recent surface treatment and is a one-step ablation that combines a reverse aspheric PRK and a phototherapeutic keratectomy (PTK). Dr. Diego de Ortueta (Recklinghausen, Germany) describes this technique with the AMARIS laser platform (Schwind eye-tech solutions, Kleinostheim, Germany).

SMILE stands for Small Incision Lenticule Extraction and is the most recent revolution in corneal refractive surgery. During the SMILE procedure, the femto laser cuts a lenticule inside the corneal stroma which is removed by a side incision. A corneal flap with all negative side effects is no longer necessary. This technique was developed by the company Zeiss together with Prof. Sekundo (Marburg, Germany), Prof. Blum (Erfurt, Germany) and Dr. Prof Meyer (Cologne, Germany). The authors describe the development of this new technique and demonstrate the surgery step-by-step.

TransPRK

2

Diego de Ortueta

Abstract

Transepithelial refractive keratectomy (TransPRK), is a more advanced surface ablation method used with the excimer laser to correct refractive errors. TransPRK with SmartSurface is a one-step ablation that combines a reverse aspheric PRK and a phototherapeutic keratectomy (PTK) with the AMARIS laser platform (Schwind eye-tech solutions, Kleinostheim, Germany). The epithelial removal matches with the ablation zone. The use of smart pulse technology (SPT) leads to a quicker return of vision. The ablation profile can be an aspherical optimized profile or, in cases with higher-order aberrations, corneal wavefront or wavefront guided. We present also results in myopia and correction of low refraction errors, astigmatism, and hyperopia. We also compare the results of the literature in comparison with other laser vision corrections as LASEK, LASIK, or lenticule extraction as SMILE. TransPRK is an efficacious and safe laser correction when we revised the literature and our results.

Keywords

Transepithelial photorefractive keratectomy · TransPRK · PRK · Schwind · AMARIS · Centration · Cornea vertex · Smart surface

TransPRK SmartSurface

TransPRK Description

An existing refractive error can be corrected, among other things, with an excimer laser by a targeted change of the corneal radii. A distinction is made between surface treatments and stromal treatments such as laser in situ keratomileusis (LASIK). Procedures based on the removal of the corneal epithelium followed by treatment of the corneal stroma with the excimer laser are referred to as "surface treatments." Surface treatments typically have a higher residual stromal thickness than LASIK. In photorefractive keratectomy (PRK), the epithelium is removed mechanically, and in laser-assisted subepithelial keratectomy (LASEK), the epithelium is pushed aside with alcohol. In LASEK, once the stroma has been ablated, the epithelium can be put back or removed, depending on the surgeon's preference.

D. de Ortueta (✉)
Aurelios, 45657 Recklinghausen, Germany
e-mail: diego.de.ortueta@augenzentrum.org

U. Spandau and G. B. Scharioth (eds.), *Cutting Edge of Ophthalmic Surgery*,
https://doi.org/10.1007/978-3-031-84204-7_2

In the late 1990s, transepithelial photorefractive keratectomy (TransPRK) was described [1]. The epithelium was ablated by excimer laser in the form of phototherapeutic keratectomy (PTK), followed by PRK. In 2009, SCHWIND eye-tech-solutions GmbH (Kleinostheim, Germany) introduced the AMARIS laser, a nomogram that allows epithelial removal and refractive correction in one step.

The conventional PRK and LASEK surface techniques have been superseded by the more advanced transepithelial photorefractive keratectomy (TransPRK) techniques, which deliver a no-touch, all-laser solution [2–4].

TransPRK is a one-step ablation that combines a reverse aspheric PRK and a phototherapeutic keratectomy (PTK) with the AMARIS laser platform (Schwind eye-tech solutions, Kleinostheim, Germany) Fig. 2.1.

The software of the laser system uses an aspherical profile with an ablation of 55 µm at the center and 65 µm at the 4 mm periphery [5] to standardize the PTK of the epithelium. The terminology "reversed single-step" describes the pseudo-sequentialization of the corneal aspheric profile, and the components of the epithelial thickness profile are achieved in a single step without interruptions. This means that, in a counterintuitive way, the refractive correction is applied first and the epithelial profile at the end [2]. Many groups have reported the efficacy and safety of TransPRK procedures [3, 4, 6, 7].

In contrast to PRK or LASEK, the TransPRK approach reduces the wound area and speeds up the healing process by calculating the diameter of epithelial removal to match the ablation zone. This leads to a quicker return of vision. According to a study by Lee et al. [8], epithelial regrowth occurred most quickly in the TransPRK-treated group with a mean time of 2.5 days, followed by the PRK group with a mean time of 3 days, and the LASEK group with a mean time of 3.5 days.

SmartSurface

The flying-spot delivery system for the laser ablation algorithm had a super-Gaussian beam profile of 0.54 mm full width-half maximum and operates at 1050 Hz [5].

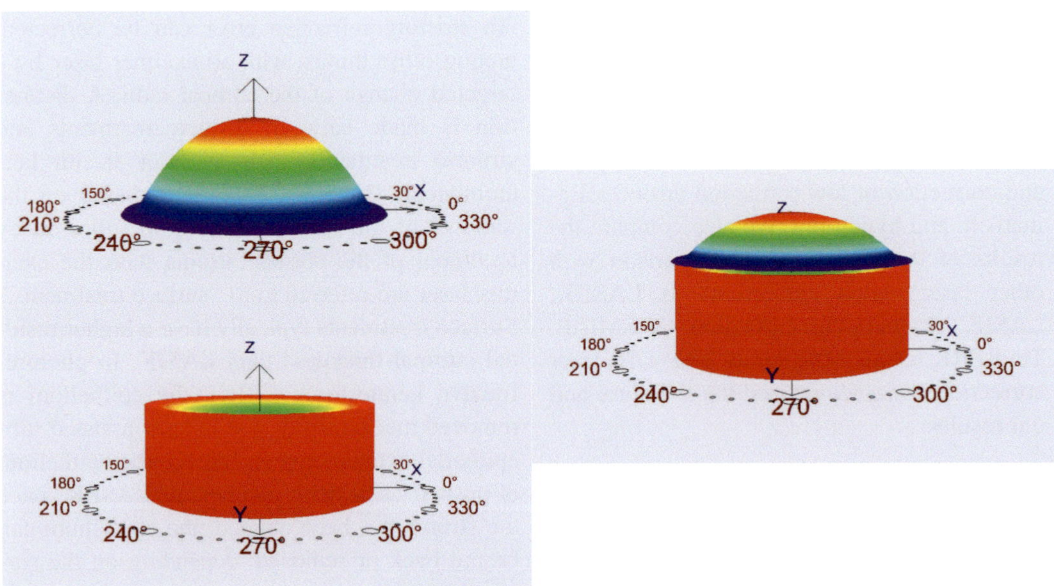

Fig. 2.1 At the top left is a photorefractive keratectomy (PRK) profile, and left is an aspherical phototherapeutic keratectomy (PTK) profile for the epithelium; both together are the profile for the transepithelial photorefractive keratectomy (TransPRK)

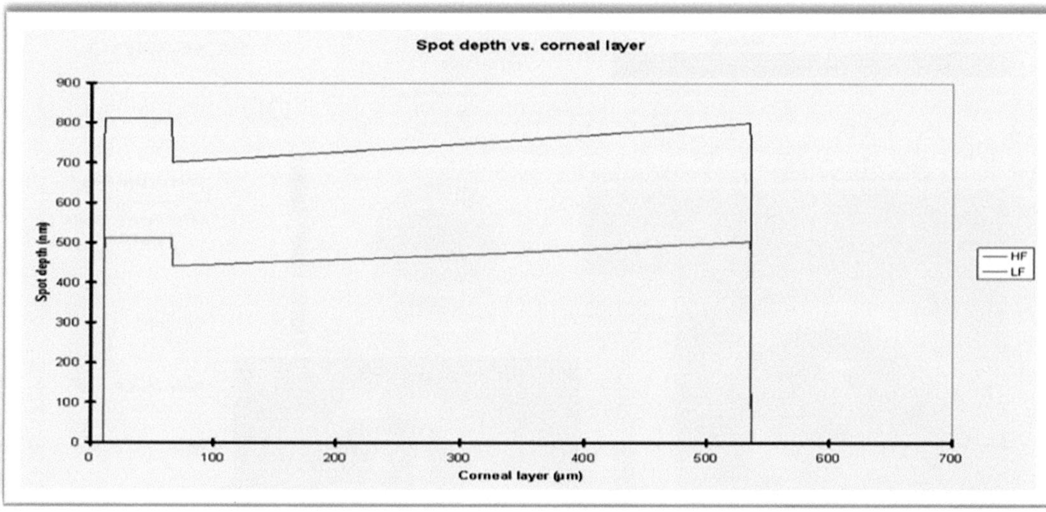

Fig. 2.2 The diagram shows the spot depth of high fluence (HF) and low fluence (LF) at the different layers of the cornea. At the epithelium, the ablation rate of the first 55 µm is higher than at the stroma; at deeper layers, the ablation depth increases. With HF, the ablation depth at the epithelium is 800 nm and at the stroma 700 nm; with LF, the ablation rate is 500 nm for the epithelium and 450 nm for the stroma

About 80% of the corneal ablation was carried out with a high fluence level (440 mJ/cm^2) depending on the planned refractive correction, and 20% was done using a low fluence level (300 mJ/cm^2) for fine correction and smoothing the ablated area [9] Fig. 2.2. In order to prevent heat buildup between laser pulses, the spot placement was randomized [10]. The application of smart pulse technology (SPT; Schwind Eye-Tech Solutions, Kleinostheim, Germany) can also be applied with the TransPRK [9, 11]. The TransPRK with SPT has the name SmartSurface. The SPT profile employs a curved corneal surface based on a fullerene structure, resulting in equally spaced ablation points. Unlike the standard ablation profile, which depicts a three-dimensional volume based on a flat corneal surface, the SPT profile employs a curved corneal surface based on a fullerene structure, resulting in equally spaced ablation points. With the SPT [9, 12], a smooth corneal surface after ablation may result in faster and better vision recovery. A smoother cornea may improve vision, particularly in the days following therapy [13]. Vincingerra et al. [9] demonstrated improved results for advanced surface ablation when comparing the Amaris 1.050-Hz excimer laser with SPT to the 750-Hz excimer laser, with higher uncorrected acuity outcomes, greater safety, and no eye losing any lines of CDVA at 6 months.

Centration

We recommend to use for centration of the ablation the vertex using the information of pupillary offset [14] (vertex corneal to pupil center) calculated by the topographer, which closely resembles the visual axis [15]. The laser system also uses a 1050 Hz infrared eye tracker to accurately align the eye under the laser. This tracker also simultaneously tracked the limbus, pupil, and torsion. The average response time of the eye tracker is 1.7 ms, and the overall latency of the system is 2.9 ms. Throughout treatment, patients were instructed to focus on a pulsing green fixation light Fig. 2.3.

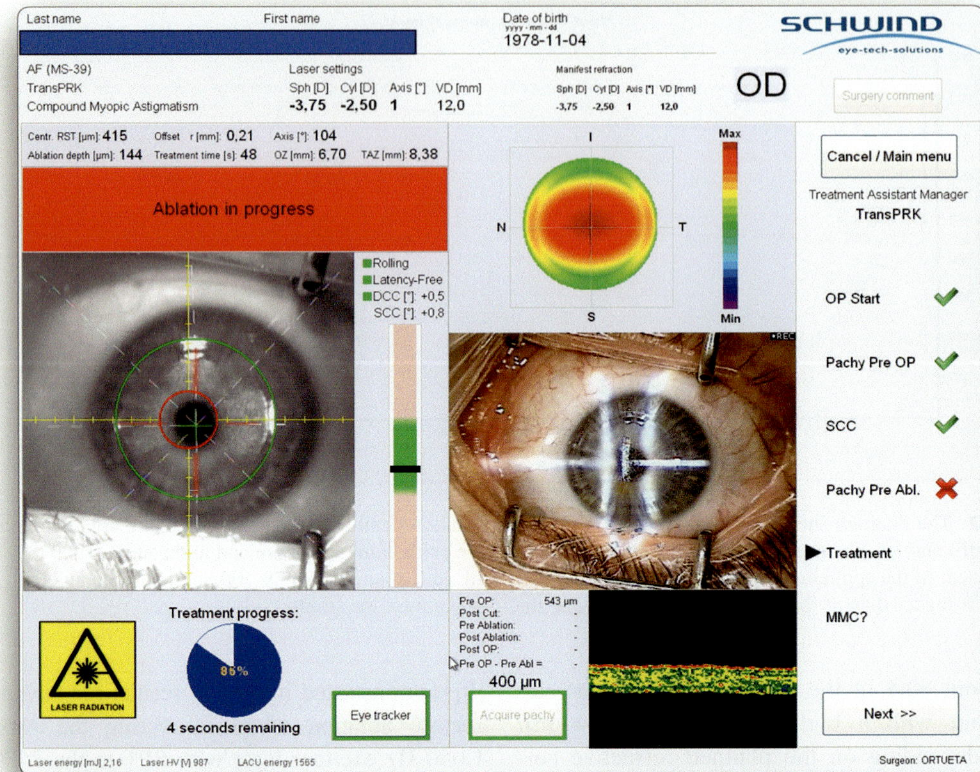

Fig. 2.3 In this graph, you can see at the left the view from the infrared camera for tracking the eye at 1050 Hz; the centration and eye tracker dynamic and static are also represented; at the right the view from the microscope; the epithelium ablation matches perfectly with the stroma ablation diameter. Downright the measurement with the OCT during the treatment and at the top the treatment type, in this case a myopic astigmatism aberration free with import of the data from the MS-39

TransPRK Profile

In most of the cases in virgin eyes we use an aspheric non-wavefront-guided treatments (aberration free), meaning that the ablations were designed to cause no change in the wavefront aberration (within the optical zone, OZ) other than the sphere and cylinder components, leaving all current high-order aberrations (HOA) unchanged [16]. The introduction of new aberrations was minimized [17]. Based on the cornea's existing shape and its keratometric values, the ideal ablation profile was then established, taking into account elements like the cosine effect, among others [18–22].

Because the patient's best-corrected visual acuity has not been affected by the pre-existing aberrations, the surgeon's overall goal when a patient is chosen for non-customized aspherical therapy should be to leave all existing high-order aberrations (HOA) untouched. [23]. We know that eyes with supervision have some aberrations [24] and that persons with the fewest aberrations did not necessarily have the highest visual acuities [16].

There is some plasticity in the brain system, so distortions in the visual field are corrected, but because patients see the world through their own wave aberration, repairs that are too far away from their "normal" experience are rejected. Furthermore, moderate levels of wavefront-aberration favour image quality stability [25] for larger visual fields.

The aberration-free profile is an aspherical optimized profile the concept is based on wavefront aberration, in which the software matches the postoperative versus preoperative wavefront by balancing the sphere and cylinder components that will be repaired within a refractive zone. In other words, there is no induced change in wavefront aberration other than the sphere and cylinder components. Thus, balancing the impacts of wavefront aberration and providing normal eyes with the greatest possible vision without compromising their ability to perceive their environment [26]. This aberration free profile is employed in 90% of our clinical instances in which the eye has good visual acuity and the HOA (higher order aberrations) at 6 mm are less than 0.3 μm under mesopic settings. We have published data demonstrating that this profile does not cause a large amount of aberrations [18, 23, 26–28].

High-order aberrations should be corrected if they are proven to be diagnostically significant by 0.5 D or 0.3 μm at 6 mm. In such cases, we suggest wavefront-guided therapies that make use of corneal and/or ocular wavefront information.

We have data from both the corneal wavefront (CW) and the ocular wavefront (OW). Subtracting this gives us information about the eye's internal aberrations (IW). If the ocular and corneal aberrations are similar, we utilize the corneal data because it covers a broader area and has no pupil influence. If the global optical difference between CW and OW is greater than 0.5 D for any eye, we consider internal wave aberration (IW) to be significant; therapy is OW-guided or IOL exchange.

Topographically guided algorithms, or Corneal Wavefront (CW), have the ability to treat highly aberrated corneas as decentered ablations or corneal diseases as scars.

The software for corneal wavefront allows for the entry of the subjective refraction. The software system takes into account the effects of higher order aberrations in refraction. As a result, based on the input manifest refraction, the expected theoretically anticipated objective impact of the HOA on refraction is evaluated and balanced. In cases that we to save tissue the TransPRK combined with the ORK-CAM Software (Schwind eye-tech, Kleinhosteim Germany) can also save tissue or volume [29] if this is necessary for example TransPRK over a LASIK flap. We have therefore the possibility to use a programme for minimizing depth or volume [29].

TransPRK for Correction of Myopia and Myopic Astigmatism

Many studies have been conducted to assess the efficacy and safety of TransPRK procedures It has been extensively demonstrated to be a successful technique for treating myopia and myopic astigmatism and astigmatism [3, 4, 6, 11, 13, 30]. The limit of treatment of myopia is in terms of spherical equivalent of 8 Diopters and cylinder of 6 diopters. The limit is given by the residual stroma that should be more than 300 μm and the predictability of the results.

TransPRK for Correction of Low Refraction Errors

With TransPRK, we altered the shape of the epithelium, and when the thickness of the epithelium matched the predetermined thickness of the software, we have a successful treatment. Arba and Awwad [22] published one of the first articles describing this technique. The capabilities of this approach are discussed in this theoretical study. The settings provided by the software's algorithms produce an epithelial thickness profile for TransPRK using the AMARIS laser system that resembles a mild hyperopic treatment (55 microns at the center and 65 microns at 4 mm of the periphery).

If the thickness of the epithelium is more than the applied epithelial ablation profile, the resulting effective optical zone (OZ) will be less. Because more stromal ablation than intended occurs when the epithelium is thinner, there is some tissue waste. As a result, when the real epithelium was thicker than what was predicted in the model, the impacts on the reduction in the obtained OZ (compared to the planned OZ) are smaller for higher refractive corrections or bigger OZs. The discrepancy between the planned and achieved OZ decreases as the planned refractive correction increases, and deeper ablation depths are accomplished as well with greater corrections or bigger OZs. The discrepancy between the planned and achieved OZ decreases as the planned refractive correction increases, and deeper ablation depths are accomplished as well with greater corrections or bigger OZs. They advise against employing TransPRK (with the default epithelium profile parameters) for myopia less than 1.00 diopter based on this theoretical calculation (D).

If it is not possible to reliably measure epithelium thickness with a diagnostic device in a clinical setting we proposed in a retrospective study of nearly 600 eyes after TransPRK [31] for low myopia (<2 D) increasing the epithelium thickness to 60 microns in the center and 70 microns at 4 mm in the periphery, as well as increasing the recommended OZ by 0.2 mm, and comparing it to a group of moderate myopia patients (> 2 D) treated with TransPRK in the standard software manner, without changing the epithelium thickness or the recommended OZ. To avoid changing the shape of the ablation profile, we have not made any adjustments to the increase in epithelium thickness from the center to the periphery. We wanted to obtain a minimum OZ of 6.5 mm because the amount of correction 2 D was little. However, we knew that if the epithelium was thicker than 55 microns at the center, we would theoretically achieve a smaller OZ or, in the worst case, no clinical correction. Therefore, we opted to utilize an OZ that was 0.2 mm larger and to design a thicker epithelial profile so that we could presume that the treatment was sufficiently deep to enter the epithelium. The only disadvantage of this choice was that some tissue was wasted because we went deeper than necessary, but this potential waste may not be clinically relevant for minor corrections. The epithelium thickness for the low myopia group has been increased to 60/70, a difference of only 5 µm from the default setting (55/65). The ablation adds a 5 µm buffer at all locations (equivalent to a flat 5 m PTK), but the profile (i.e., the refractive correction) remains unchanged. Similarly when we expand the OZ in diameter by 0.2 mm, representing only a 2 µm increase in ablation depth [31]. The ablation adds a 2 µm buffer at all locations and expands the ablation zone by 0.2 mm like a 2 µm flat PTK with a tapered TZ), but the profile (i.e., the refractive correction) remains unchanged. This modification is analogous to carrying out an aspherical phototherapeutic change in the cornea, which can result in the wastage of more tissue than is strictly required because we may go deeper than is strictly required while still achieving the desired optical zone. If we increase the thickness of the epithelium by 5 microns, it will theoretically ablate stroma when it should be ablating epithelium. Because this happens across the entire surface, the surface's overall curvature will end up being the same.

The software makes its recommendation for epithelium thickness after analyzing previously published research. It has been demonstrated by confocal microscopy [32], optical coherence tomography [33], and high-frequency ultrasound [34] that the epithelium has a central thickness that ranges from 52 to 54 microns, with a standard deviation of 7 microns. These findings come from a variety of studies that have been conducted.

Furthermore, additional refractive errors may be induced when the actual difference center-to-periphery in the corneal epithelial profile differs from the applied epithelial ablation profile. Jun et al. [35] compared the outcomes of mechanical PRK and TransPRK for myopia of 2 D or less, using a mean OZ of 7.1 mm; there were no significant differences in postoperative visual acuity or refractive error. According to the authors, using a large OZ in cornea refractive surgery has several advantages, including reduced postoperative night vision disturbances and halos, fewer optical aberrations, and fewer regressions.

Transepithelial approaches modify the cornea across the epithelium, allowing, theoretically, greater correspondence between the anterior corneal surface and corneal topography and the ablation profile than other refractive surgery techniques performed on deeper stromal layers of the cornea [11]. As a result, the possibility of inaccuracy is reduced to the differential in photoablation rates between stroma and epithelial tissue. When only small amount of tissue is involved, this difference (about 20% greater in epithelium [36]) is insignificant. Jun et al. recently published a study on transepithelial PRK and the inter-individual epithelial thickness profile variability and the associated refractive effect if the standard epithelial thickness was used for all cases; they discovered that the results were effective for both thin and thick epithelium corneas, but astigmatism was less corrected in eyes with thicker epithelium corneas [35].

Astigmatism Correction

In terms of astigmatic corrections, the normal population's mean asymmetry for epithelial thickness (if not considered in the profile) corresponds to 0.24 D of residual astigmatism [11]. In corneas with significant toricity (resulting in corneal astigmatism), the epithelial layer may have a different toricity than the underlying Bowman's membrane. In an in vivo study using slit scanning topography, moving from the anterior epithelial (air/tear film) interface to the Bowman's layer surface resulted in a clinically significant reduction in the amount of anterior astigmatism. This partial compensation demonstrates that the epithelial thickness distribution has azimuthal differences [31]. Because the thickness profile of the epithelial layer along the steepest meridian may differ from the thickness profile along the flattest meridian. The underlying epithelial toricty and the epithelial ablation profile would determine this. The use of a rotationally symmetrical transepithelial profile on a toric corneal surface may result in lenticules of wasted tissue with an oval perimeter (or variations in the achieved OZ) [11]. All these uncertainties may reduce astigmatic correction precision and limit the benefit provided by TransPRK ablations. While this is not a significant issue for the spherical component, small amounts of coma and astigmatism may be induced (with a mean value of 0.25 D worse astigmatism correction with TransPRK for normal populations, but peaks of up to 0.63 D). The risk of an extra 0.25 D of residual astigmatism (up to 0.5 D) should be considered when using radial symmetric epithelial ablation profiles [31]. In a retrospective study on eyes with astigmatism > 2 D we demonstrated with TransPRK an excellent angle matching by the laser in this population and confirming the refractive changes at the topographic level (keratometries) perfectly matched the measured change in manifest refraction [11]. The development of high-resolution OCT techniques allows us proper representation of the epithelial layer and measure the epithelial thickness, leading to customized epithelial ablations if we use the data of the epithelium thickness [37].

Epithelium Customized Ablations with TransPRK

We can now measure epithelial thickness with high repeatability and reproducibility using anterior segment coherence tomography (AS-OCT) [38, 39]. On the market, there are several AS-OCT instruments that can provide good reproducibility and reliability [40]. We used the MS-39 (Costruzione Strumenti Oftalmici, Florence, Italy), which combines AS-OCT with Placido Rings technology using spectral-domain anterior segment OCT combined with Placido-based topography, has an axial resolution of 3.5 microns for tissue and can calculate epithelial and stromal thickness maps over an 8 mm diameter [41]. So it can detect different corneal layers separately with a very high resolution and a wide-field epithelial thickness map [42]. We perform a retrospective study to compare the outcomes of TransPRK in a group of low-myopic eyes treated with an optimized standard corneal epithelium thickness to outcomes in a group of eyes treated with a customized epithelium thickness [37]. An optimized standard corneal epithelium thickness denotes an epithelium of 60 microns rather than the software's proposed epithelium of 55 microns, and it enlarges the optical zone (OZ) by at least 0.2 mm. The mean central thickness was entered in the laser to customized epithelium and at 4 mm an increment of 10 μm was entered for the periphery data of the epithelium.

Using OCT, Sin et al. [33] discovered that the epithelial thickness of normal eyes was 52 + /3 mm, with 5th and 95th percentiles for central epithelial thickness of 48 and 57 microns, respectively. Eckard et al. [32] used confocal laser scanning and reported a central mean thickness of 54 + /7 m and a peripheral mean thickness of 61.5 m. Reinstein et al. [34] used high-frequency digital ultrasound techniques to report a mean epithelial thickness at the corneal vertex of 53.4 + /4.6 microns, and the average epithelial thickness map revealed that the corneal epithelium was significantly thicker inferiorly rather than superiorly (5.9 μm at the 3.0 mm radius) and nasally rather than temporally (1.3 μm at the 3.0 mm radius). The epithelium's thinnest point was 0.33 mm temporally and 0.90 mm superiorly, with reference to the corneal vertex.

Both groups' accuracy was good. More eyes in the customized epithelium profile group had UDVAs greater than 20/20 and more eyes gained one line of CDVA post-operatively, indicating greater safety and effectiveness. In the new future it will be possible to customize even more the epithelium as we could probably enter also peripherally the data of the epithelium, and even maybe import an epithelium map.

Remodeling of the Epithelium After TransPRK

We also wanted to know how epithelium is remodeling after TransPRK with SPT. Although there have been attempts to distinguish (topographic or corneal) regression (i.e., the modified corneal curvature changes back towards its preoperative curvature) from refractive progression, the evolution of the postoperative refraction back towards the initial refraction has typically been referred to as (refractive) regression (i.e. the refraction changes back towards its preoperative values, by e.g. continued axial elongation). Topographic or corneal regression has been often associated to changes in the morphology epithelium induced by the changed in curvature imposed to the stroma [43, 44]. The refractive effect of epithelial remodelling following aberration-neutral Transepithelial Photorefractive Keratectomy [45] remained within 0.25 D for all measured locations along both meridian axes. The overall refractive effect of epithelial remodelling after aberration-neutral Transepithelial Photorefractive Keratectomy can be estimated as 0.09 D spherical equivalent component (average of the horizontal and vertical meridional effects), 0.19 D astigmatism component (difference between the horizontal and vertical meridional effects), and 0.49 D coma component (peak to valley refractive difference along the meridians).

TransPRK for Corrections After Other Refractive Treatments as Lens Exchange, SMILE or LASIK

In the refractive office the patients will not tolerate some degree of residual refractive error, therefore in some circumstances, a second surgery is required to enhance patient satisfaction and achieve good postoperative uncorrected visual acuity (UCVA).

In cases where we perform a lens exchange and after that If the ametropia is severe, we can replace the implanted intraocular lens or add a second intraocular lens (piggyback procedure). A third option is refractive corneal surgery. Laser vision correction has been demonstrated to be predictable and effective for correcting minor spherical and cylindrical errors [46, 47].

We also perform a study is to assess the efficiency of transepithelial photorefractive keratectomy (TransPRK) after clear lens exchange in correcting residual refractive error [48]. In alle cases we perform a TransPRK with a minimum optical zone of 7.2 mm entering on the vertex of the cornea. The average of eyes treated was 57 years old with a range between 48 to 68 years. The mean treated sphere was 0.42 D with a range between −1.0 and + 1.75 D. The mean astigmatism was 1.06 D. Postoperatively after Touch up we reduced the sphere 0.11 D (range −0.5 to + 0.75 D) and the mean astigmatism was 0.25 D (range −0.75 to 0 D). The predictability was for a SEQ (spheric equivalent) of 0.5 D 91% and for 1 D 100% of the cases. No eye loses more than 1 line.

Corrections after clear lens extraction. We used in most of the cases lenses with extended depth of focus, bifocal, and trifocal lenses in our center. We noticed that trifocal lenses required the most laser vision correction. A recent work by Seiler et al. [49] revealed that trifocal lenses in a population of cataract patients required laser vision correction in 26% of the instances. One of the challenges of utilizing multifocal lenses is measuring ametropia; measurements taken in individuals with diffractive IOLs may not be reliable.

Many aberrometers are incapable of obtaining an accurate measurement through these lenses. In multifocal IOLs, refraction may vary based on lighting conditions and pupil size. To avoid postoperative predictability issues [50], a reference point for spherical subjective refraction should be set when refracting patients with multifocal IOLs, as the midway of the clear vision interval afforded by the depth of field of the IOL. For Astigmatism, we employ Topography and Ocular Wavefront data to determine which is the best accepted astigmatism for distant and near vision.

We published the first correction with TransPRK for small incision lenticule extraction (SMILE) [51]. Surface ablation has advantages over intrastromal ablations, especially when the goal is to repair the generated aberrations [52]. We can treat the induced aberrations and the refractive error after SMILE, the advantage over other surface techniques is the faster recovery of the visual acuity [8]. Gab-Alla [53] published recently a bigger group of eyes treated with TransPRK after SMILE showing also good results. For enhancements after stromal ablation, we recommend using Mitomycin C 0.02% for at least 20 s.

TransPRK Medication

After the eyes were treated with TransPRK, the interface was irrigated with balanced salt solution, for removing any debris. At the end of the procedure one Ofloxacin drop (3 mg pro ml), one Dexamethason drop (0.5 mg pro 0.5 ml), and one Phenylephrin drop (82.1 mg pro ml) were applied and bandage contact lenses were placed before discharging the patient. Patients received Dexamethason eye drops and Orfloxacin for 1 week 4 times and Fluormetholon (Fluoropos Ursapharm GmbH, Germany) 3 times per day for another 6 weeks, preservative free lubricants for 2 months as needed, and beyond as per the need.

We use Mitomycin C 0,02% for 20 s only for Hyperopia treatments of 2 Dioptres or ablation of stroma higher than 100 µm and after retreatments.

TransPRK Versus Other Laser Refractive Techniques

TransPRK is an advanced surface ablation technique with similar results versus PRK and LASEK, the mean difference is the visual recovery time that have been showed in different studies to be better with TransPRK as the ablation treats only the necessary epithelium diameter and therefore as showed be Lee et al. [8] the epithelium is earlier closed. The group of Aslanides [2] found that TransPRK offers faster epithelial healing, lower pain scores, and significantly less haze formation than LASEK.

Other advantage is that the topography or aberrometry that we measured is that we treat with customized ablation. Transepithelial approaches aim to modify the cornea across the epithelium, allowing for greater correspondence between corneal topography and ablation profile than other refractive surgery techniques performed on deeper stromal layers of the cornea. The epithelium map is included in the topography if we use an optical coherence tomography [37] and therefore the customization could be more effective. We have used customized epithelium thickness [37] for TransPRK and got better results than without customization. We customized the center and give at the periphery the 10 μm proposed by the software. Nowadays we can export the epithelium map and the software imports the data and the periphery at 4 mm with a mean value.

LASIK with Microkeratome or with Femtosecond Laser (Femto-LASIK) get similar results as diverse metaanalysis [54, 55] show in terms of effectivity but in terms of safety TransPRK is superior.

The group of Luger et al. [56] compared TransPRK with Femto-LASIK in correction of myopia in 196 eyes for each group, the outcomes 1 year postoperatively were equivalent to those of femtosecond-assisted LASIK. Transepithelial PRK was efficacious and safe; however, the procedure had a longer recovery time than the femtosecond-assisted LASIK. The UCDVA was better with TransPRK.

Similar results had the group Aslanides et al. [57] compared the outcomes of single-step modified transepithelial PRK with those of conventional alcohol-assisted PRK and LASIK to correct myopia of 6.00 D or more. Refractive outcomes and regression at 12 months did not vary between groups (P O 0.05). the found a significantly better vision in the transepithelial PRK group than in the LASIK group and the PRK group.

The lenticule extraction procedure (SMILE) and the surface ablation technique (PRK) may be considered equivalent in terms of biomechanical stability when measured experimentally in ex vivo human fellow eye corneas. [58] In terms of preserving corneal biomechanical strength after surgeries, SMILE was superior to either FS-LASIK or LASIK, while comparable to PRK/LASEK group based on the results from ocular response analyzer [59].

Difficult is to compare TransPRK with lenticule extraction, most studies compare SMILE with Femto-LASIK but there are few comparing refractive results TransPRK with SMILE.

When compared to Trans-PRK and LASIK, SMILE has an intermediate vision recovery time and no flap-related problems. However, it is missing the eye-tracking system, cyclotorsion-compensation system, and personalized treatment profile for high astigmatism or an uneven corneal surface.

If we look at the SMILE results, there is an interesting editorial from Lietman et al. [60] the authors that most of the studies show that there is a non inferiority of SMILE versus Femto-LASIK or PRK but they not showing superiority at least at the moment that I am writing this chapter. Non inferiority studies use a margin (the non-inferiority margin) a predetermined margin of difference between the new and standard treatment that is considered acceptable or tolerable for the new treatment to be considered 'similar' or 'not worse'. The problem with essays of non-inferiority is that if the sample size is small, we will not see differences and then at least the new method is not worse or similar.

So the study from Ang et al. [61] compared SMILE versus LASIK with an non inferiority margin of 10% and used for this randomized study of 70 patients undergoing in 1 eye LASIK and in the other SMILE. The efficacy index was calculated by dividing the mean postoperative UDVA by the mean preoperative CDVA (0.97 SMILE vs. 0.99 LASIK P 1⁄4 0.56), UDVA of 20/20 or better (84% vs. 87%); In terms of the percentage of eyes within ± 0.5 D of attempted correction, 87% of SMILE and 92% of LASIK eyes achieved this.

In other words, TransPRK was the most efficacious and safe laser correction when we revised the literature. SMILE has not demonstrated to be superior to Femto-LASIK or TransPRK; it has only demonstrated to not be inferior.

References

1. Clinch TE, Moshirfar M, Weis JR, Ahn CS, Hutchinson CB, Jeffrey JH. Comparison of mechanical and transepithelial debridement during photorefractive keratectomy. Ophthalmology. 1999;106(3):483–9.https://doi.org/10.1016/S0161-6420(99)90135-5.
2. Aslanides IM, Padroni S, Arba Mosquera S, Ioannides A, Mukherjee A. Comparison of single-step reverse transepithelial all-surface laser ablation (ASLA) to alcohol-assisted photorefractive keratectomy. Clin Ophthalmol. 2012;6:973–80. https://doi.org/10.2147/OPTH.S32374.
3. Kaluzny BJ, Cieslinska I, Mosquera SA, Verma S. Single-step transepithelial PRK vs alcohol-assisted PRK in myopia and compound myopic astigmatism correction. Medicine (Baltimore). 2016;95(6): e1993. https://doi.org/10.1097/MD.0000000000001993.
4. Antonios R, Abdul Fattah M, Arba Mosquera S, Abiad BH, Sleiman K, Awwad ST. Br J Ophthalmol. 2017;101(8):1106–12. https://doi.org/10.1136/bjophthalmol-2016-309409.
5. Arba-Mosquera S, Hollerbach T. Ablation resolution in laser corneal refractive surgery: the dual fluence concept of the AMARIS platform. Adv Opt Technol. 2010;2010:1–13. https://doi.org/10.1155/2010/538541.
6. Adib-Moghaddam S, Soleyman-Jahi S, Sanjari Moghaddam A, et al. Efficacy and safety of transepithelial photorefractive keratectomy. J Cataract Refract Surg. 2018;44(10):1267–1279. https://doi.org/10.1016/j.jcrs.2018.07.021
7. de Ortueta D, von Rüden D. Transepithelial photorefractive keratectomy : results and clinical experiences. Ophthalmologe. 2018;116(6):534–41. https://doi.org/10.1007/s00347-018-0814-x.
8. Lee HK, Lee KS, Kim JK, Kim HC, Seo KR, Kim EK. Epithelial healing and clinical outcomes in excimer laser photorefractive surgery following three epithelial removal techniques: mechanical, alcohol, and excimer laser. Am J Ophthalmol. 2005;139(1):56–63. https://doi.org/10.1016/j.ajo.2004.08.049.
9. Vinciguerra P, Camesasca FI, Vinciguerra R, et al. Advanced surface ablation with a new software for the reduction of ablation irregularities. J Refract Sur g. 2017;33(2):89–95. https://doi.org/10.3928/1081597X-20161122-01.
10. de Ortueta D, Magnago T, Triefenbach N, Arba Mosquera S, Sauer U, Brunsmann U. In vivo measurements of thermal load during ablation in high-speed laser corneal refractive surgery. J Refract Surg. 2012;28(1):53–8. https://doi.org/10.3928/1081597X-20110906-01.
11. de Ortueta D, von Rüden D, Verma S, Magnago T, Arba-Mosquera S. Transepithelial photorefractive keratectomy in moderate to high astigmatism with a non-wavefront–guided aberration-neutral ablation profile. J Refract Surg. 2018;34(7):466–74. https://doi.org/10.3928/1081597X-20180402-04.
12. Lin DTC, Holland SP, Verma S, Hogden J, Arba-Mosquera S. Immediate and short term visual recovery after SmartSurf(ACE) photorefractive keratectomy. J Optom. 2019;12(4):240–7. https://doi.org/10.1016/j.optom.2019.04.003.
13. Aslanides IM, Kymionis GD. Trans advanced surface laser ablation (TransPRK) outcomes using SmartPulseTechnology. Cont Lens Anterior Eye. 2017;40(1):42–6. https://doi.org/10.1016/j.clae.2016.11.004.
14. de Ortueta D, Schreyger FD. Centration on the cornea vertex normal during hyperopic refractive photoablation using videokeratoscopy. J Refract Surg. 2007;23(2):198–200
15. Arbelaez MC, Vidal C, Arba-Mosquera S. Clinical outcomes of corneal vertex versus central pupil references with aberration-free ablation strategies and LASIK. Invest Ophthalmol Vis Sci. 2008;49(12):5287–94. https://doi.org/10.1167/iovs.08-2176.
16. Artal P, Chen L, Fernández EJ, Singer B, Manzanera S, Williams DR. Neural compensation for the eye's optical aberrations. J Vis. 2004;4(4):4. https://doi.org/10.1167/4.4.4.
17. Marcos S, Cano D, Barbero S. Increase in corneal asphericity after standard laser in situ keratomileusis for myopia is not inherent to the munnerlyn algorithm. J Refract Surg. 2003;19(5):S592-6. https://doi.org/10.3928/1081-597X-20030901-17.
18. Arba-Mosquera S, de Ortueta D. Geometrical analysis of the loss of ablation efficiency at non-normal incidence. Opt Express. 2008;16(6):3877–95. https://doi.org/10.1364/oe.16.003877.
19. Mrochen M, Seiler T. Influence of corneal curvature on calculation of ablation patterns used in photorefractive laser surgery. J Refract Surg. 2001;17(5):S584-7. https://doi.org/10.3928/1081-597X-20010901-15.
20. Jiménez JR, Anera RG, Barco LJ, Hita E, Pérez-Ocón F. Correction factor for ablation algorithms used in corneal refractive surgery with gaussian-profile beams. Opt Express. 2005;13(1):336–43. https://doi.org/10.1364/OPEX.13.000336.
21. Anera RG, Jiménez JR, Jiménez del Barco L, Hita E. Changes in corneal asphericity after laser refractive surgery, including reflection losses and non-normal incidence upon the anterior cornea. Opt Lett. 2003;28(6):417–9. https://doi.org/10.1364/OL.28.000417
22. Arba Mosquera S, Awwad ST. Theoretical analyses of the refractive implications of transepithelial PRK ablations. Br J Ophthalmol. 2013;97(7):905–11. https://doi.org/10.1136/bjophthalmol-2012-302853.
23. Arba-Mosquera S, Arbelaez MC, de Ortueta D. Laser corneal refractive surgery in the twenty-first century: a review of the impact of refractive surgery on high-order aberrations (and vice versa). J Mod Opt. 2010;57(12):1041–74. https://doi.org/10.1080/09500340.2010.493243.
24. Levy Y, Segal O, Avni I, Zadok D. Ocular higher-order aberrations in eyes with supernormal vision.

Am J Ophthalmol. 2005;139(2):225–8. https://doi.org/10.1016/j.ajo.2004.08.035.
25. Bará S, Navarro R. Wide-field compensation of monochromatic eye aberrations: expected performance and design trade-offs. J Opt Soc Am A. 2003;20(1):1–10. https://doi.org/10.1364/JOSAA.20.000001.
26. Arba-Mosquera S, de Ortueta D. Analysis of optimized profiles for "aberration-free" refractive surgery. Ophthalmic Physiol Opt. 2009;29(5):535–48. https://doi.org/10.1111/j.1475-1313.2009.00670.x.
27. de Ortueta D, Arba Mosquera S, Baatz H. Aberration-neutral ablation pattern in hyperopic LASIK with the ESIRIS laser platform. J Refract Surg. 2009;25(2):175–84. https://doi.org/10.3928/1081597X-20090201-02.
28. de Ortueta D, Arba Mosquera S, Baatz H. Comparison of standard and aberration-neutral profiles for myopic LASIK with the SCHWIND ESIRIS platform. J Refract Surg. 2009;25(4):339–49. https://doi.org/10.3928/1081597X-20090401-03.
29. Arba Mosquera S, de Ortueta D. Optimized zernike term selection in customized treatments for laser corneal refractive surgery: case report. J Refract Surg. 2010;27(2):148–52. https://doi.org/10.3928/1081597X-20100224-01.
30. Fadlallah A, Fahed D, Khalil K, et al. Transepithelial photorefractive keratectomy: clinical results. J Cataract Refract Surg. 2011;37(10):1852–7. https://doi.org/10.1016/j.jcrs.2011.04.029.
31. de Ortueta D, von Rüden D, Arba-Mosquera S. Comparison of refractive and visual outcomes after transepithelial photorefractive keratectomy (TransPRK) in low versus moderate myopia. Photonics. 2021;8(7):262. https://doi.org/10.3390/photonics8070262.
32. Eckard A, Stave J, Guthoff RF. In vivo investigations of the corneal epithelium with the confocal Rostock Laser Scanning Microscope (RLSM). Cornea. 2006;25(2):127–31. https://doi.org/10.1097/01.ico.0000170694.90455.f7.
33. Sin S, Simpson TL. The repeatability of corneal and corneal epithelial thickness measurements using optical coherence tomography. Optom Vis Sci. 2006;83(6):360–5. https://doi.org/10.1097/01.opx.0000221388.26031.23.
34. Reinstein DZ, Archer TJ, Gobbe M, Silverman RH, Coleman DJ. Epithelial thickness in the normal cornea: three-dimensional display with Artemis very high-frequency digital ultrasound. J Refract Surg. 2008;24(6):571–81. https://doi.org/10.3928/1081597X-20080601-05.
35. Jun I, Yong Kang DS, Arba-Mosquera S, et al. Clinical outcomes of mechanical and transepithelial photorefractive keratectomy in low myopia with a large ablation zone. J Cataract Refract Surg. 2019;45(7):977–84. https://doi.org/10.1016/j.jcrs.2019.02.007.
36. Seiler T, Kriegerowski M, Schnoy N, Bende T. Ablation rate of human corneal epithelium and Bowman's layer with the excimer laser (193 nm). Refract Corneal Surg. 1990;6(2):99–102.
37. de Ortueta D, von Rüden D, Arba-Mosquera S. Customized versus standard epithelium profiles in transepithelial photorefractive keratectomy. Optics. 2021;2(4):266–75. https://doi.org/10.3390/opt2040025.
38. Hashmani N, Hashmani S, Saad CM. Wide corneal epithelial mapping using an optical coherence tomography. Invest Ophthalmol Vis Sci. 2018;59(3):1652. https://doi.org/10.1167/iovs.17-23717.
39. Haque S, Jones L, Simpson T. Thickness mapping of the cornea and epithelium using optical coherence tomography. Optom Vis Sci. 2008;85(10):E963–76. https://doi.org/10.1097/OPX.0b013e318188892c.
40. Savini G, Schiano-Lomoriello D, Hoffer KJ. Repeatability of automatic measurements by a new anterior segment optical coherence tomographer combined with Placido topography and agreement with 2 Scheimpflug cameras. J Cataract Refract Surg. 2018;44(4). https://journals.lww.com/jcrs/Fulltext/2018/04000/Repeatability_of_automatic_measurements_by_a_new.10.aspx
41. Khamar P, Rao K, Wadia K, et al. Advanced epithelial mapping for refractive surgery. Indian J Ophthalmol. 2020;68(12):2819. https://doi.org/10.4103/ijo.IJO_2399_20.
42. Mohammadpour M, Heidari Z. MS-39®. In: Mohammadpour M, editor. Diagnostics in ocular imaging. Springer International Publishing; 2021. p. 265–84. https://doi.org/10.1007/978-3-030-54863-6_6
43. Lohmann CP, Guell JL. Regression after LASIK for the treatment of myopia: the role of the corneal epithelium. Semin Ophthalmol. 1998;13(2):79–82. https://doi.org/10.3109/08820539809059822.
44. Reinstein DZ, Archer TJ, Gobbe M. Rate of change of curvature of the corneal stromal surface drives epithelial compensatory changes and remodeling. J Refract Surg. 2014;30(12):800–2. https://doi.org/10.3928/1081597X-20141113-02.
45. de Ortueta D, von Rüden D, Arba-Mosquera S. Refractive effect of epithelial remodelling in myopia after transepithelial photorefractive keratectomy. Vision. 2022;6(4):74. https://doi.org/10.3390/vision6040074.
46. Sáles CS, Manche EE. Managing residual refractive error after cataract surgery. J Cataract Refract Surg. 2015;41(6):1289–99. https://doi.org/10.1016/j.jcrs.2015.05.001.
47. Moshirfar M, McCaughey MV, Santiago-Caban L. Corrective techniques and future directions for treatment of residual refractive error following cataract surgery. Expert Rev Ophthalmol. 2014;9(6):529–37. https://doi.org/10.1586/17469899.2014.966817.
48. de Ortueta D. Transepithelial photorefractive keratektomy after a clear lens exchange. Vision (Basel). 2021;5(1). https://doi.org/10.3390/vision5010008
49. Seiler TG, Wegner A, Senfft T, Seiler T. Dissatisfaction after trifocal IOL implantation and its

improvement by selective wavefront-guided LASIK. J Refract Surg. 2019;35(6):346–52. https://doi.org/10.3928/1081597X-20190510-02.
50. Piñero DP, Espinosa MJA, Alió JL. LASIK outcomes following multifocal and monofocal intraocular lens implantation. J Refract Surg. 2010;26(8):569–77. https://doi.org/10.3928/1081597X-20091030-02.
51. de Ortueta D, von Rüden D, Verma S, Arba-Mosquera S. TransPRK treatment for residual refractive error and induced aberrations in eye undergone SMILE treatment. Eur J Ophthalmol. 2021;31(6):NP22–5. https://doi.org/10.1177/1120672120934393
52. Siedlecki J, Luft N, Kook D, et al. Enhancement after myopic small incision lenticule extraction (smile) using surface ablation. J Refract Surg. 2017;33(8):513–8. https://doi.org/10.3928/1081597X-20170602-01.
53. Gab-Alla AA. SmartSurfACE transepithelial photorefractive keratectomy with mitomycin C enhancement after small incision lenticule extraction. Eye Vis (Lond). 2021;8(1):28. https://doi.org/10.1186/s40662-021-00254-2.
54. Peñarrocha-Oltra S, Soto-Peñaloza R, Alonso-Arroyo A, Vidal-Infer A, Pascual-Segarra J. Laser-based refractive surgery techniques to treat myopia in adults. An overview of systematic reviews and meta-analyses. Acta Ophthalmologica. 2022;100(8):878–93. https://doi.org/10.1111/aos.15160
55. Chang JY, Lin PY, Hsu CC, Liu CJL. Comparison of clinical outcomes of LASIK, Trans-PRK, and SMILE for correction of myopia. J Chin Med Assoc. 2022;85(2):145–51. https://doi.org/10.1097/JCMA.0000000000000674.
56. Luger MHA, Ewering T, Arba-Mosquera S. Myopia correction with transepithelial photorefractive keratectomy versus femtosecond-assisted laser in situ keratomileusis: one-year case-matched analysis. J Cataract Refract Surg. 2016;42(11):1579–87. https://doi.org/10.1016/j.jcrs.2016.08.025.
57. Aslanides I, Georgoudis P, Selimis V, Mukherjee A. Single-step transepithelial ASLA (SCHWIND) with mitomycin-C for the correction of high myopia: long term follow-up. OPTH. 2014;33. https://doi.org/10.2147/OPTH.S73424
58. Spiru B, Torres-Netto EA, Kling S, Lazaridis A, Hafezi F, Sekundo W. Biomechanical properties of human Cornea tested by two-dimensional extensiometry Ex Vivo in fellow eyes: PRK versus SMILE. J Refract Surg. 2019;35(8):501–5. https://doi.org/10.3928/1081597X-20190730-02.
59. Guo H, Hosseini-Moghaddam SM, Hodge W. Corneal biomechanical properties after SMILE versus FLEX, LASIK, LASEK, or PRK: a systematic review and meta-analysis. BMC Ophthalmol. 2019;19(1):167. https://doi.org/10.1186/s12886-019-1165-3.
60. Lietman TM, Oldenburg CE, O'Brien KS. Noninferiority: it's all in the margins. Ophthalmology. 2020;127(6):711–2. https://doi.org/10.1016/j.ophtha.2020.04.010.
61. Ang M, Farook M, Htoon HM, Mehta JS. Randomized clinical trial comparing femtosecond LASIK and small-incision lenticule extraction. Ophthalmology. 2020;127(6):724–30. https://doi.org/10.1016/j.ophtha.2019.09.006.

3 Historical Overview of the Clinical Development of "All in One" Femtosecond Refractive Laser Surgery

Marcus Blum and Walter Sekundo

Abstract

Corneal resectional refractive procedures for the correction of myopia were pioneered by Barraquer and Ruiz in the 60s and 70s (Barraquer in Int Ophthalmol Clin 36:1–7, 1996). They removed a layer of intrastromal tissue utilizing a microkeratome and called this procedure "in situ keratomileusis". However, the results of the procedure performed with mechanical devices were not entirely satisfactory (Ibrahim et al. in J Refract Surg 11:431–41, 1995; Wiegand et al. in Erste Ergebnisse. Ophthalmologe 92:402–9, 1995).

Keywords

Femtosecond laser · Excimer laser · Femtosecond laser system · Myopic astigmatism · Corneal flap

SMILE stands for small incision lenticule extraction and is the most recent revolution in corneal refractive surgery. During the SMILE procedure, the femtosecond laser cuts a lenticule inside the corneal stroma which is removed by a side incision. A corneal flap with all the negative side effects is no longer necessary. This technique was developed by the company Zeiss together with Prof. Sekundo (Marburg, Germany), Prof. Blum (Erfurt, Germany), and Prof. Meyer (Cologne, Germany). The authors describe the development of this new technique and demonstrate the surgery step by step.

M. Blum (✉)
Department of Ophthalmology, Helios Hospital Erfurt, Erfurt, Germany
e-mail: marcus.blum@helios-gesundheit.de

W. Sekundo
Department of Ophthalmology, Phillips Universität Marburg, Marburg, Germany

Corneal resectional refractive procedures for the correction of myopia were pioneered by Barraquer and Ruiz in the 60s and 70s [1]. They removed a layer of intrastromal tissue utilizing a microkeratome and called this procedure "in situ keratomileusis". However, the results of the procedure performed with mechanical devices were not entirely satisfactory [2, 3].

Few years later, lasers entered the field of refractive surgery, and in 1989, Stern reported the use of lasers to ablate the cornea [4]. For many years a number of sophisticated excimer laser systems have been available to perform laser in situ keratomileusis (LASIK) with a very high accuracy. The microkeratome was used to create the corneal flap. The first use of a laser instead of a microkeratome to achieve an intrastromal lenticule was described in 1996 [5]. Using a picosecond laser an intrastromal lenticule was generated and was then removed manually after lifting the flap. In two highly myopic eyes a fair amount of manual dissection was required resulting in an irregular surface [6]. Its use was therefore limited to animal studies [7, 8]. It is noteworthy that in the early 90s of the

U. Spandau and G. B. Schariothn(eds.), *Cutting Edge of Ophthalmic Surgery*,
https://doi.org/10.1007/978-3-031-84204-7_3

last century, the idea of full femtosecond laser system based refractive correction had already been born.

First clinical results with a laser induced extraction of a refractive lenticule were reported with five blind or amblyopic eyes in 2003 [9]. Unfortunately, these first studies lack a sufficient number of eyes and a detailed analysis of the achieved refractive data. The studies have not been continued with a representative study cohort.

For several years femtosecond laser technology was used solely to the creation of flaps and thus to take the place of the microkeratome. The actual refractive procedure was still performed with the 193 nm excimer laser [10]. With regard to the quality of the surgical outcome, femtosecond laser microkeratomes have advantages over mechanical devices [11–13].

After a series of experiments in the laboratory and in animal models as well as after some initial treatments of blind eyes a prototype femtosecond laser system—now known as VisuMax® (Carl Zeiss Meditec, Jena, Germany) came on the market. To prove the function of the fs-laser a study combining the fs-flap cut with the MEL 80 Excimer laser was performed first [14]. During the same time a series of studies (unpublished data) with animals and blind eyes underwent a new refractive procedure which no longer required an excimer laser (Fig. 3.1a–e). The

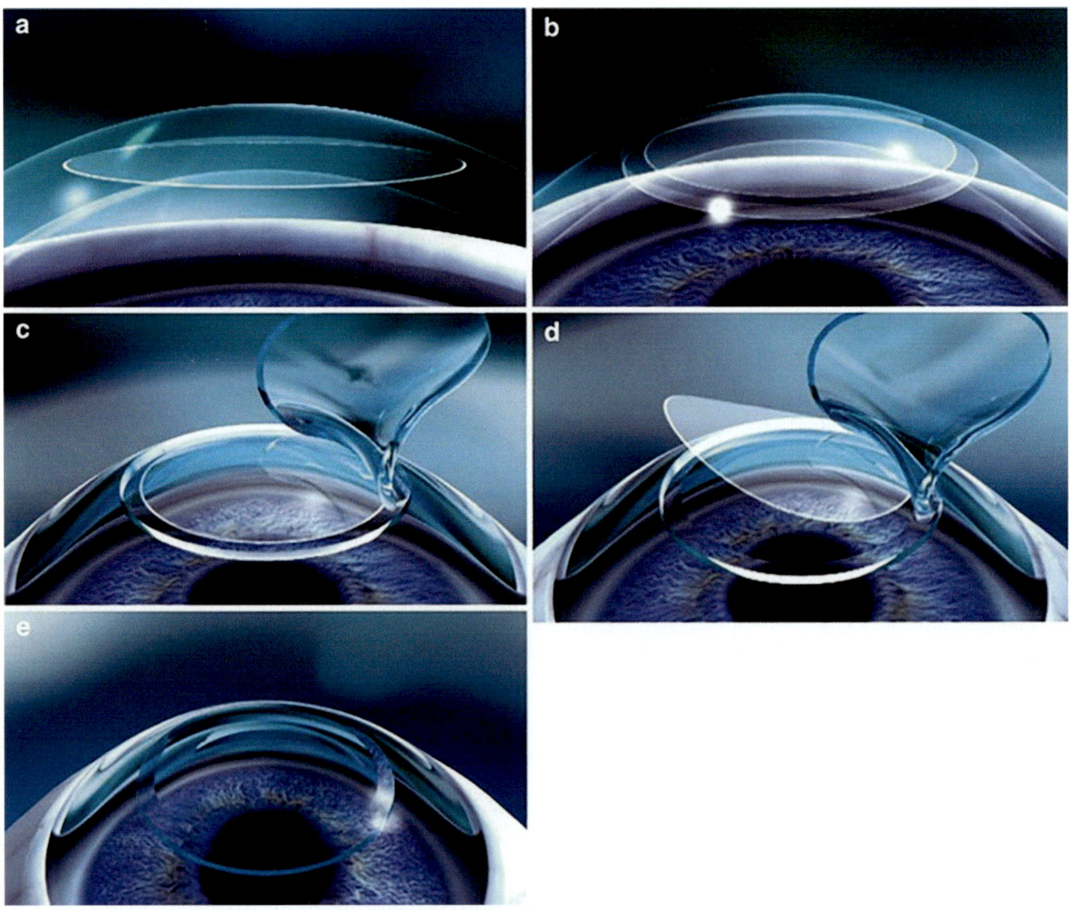

Fig. 3.1 (**a**–**e**) A schematic drawing of the FLEx-procedure. The VisuMax® femtosecond laser system cuts the back of the refractive lenticule (**a**) followed by its front surface incision (**b**) followed by a vertical incision leaving an arc of 50° untouched (hinge) (**c**). The final step is performed manually, with the flap being lifted with the spatula and the lenticule removed manually using forceps (**d**). The flap is then repositioned (**e**)

procedure was called Femtosecond Lenticule Extraction (FLEx) in order to distinguish it from other known refractive procedures. When performing FLEx, both the flap and the refractive lenticule are cut in a "one step"-procedure by the femtosecond laser. The first ten cases were presented by Sekundo at the 2006 annual meeting of the American Academy of Ophthalmology (AAO) and published in 2008 [15].

This very first report was followed by a cohort of fully seeing eyes treated for myopia. A total of 108 eyes had been recruited and treated from 56 patients with spherical myopia between − 2 and − 8.5 D and myopic astigmatism up to − 6 D cyl. The eyes were followed up for 6 months and—on a voluntary basis—for 12 months [16, 17]. Meanwhile 5 year results were published [18].

The consequent improvement of the FLEx technique which requires a flap was the development of a flapless technique. A flapless technique would enable a mechanic stable cornea. FLEx turned out to be just one step towards developing a new technique without lifting the flap—made possible by continuous improvements in surgical performance, energy settings, and laser technology [19–21]. This procedure was named Small Incision Lenticule Extraction (SMILE): by passing a dissector through a small 2–3 mm incision the anterior and posterior lenticular interfaces are separated and the lenticule is than removed through the incision (Fig. 3.2a–c). This eliminates the need to create a flap and the cornea above the upper interface of the lenticule is now referred to as the cap.

First results of this minimally invasive procedure have been published by our group in 2011 [22]. The potential advantages of this refined technique have encouraged a number of international groups to employ the newly developed 500 kHz femto second laser for refractive lenticule extraction [23–25]. In order to avoid confusion, the "all in one" femtosecond laser alone procedures have been patented by the manufacturer of the VisuMax laser as refractive lenticule extraction (ReLEx®) with two possible techniques: the ReLEx® flex and ReLEx® smile. Meanwhile the small incision lenticule

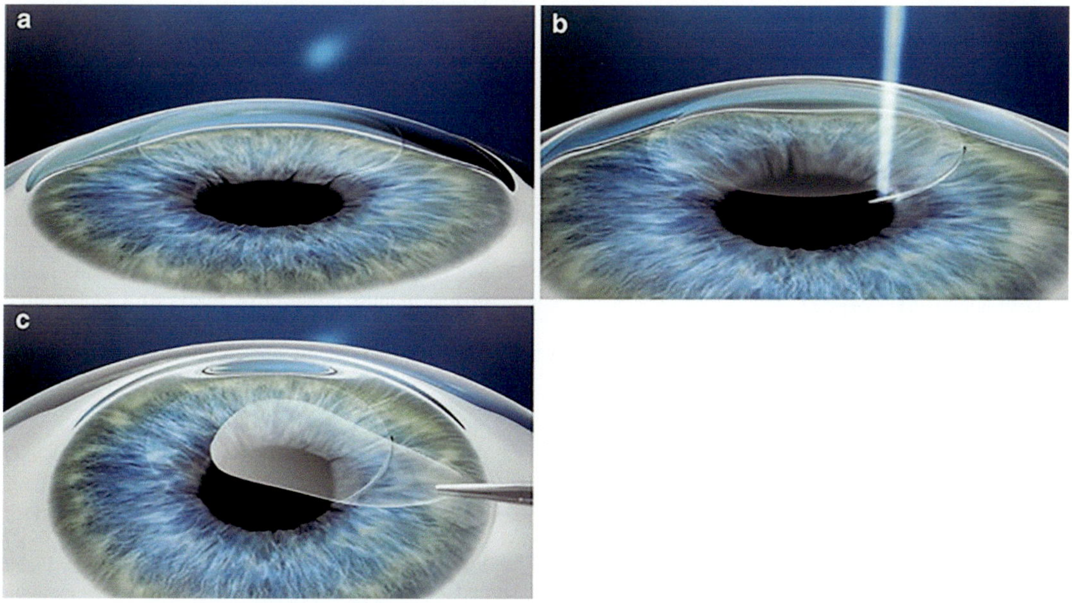

Fig. 3.2 (**a–c**) A schematic drawing of the SMILE procedure. The fs-Laser cuts the posterior and anterior surface of the lenticule in the corneal stroma (**a**), followed by a small incision of the epithelium (**b**). The lenticule is removed through this small incision (**c**) by the use of forceps without lifting a flap. The tissue above the lenticule is therefore referred to as the "cap"

extraction (SMILE) became a well-known term, which in our opinion will remain irrespective of the manufacturer of the laser.

The rapid increase in available clinical data has led to an ongoing discussion about the advantages and disadvantages of ReLEx femtosecond lenticule extraction [26–36]. We will now describe the technique in its different stages and its current clinical applications.

References

1. Barraquer JI. The history and evolution of keratomileusis. Int Ophthalmol Clin. 1996;36:1–7.
2. Ibrahim O, Waring GO, Salah T, el Maghraby A. Automated in situ Keratomileusis for myopia. J Refract Surg. 1995;11:431–41.
3. Wiegand W, Krusenberg B, Kroll P. Keratomileusis in situ bei hochgradiger Myopie. Erste Ergebnisse. Ophthalmologe. 1995;92:402–9.
4. Stern D, Schoenlein RW, Puliafito CA. Corneal ablation by nanosecond, picoseconds, and femtosecond lasers at 532 and 625 nm. Arch Ophthalmol. 1989;107:567–92.
5. Ito M, Quantock AJ, Malhan S, Schanzlin DJ, Krueger RR. Picosecond laser in situ keratomileusis with a 1053-nm Nd:YFL laser. J Refract Surg. 1996;12:721–8.
6. Krueger RR, Juhasz T, Gualano A, Marchi V. The picosecond laser for nonmechanical laser in situ keratomileusis. J Refract Surg. 1998;14:467–9.
7. Kurtz RM, Horvath C, Liu HH, Krueger RR, Juhasz T. Lamellar refractive surgery with scanned intrastromal picoseconds and femtosecond laser pulses in animal eyes. J Refract Surg. 1998;14:541–8.
8. Heisterkamp A, Mamon T, Kermani O, Drommer W, Welling H, Ertmer W, Lubatschowski H. Intrastromal refractive surgery with ultrashort laser pulses: in vivo study on the rabbit eye. Graefes Arch Clin Exp Ophthalmol. 2003;241:511–7.
9. Ratkay-Traub I, Ferincz IE, Juhasz T, Kurtz RM, Krueger RR. First clinical results with the femtosecond neodymium-glass laser in refractive surgery. J Refract Surg. 2003;19:94–103.
10. Nordan LT, Slade SG, Baker RN. Femtosecond laser flap creation for laser in situ keratomileusis: six-months follow-up of the initial US clinical series. J Refract Surg. 2003;19:8–14.
11. Kezirian GM, Stonecipher KG. Comparison of the IntraLase femtosecond laser and mechanical microkeratome for laser in situ Keratomileusis. J Cataract Refract Surg. 2004;30:26–32.
12. Durrie DS, Kezirian GM. Femtosecond laser versus mechanical keratome flaps in wavefront-guided laser in situ keratomileusis: prospective contralateral eye study. J Cataract Refract Surg. 2005;31:120–6.
13. Tran DB, Sarayba MA, Bor Z, et al. Randomized prospective clinical study comparing induced aberrations with IntraLase and Hansatome flap creation in fellow eyes: potential impact on wavefront-guided laser in situ keratomileusis. J Cataract Refract Surg. 2005;31:97–105.
14. Blum M, Kunert K, Gille A, Sekundo W. First experience in Femtosecond LASIK with the Zeiss VISUMAX® Laser. J Refract Surg. 2009;25:350–6.
15. Sekundo W, Kunert K, Russmann C, Gille A, Bissmann W, Strobrawa G, Stickler M, Bischoff M, Blum M. First efficacy and safty study of femtosecond lenticule extraction for the correction of myopia. J Cataract Refract Surg. 2008;34:1513–20.
16. Blum M, Kunert K, Schröder M, Sekundo W. Femtosecond Lenticule Extraction (FLEX) for the correction of myopia: 6 months results. Graefe's Arch Clin Exp Ophthalmol. 2010;248:1019–27.
17. Blum M, Kunert KS, Engelbrecht C, Dawczynski J, Sekundo W. Femtosekunden-Lentikel-Extraktion (FLEX) – Ergebnisse nach 12 Monaten bei myopem Astigmatismus. Klin Monatsbl Augenheilkd. 2010;227:961–5.
18. Blum M, Flach A, Kunert KS, Sekundo W. Five-year results of refractive lenticule extraction. J Cataract Refract Surg. 2014;40:1425–9.
19. Shah R, Shah S. Effect of scanning patterns on the results of femtosecond laser lenticule extraction refractive surgery. J Cataract Refract Surg. 2011;37:1636–47.
20. Kunert KS, Blum M, Duncker GIW, Sietmann R, Heichel J. Surface quality of human corneal lenticules after femtosecond laser surgery for myopia comparing different laser parameters. Graefe's Arch Clin Exp Ophthalmol. 2011;249:1417–24.
21. Heichelt J, Blum M, Duncker GIW, Sietmann R, Kunert KS. Surface quality of porcine corneal lenticules after Femtosecond Lenticule extraction. Ophthalmic Res. 2011;46:107–12.
22. Sekundo W, Kunert K, Blum M. Small incision femtosecond lenticule extraction (SMILE) for the correction of myopia and myopic astigmatism: results of a 6 months prospective study. Br J Ophthalmol. 2011;95:335–9.
23. Shah R, Shah S, Segupta S. Results of small incision lenticule extraction: all-in-one femtosecond laser refractive surgery. J Cataract Refract Surg. 2011;37:127–37.
24. Hjortdal JO, Vestergaard AH, Ivarsen A, Ragunathan S, Asp S. Predictors for the outcome of small-incision lenticule extraction for myopia. J Refract Surg. 2012;28:865–71.
25. Kamiya K, Shimizu K, Igarashi A, Kobashi H. Visual and refractive outcomes of femtosecond lenticule extraction and small-incision lenticule extraction for myopia. Am J Ophthalmol. 2014;157:128–34.
26. Ivarsen A, Asp S, Hjortdal J. Safty and complications of more than 1500 small incision lenticule extraction procedures. Ophthalmology. 2014;121:822–82.

27. Sekundo W, Gertnere J, Bertelmann T, Solomatin I. One-year refractive results, contrast sensitivity, high-order aberrations and complications after myopic small-incision lenticule extraction (ReLEx SMILE). Graefes Arch Clin Exp Ophthalmol. 2014;252(5):837–43.
28. Vestergaard AH, Gronbech KT, Grauslund J, et al. Subbasal nerve morphology, corneal sensation, and tear film evaluation after refractive femtosecond laser lenticule extraction. Graefes Arch Clin Exp Ophthalmol. 2013;251:2591–600.
29. Demirok A, Ozgurhan EB, Agca A, et al. Corneal sensation after corneal refractive surgery with small incision lenticule extraction. Optom Vis Sci. 2013;90:1040–7.
30. Li M, Zhou Z, Shen Y, et al. Comparison of corneal sensation between small incision lenticule extraction (SMILE) and femtosecond laser-assisted LASIK for myopia. J Refract Surg. 2014;30:94–100.
31. Mohamed-Noriega K, Riau AK, Lwin NC, et al. Early corneal nerve damage and recovery following small incision lenticule extraction (SMILE) and laser in situ keratimileusis (LASIK). Invest Ophthalmol Vis Sci. 2014;55:1823–34.
32. Xu Y, Yang Y. Dry eye after small incision lenticule extraction and LASIK for myopia. J Refract Surg. 2014;30:186–90.
33. Reinstein DZ, Archer TJ, Randleman JB. Mathematical model to compare the relative tensile strength of the cornea after PRK, LASIK and small incision lenticule extraction. J Refract Surg. 2013;29:454–60.
34. Wu D, Wang Y, Zhang L, et al. Corneal biomechanical effects: small incision lenticule extraction versus fetosecond laser-assisted laser in situ keratomileusis. J Cataract Refract Surg. 2014;40:954–62.
35. Kamiya K, Shimizu K, Igarashi A, et al. Intraindividual comparison of changes in corneal biomechanical parameters after femtosecond lenticule extraction and small incision lenticule extraction. J Cataract Refract Surg. 2014;40:963–70.
36. Roy A, Dupps WJ, Roberts CJ. Comparison of biomechanical effects of small-incision lenticule extraction and laser in situ keratomileusis: finite-element analysis. J Cataract Refract Surg. 2014;40:971–80.

SMILE: Small Incision Lenticule Extraction—A Basic Guideline

4

Bertram Meyer

Abstract

Flapless and all femto—SMILE is the first minimal invasive procedure in laser refractive surgery.

Keywords

Corneal surface · Refractive outcome · Refractive correction · Optical zone · Excimer laser ablation

Flapless and all femto—SMILE is the first minimal invasive procedure in laser refractive surgery.

The significant difference between SMILE and traditional Femto-Lasik is that with the femtosecond laser an intrastromal lenticule is created which is removed manually throughout a small incision in a second step. That way refractive correction is not achieved by laser ablation but by tissue removal. The predictability of the refractive outcomes depends on the accuracy of the femtosecond laser only.

At the moment the VISUMAX femtosecond laser from ZEISS (Fig. 4.1) is the only device worldwide which enables to perform SMILE.

Practical Advices

Treatment range for SMILE:

Currently the SMILE treatment range is for pure myopia from − 0.50 D to − 10.0 D (SEQ) and for myopic astigmatism up to − 5.0 D. Hyperopic SMILE treatments are not commercially available yet (Fig. 4.2).

General preparation of the patient:

- low-dose tranquilizer 1 h before surgery
- local anesthesia with eye drops
- local routine periocular disinfection
- covering of eye lashes with drape

Samples of surgical instruments for SMILE from GENDER and MALOSA are shown in Figs. 4.21, 4.22, 4.23 and 4.24.

- aspirating lid speculum (e.g. Knorz)
- curved dissector (e.g. Chansue, Blum, Guell, Pfaeffl and others)

Supplementary Information The online version contains supplementary material available at https://doi.org/10.1007/978-3-031-84204-7_4.

B. Meyer (✉)
Eye Center Cologne, Cologne, Germany
e-mail: Bertram.Meyer@t-online.de

U. Spandau and G. B. Scharioth (eds.), *Cutting Edge of Ophthalmic Surgery*,
https://doi.org/10.1007/978-3-031-84204-7_4

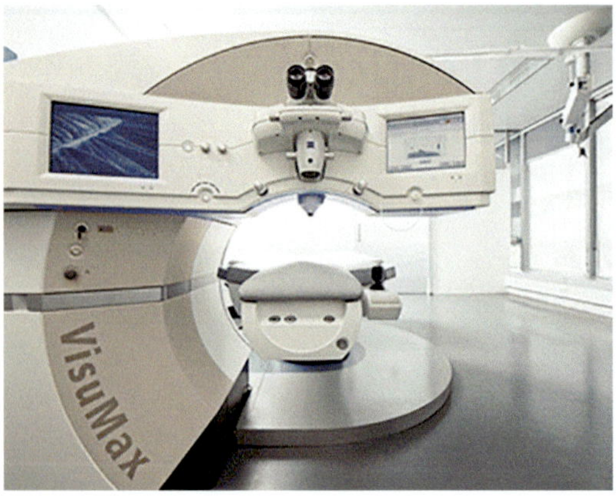

Fig. 4.1 VISUMAX femtosecond laser

- colibri style forceps for stabilizing the globe (if necessary)
- crocodile-style micro-forceps for removal of the lenticule (e.g.Shah).

SMILE Surgery Step-By-Step (Videos 4.1 and 4.2)

A curved contact glass (size S or M; mostly S depending on the corneal size) is fixed at the laser opening and automatically calibrated. Next steps: Routine local disinfection periocular, application of local anesthetic drops, coverage of eyelashes with sterile drape, placement of eyelid speculum, flushing with BSS and aspiration of pooled fluids and secrets out of the fornix for a clean corneal surface. Then the patient's eye is moved towards to the contact glass by lifting the bed, and the contact glass is gently docked on the corneal surface (Fig. 4.3). Be sure that the contact glass has free access to the cornea and that there is no touch with a prominent nose, the speculum or orbital bones. If there is need you can move the head rest of the bed up and down, elevate the chin or turn the face in the opposite direction. Watch out that the patient's head is lying straight and comfortable.

The big advantage of the curved contact glass (Fig. 4.4) is that there is no strong applanation but only soft acurvation of the corneal surface. Thus we have only a low increase of the intraocular pressure and a minimized tissue distortion during the whole suction procedure. Moreover, the advantage is that with this soft docking the patient fixation is maintained during the whole laser procedure but with the risk of suction loss if the contact glass is not docked properly.

During the docking procedure the patient has to cooperate by fixating a green blinking light (Fig. 4.5); this guarantees a perfect centration of the contact glass and consequently an exact centration of the lenticule onto the visual axis. After more than 90% of contact between cornea and contact glass you press the suction button; be sure that there is hardly any fluid and Meibom's secret between cornea and contact glass.

After the VISUMAX confirms the end of a correct suction procedure with the word "ready" you press the foot switch and the laser application is starting. First the laser prepares the refractive part of the lenticule (= backside of the lenticule) with a spiral starting from outside (Fig. 4.6) followed by the lenticule's side cut. Typically the optical zone of the lenticule is between 6 and 7 mm (standard is 6.5 mm).

Second, the VISUMAX is preparing the front side of the lenticule (Fig. 4.7) which is a plane-parallel spiral cut starting from inside (Fig. 4.7). The laser procedure is finished by the incision preparation with a size of 2–4 mm (free choice). Normally the cap diameter is chosen between 7.3 and 7.8 mm (Figs. 4.8 and 4.9). When the procedure is finished suction is released automatically. The whole suction time including the laser application takes not more than 30–35 s depending on the diameter.

Be sure that you have the correct spot and track distance and an optimized spot energy; this guarantees a minimum of opaque bubble layer (OBL) and consequently an easy mechanical dissection of the residual micro-bridges of the lenticule. As the energy levels are specific and different for each device your application specialist from ZEISS will instruct you at the beginning (standard energy levels are between 150 and 170 nJ per spot depending on each single device).

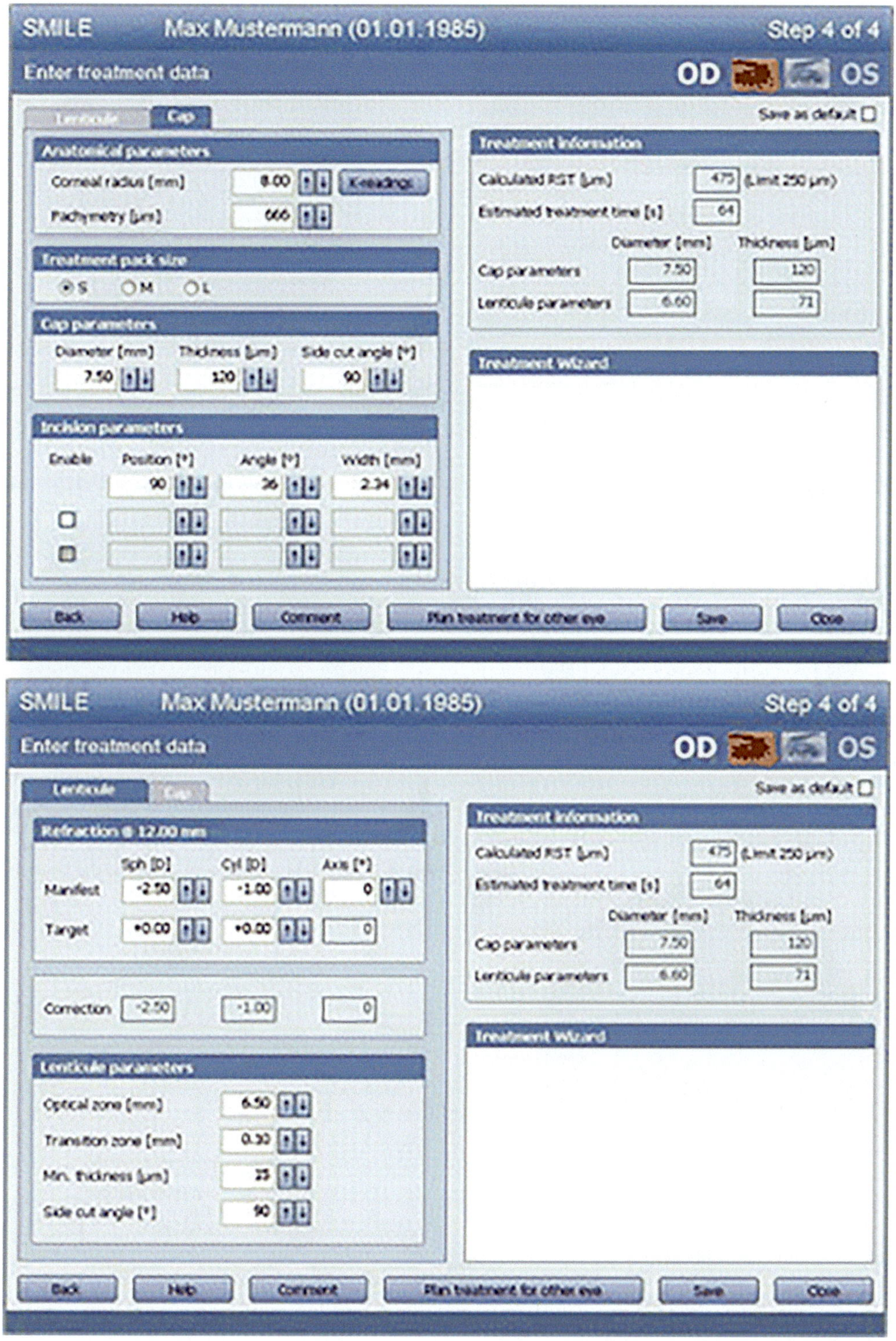

Fig. 4.2 Treatment data display

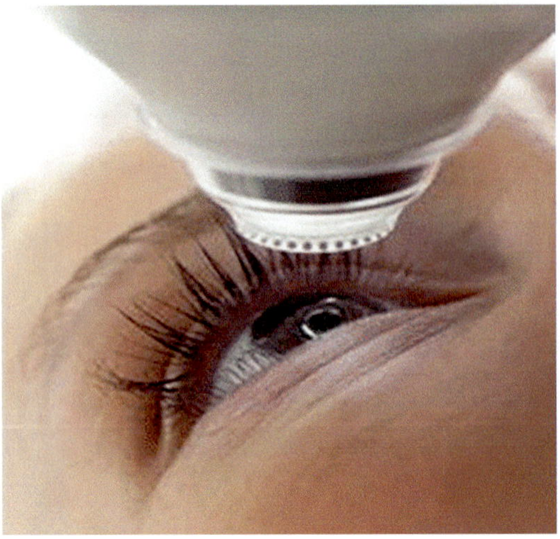

Fig. 4.3 Docking procedure

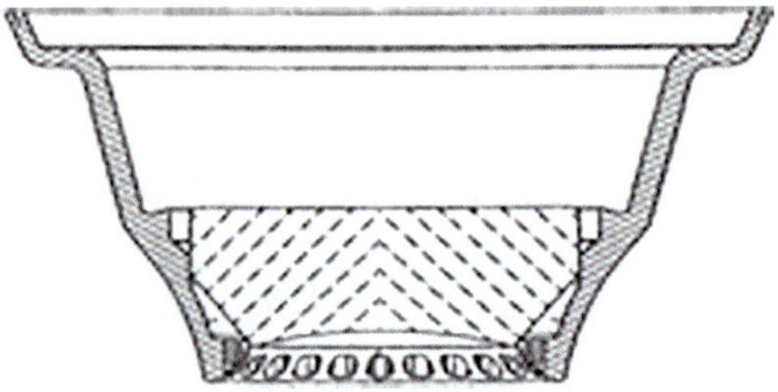

Fig. 4.4 Curved contact glass

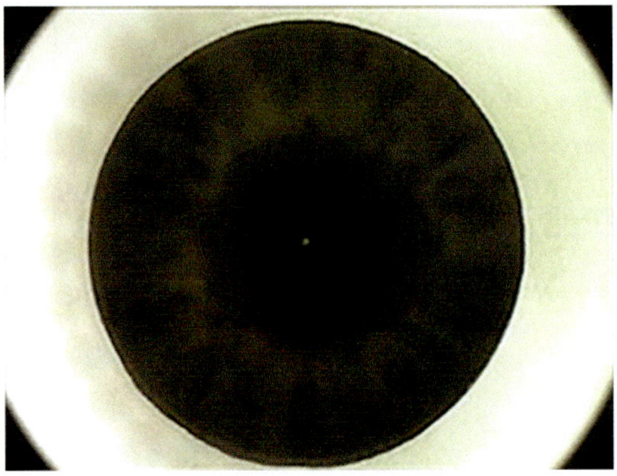

Fig. 4.5 Centration onto optical axis

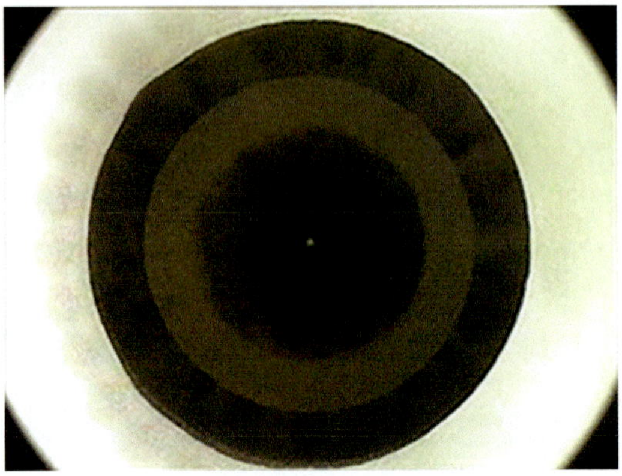

Fig. 4.6 Preparation of the refractive part of the lenticule

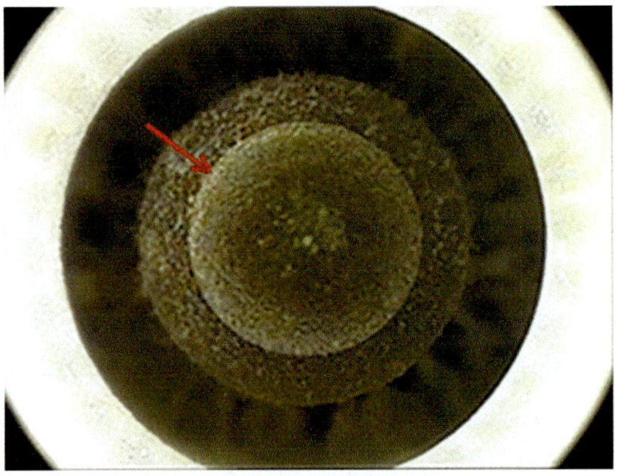

Fig. 4.7 Preparation of the frontside of the lenticule

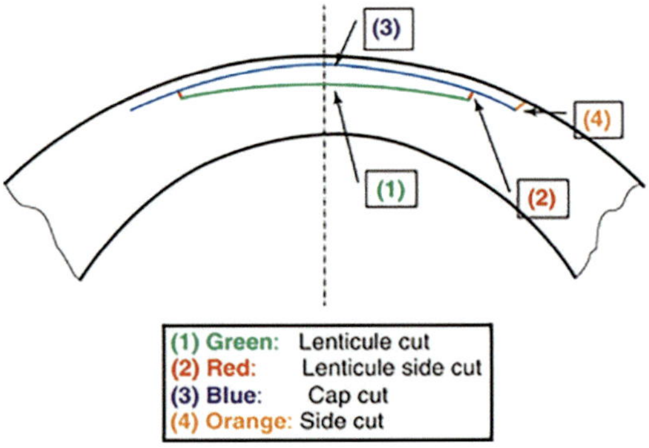

Fig. 4.8 SMILE: Drawing of corneal cut

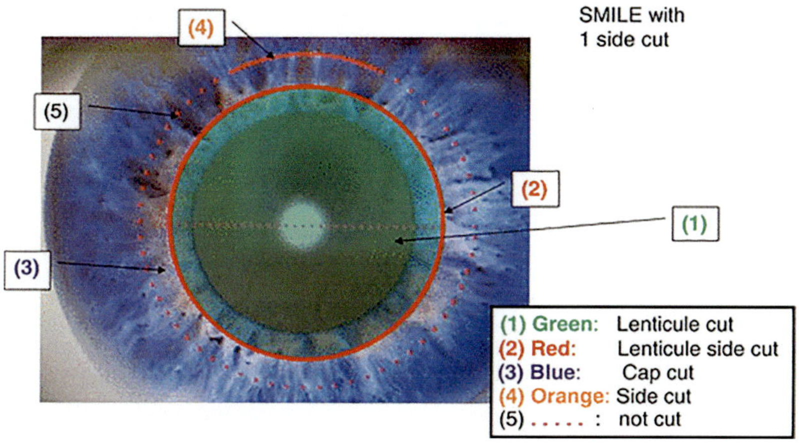

Fig. 4.9 SMILE: Drawing of corneal cut

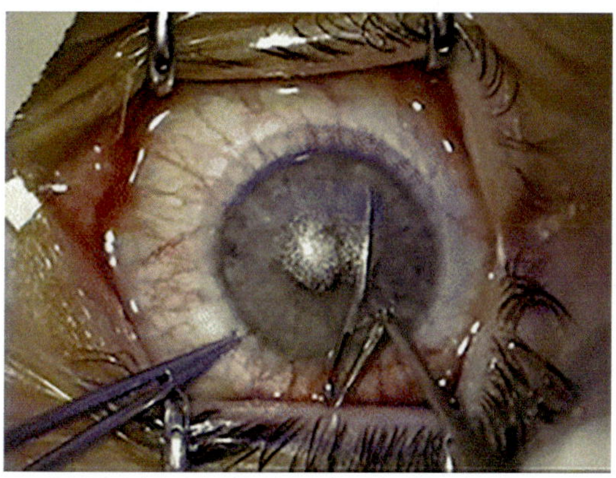

Fig. 4.10 Lenticule dissection

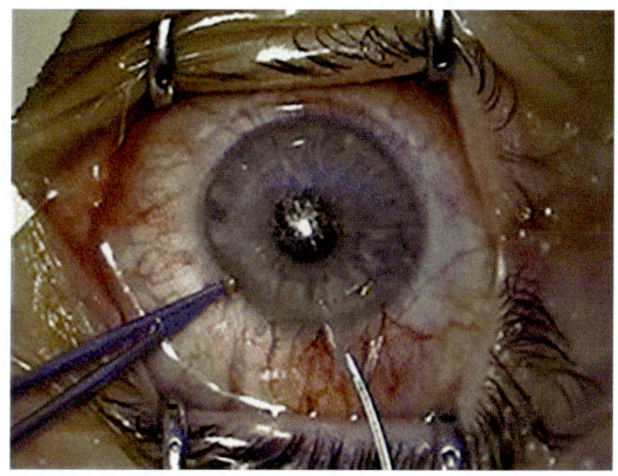

Fig. 4.11 Lenticule extraction

For an easy lenticule dissection you first open the incision with a Sinskey hook or similar. Next you prepare two small pockets (1 × 1 mm) with the hook—one in the front and one in the back plane of the lenticule. This is most important. For an uncomplicated dissection of the lenticule you have to ensure to start the dissection with the front side of the lenticule first followed by the backside. The dissection is to be done with gender swinging moves all over the whole expanse of the pocket (Fig. 4.10). If there is need you can fix the bulb with a scleral micro-forceps.

After a complete dissection the lenticule is easily extracted with a forceps (Fig. 4.11). Please check that the lenticule is removed in total (you can place it on the cornea and spread it out and check whether edges are intact and circular). Few surgeons prefer to irrigate the interface with BSS, others don't. Post-operative application of combined antibiotic and steroid eye drops is recommended four times per day for 1 week. As SMILE is a flapless procedure there is no need for eye patches or eye shields after surgery. Regular follow ups are recommended after 1 day, 1 week and 1 month.

Re-treatment Options After ReLEx-Smile

With an incidence of less than 2%, re-treatments after SMILE are rare. The reason is a very high stability of refractive outcomes and a high tolerance of small refractive errors post-operatively. If a touchup is required we have different options:

1. **Surface ablation (= PRK/LASEK)**:
   - corneal abrasion, refractive correction done by excimer laser ablation
   - use of Mitomycin C
   - advantage: preservation of corneal stability
   - disadvantage: painful healing, prolonged visual recovery time (up to 3 or even 6 months)
2. **Standard Femto-flap procedure**:
   - same parameters, same size of contact glass and laser settings to convert the cap into a flap
   - refractive correction done by excimer laser ablation
   - advantage: fast visual recovery time
   - disadvantage: reduction of corneal stability generating the flap side cut.
3. **Thin flap Femto-LASIK** (off label) with a 100 μ thick flap:
   - only advised if the cap created in the initial treatment is thick enough (>140 μ) and only a small refractive error is to be corrected
   - refractive correction done by excimer laser ablation
   - advantage: fast visual recovery time
   - disadvantage: reduction of corneal stability generating a flap side cut, risk of gas breakthrough or cryptic button hole
4. **Circle procedure**:
   - "Circle" was invented by Carl Zeiss Meditec for touch up after SMILE and extends the previous SMILE interface to a flap (Fig. 4.12).
   - refractive correction done by excimer laser ablation
   - advantage: fast visual recovery time; no risk of an additional sectional plane
   - disadvantage: reduction of corneal stability generating a side cut.
5. **Capless SMILE** (off label):
   - First published by David Donate (Lyon) in 2015
   - preparation of a second lenticule while taking advantage of the initial interface and initial incision (Fig. 4.13)
   - advantage: innovative option which preserves all SMILE advantages, fast visual recovery time and preservation of corneal stability

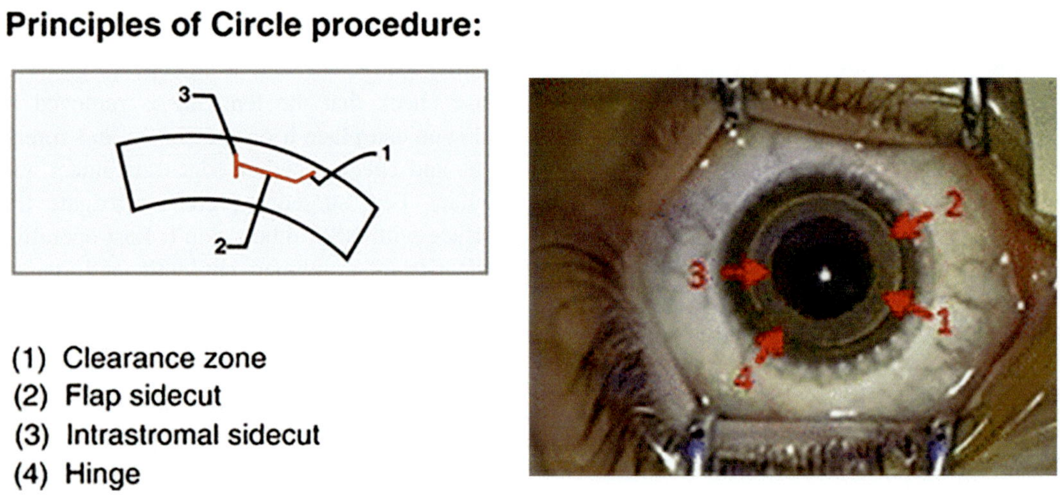

Fig. 4.12 Circle procedure

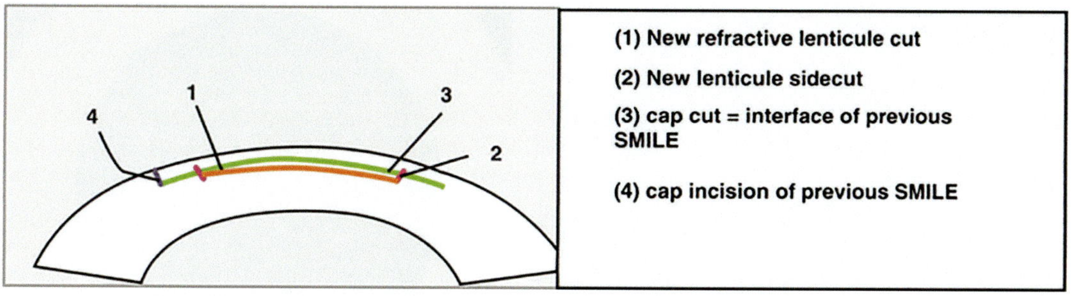

Fig. 4.13 Drawing of corneal cut of "capless SMILE"

- disadvantage: risk of distorted lenticule, very small corrections (< −1,0 D) not possible

The advantages of the second, third and fourth option benefit in a short recovery time and absence of pain. At the same time the advantages of SMILE (e. g. better corneal stability and less cut nerves with reduced dry-eye-symptoms) are becoming obsolete, as you would cut a flap and do the refractive correction using an excimer laser.

Complications and Complication Management

1. **Suction-loss during lenticule and side cut preparation** (Video 4.3)**:**

If suction loss occurs during laser preparation of the refractive part (posterior cut) of the lenticule it is not advisable to continue (Fig. 4.14). Abort the procedure and perform a Femto-Lasik or a PRK after 4–6 weeks.

In case of suction loss during the cap cut (anterior cut), which is a non-refractive plane-parallel cut, you can immediately re-dock and easily proceed with the laser preparation. A perfect centration in respect of the initial cuts is a matter of course. There will be no negative effects on the refractive outcomes.

In all situations the VISUMAX software will automatically recommend how to proceed.

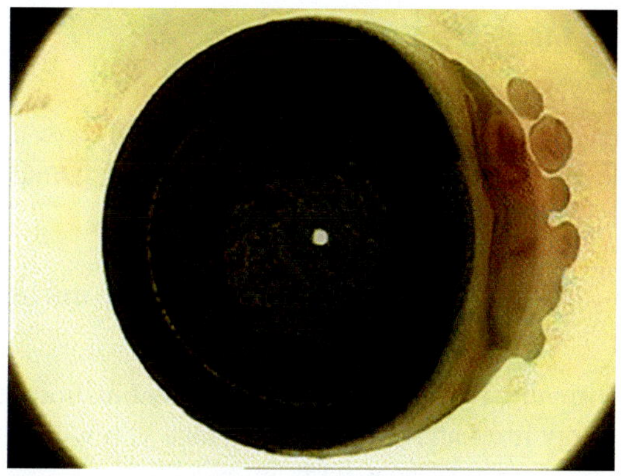

Fig. 4.14 Suction loss

2. **Dissection in wrong layer**:

The golden rule is: front side first than backside. In case of preparing the deeper plane first the lenticule is sticking on the posterior part of the cap. If so, the anterior layer is not easy to be prepared as there is a lack of resistance. Try to find the edge of the lenticule by moving the hook pointed slightly up carefully and dissect with slow moves.

If you cannot manage the dissection through the small incision convert to ReLEx-Flex with a side cut procedure (Circle: side cut only), open the "new" flap and carefully strip the lenticule from the backside of the flap.

To avoid this critical situation you should first prepare two small pockets (1 × 1 mm) in both sectional planes after opening the incision to identify each layer (Fig. 4.15). For the

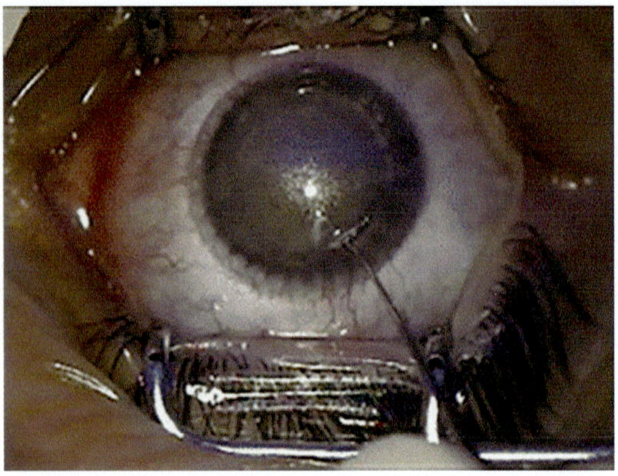

Fig. 4.15 Pocket preparation

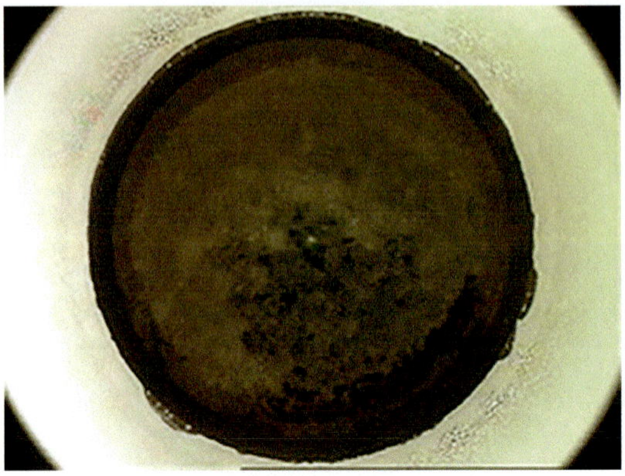

Fig. 4.17 Confluent black spot area

anterior plane you turn the hook slightly upside down; for the posterior plane the hook is pointed down towards the center of the globe.

3. **Black spots and incomplete cut during laser preparation**

Normally, by choosing the right combination of energy level and spot/track distance you will get a homogenous layer with an excellent cut quality and easy tissue separation. Only if the tear film between contact glass and cornea is not clear but oily and dirty caused by e.g. Meibom's secret or filaments you will get areas of low cut quality (looks like an untouched "black" spot; Fig. 4.16). Small local areas outside the visual axis or in the periphery of the optical zone are without consequences. If these small spots conflate to larger areas troubles during the followed mechanical tissue separation are to be expected (Fig. 4.17). Depending on the size of the "black spots" you have to go for a second laser run or you have to abort and to convert the procedure to Femto-LASIK or PRK later.

Advice: If you see an oily liquid film or other dirt on the corneal surface after the docking procedure, do not start the laser application. Drop the suction and clean the corneal surface by irrigating with BSS, take advantage of the aspirating lid speculum and re-dock with a new contact glass.

4. **Epithelium in the interface**

Epithelium is rarely "growing" into the interface but mostly left iatrogenic by the surgeon (Fig. 4.18). It causes topography irregularities

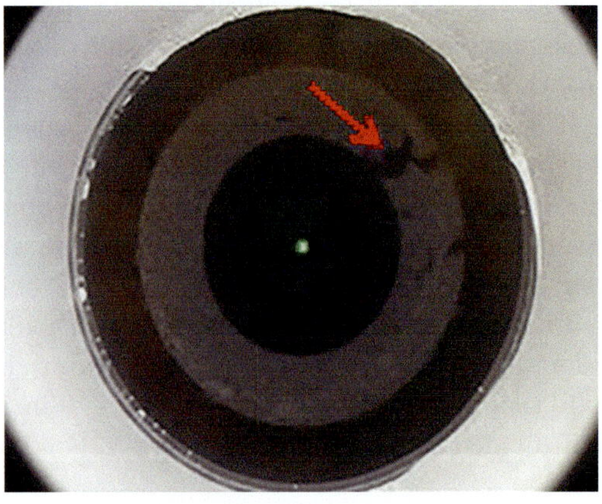

Fig. 4.16 Localized black spot

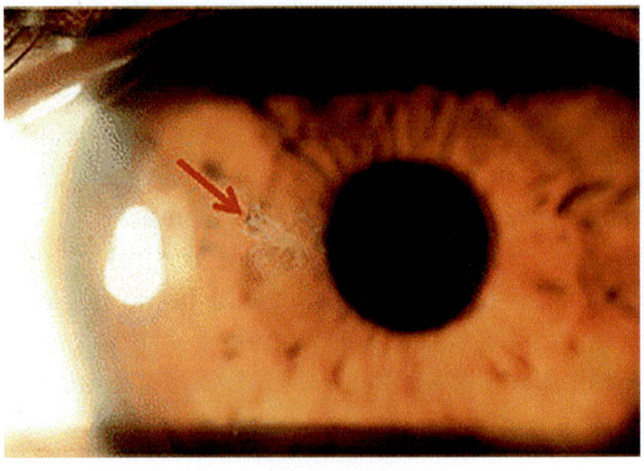

Fig. 4.18 Epithelium in interface

and—if in the center-reduces visual acuity. It has a consistency like jelly and can easily be removed with a hook or a spatula before corneal melting effects are initiated.

5. **SMILE in low myopia**

Also for low myopic diopters SMILE has become an excellent option. During the last years we have performed SMILE on low myopic eyes between − 0.75 and − 3.0 diopters. To simplify the management of the thin lenticule we have decided for a larger optical zone (7.0 mm) and added an additional and refraction neutral corneal tissue base; the minimal thickness of the lenticule has to be at least 40 µm. Safety and refractive outcomes are excellent (Fig. 4.19).

Clinical Results

Since 2010 we performed more than 2500 SMILE procedures, using the ZEISS solution ReLEx SMILE, on myopic and myopic-astigmatic eyes between − 0.75 and − 12.5 diopters (SEQ). The clinical outcomes are outstanding and even slightly better compared with those after traditional Femto-LASIK (Fig. 4.20): After

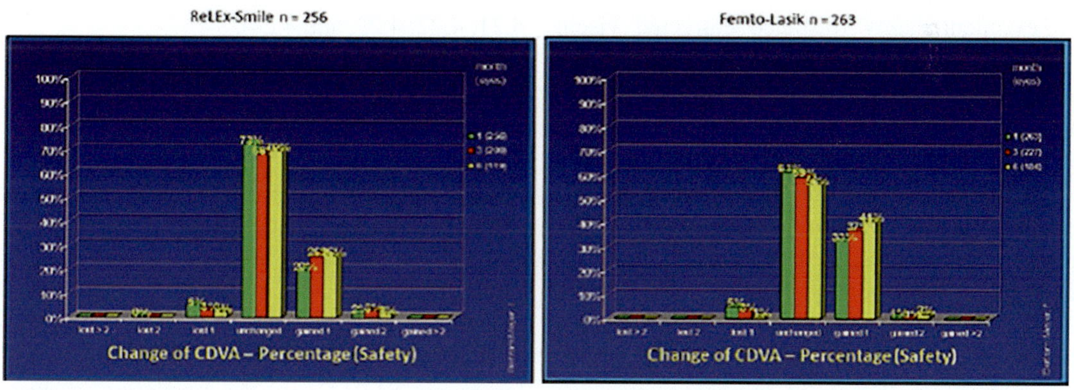

Fig. 4.19 Correction of high myopia: –6, 0 D to –9, 0 D (SEQ): Advantage of ReLEx-Smile versus F-Lasik: high safety

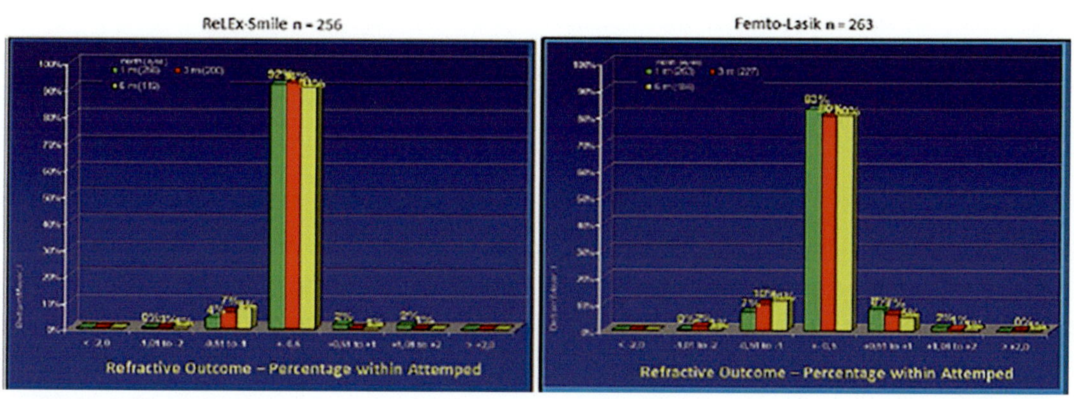

Fig. 4.20 Correction of high myopia: –6, 0 D to –9, 0 D (SEQ): Advantage of ReLEx-Smile versus F-Lasik: high accuracy, high predictability

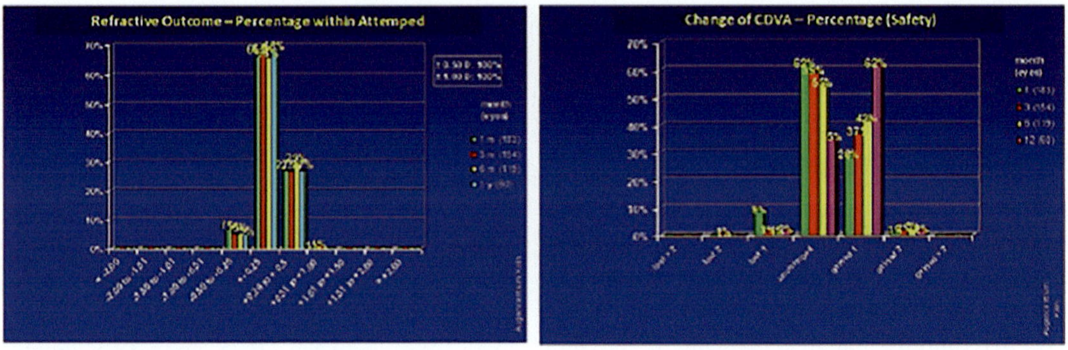

Fig. 4.21 SMILE in low myopia: high accuracy, high safety

3 months, more than 92% are within + 0.5 diopters. There is an excellent stability over time and an excellent safety (distance corrected visual acuity preop versus distance corrected visual acuity postop). The recovery of post-operative visual acuity takes slightly longer compared to conventional Femto-Lasik, however most of our patients fulfill the requirements for car driving 1 day after surgery. Post-operative corneal topographies show a large and homogeneous optical zone with a slightly prolate shape. The achieved effective optical zone is identical to the laser setting independent of the refractive correction. Wavefront measurements have confirmed that there is no significant change in aberrations prior and after surgery, especially no spherical aberrations (Z 4/0) have been induced by the lenticule creation and extraction (Figs. 4.21, 4.22, 4.23, and 4.24).

Summary

SMILE represents the 3rd generation of laser refractive surgery beyond PRK and LASIK. SMILE is the first minimal invasive keyhole procedure with excellent refractive and visual outcomes combined with a maximum of safety. To round up the treatment range, hyperopic SMILE and the correction of myopia with more than − 10 diopters are currently investigated.

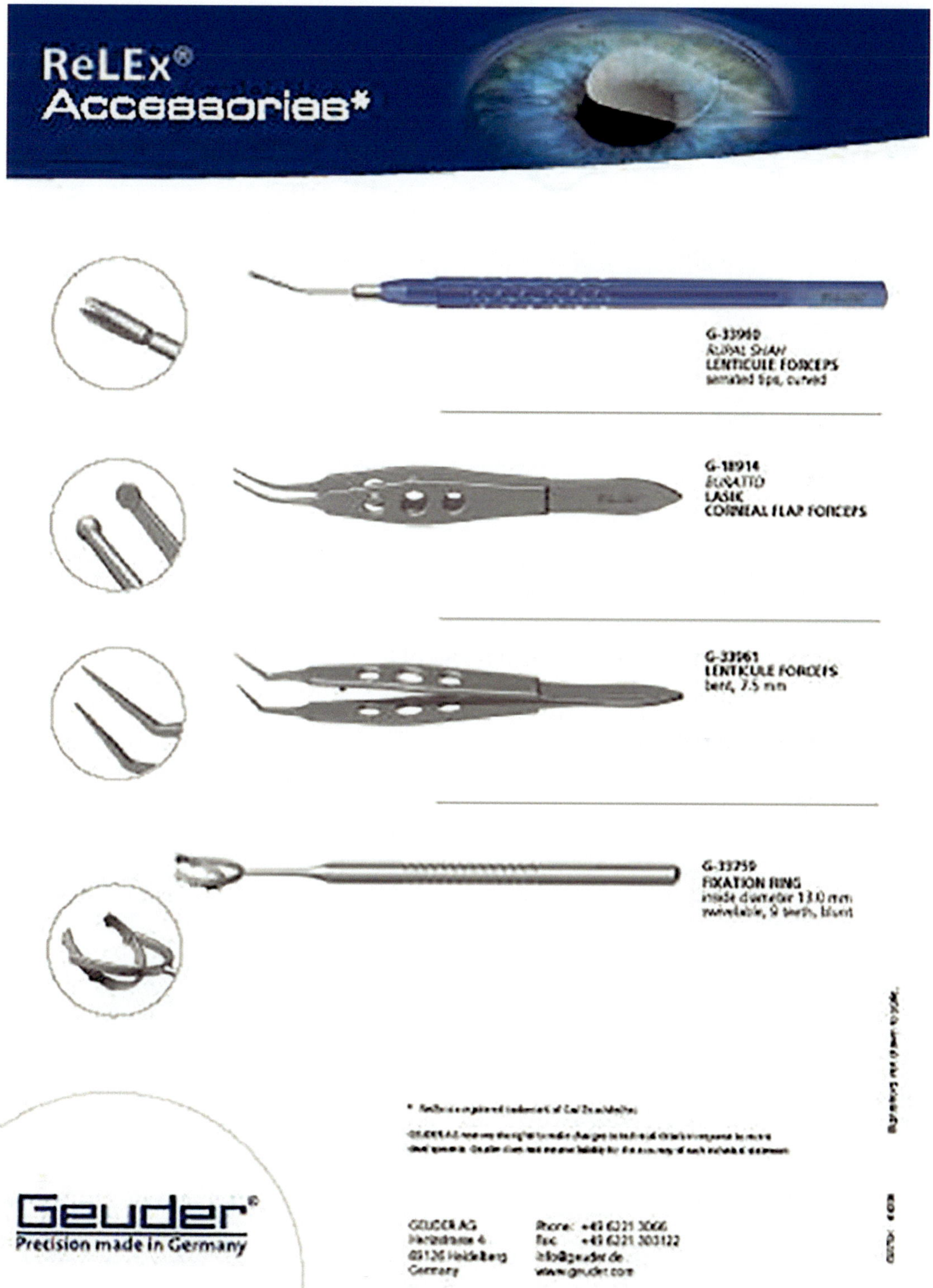

Fig. 4.22 Surgical instruments for SMILE from Geuder, Germany. Part 2

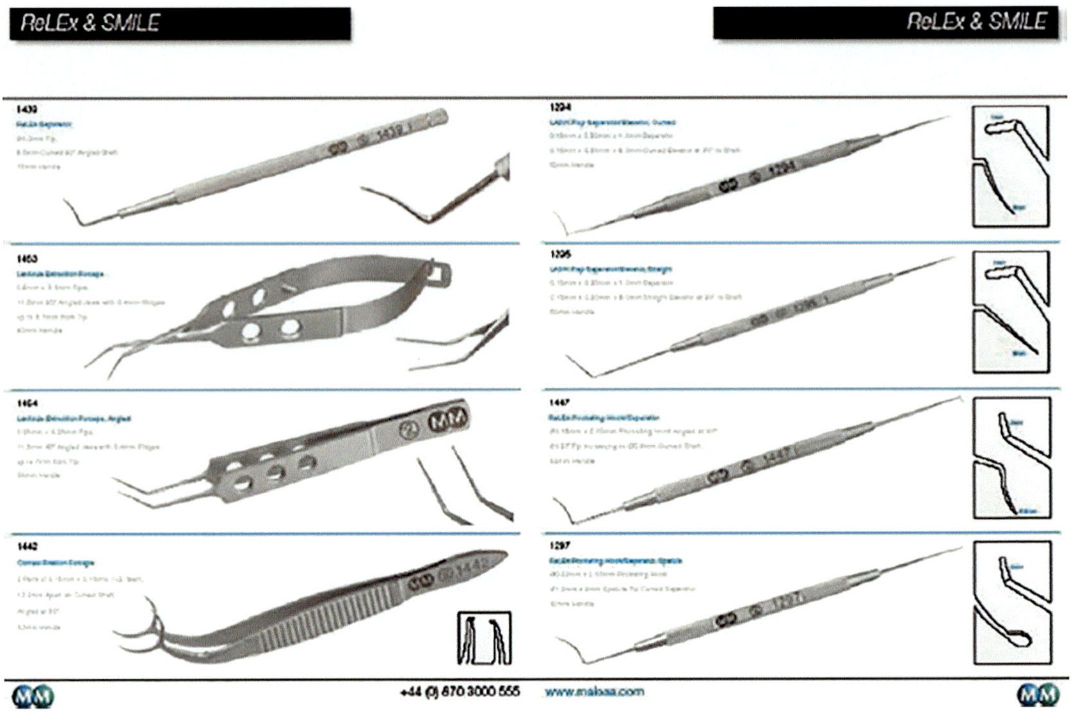

Fig. 4.23 Surgical instruments for SMILE from Malosa, UK. Part 1

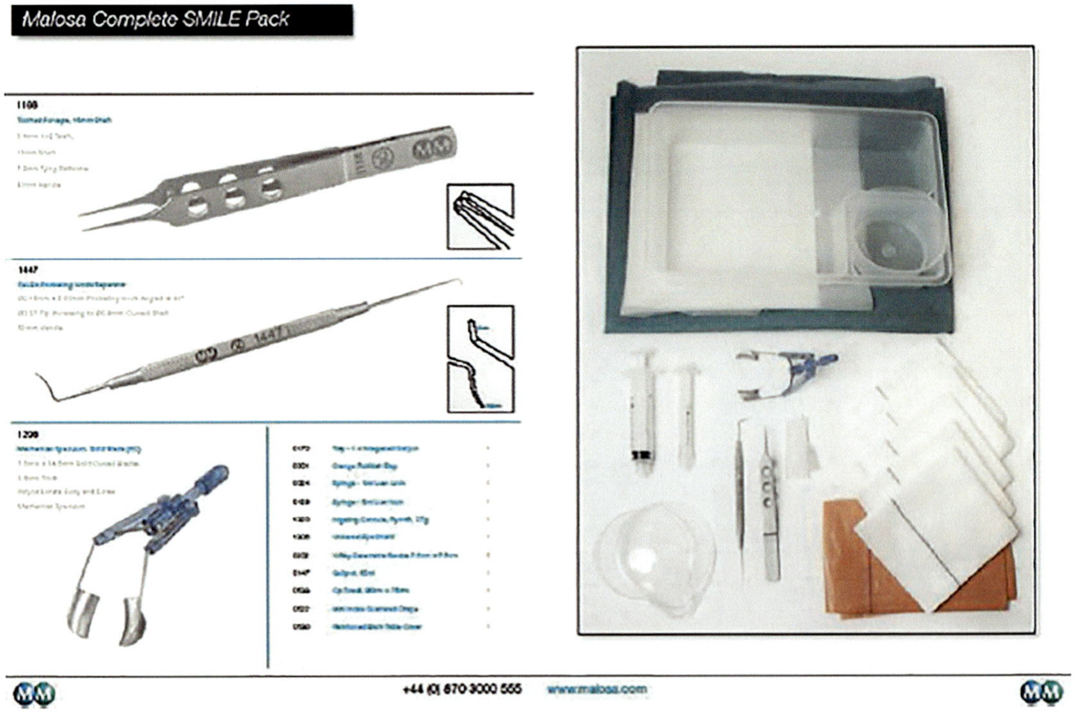

Fig. 4.24 Surgical instruments for SMILE from Malosa, UK. Part 2

Material and Companies Address

Geuder AG

Hertzstr. 4
69126 Heidelberg
Phone: 06221/3066
Fax: 06221/303 122
info@geuder.de
www.geuder.de

Malosa Medical

Contact us +44 (0)870 3000 555
mailto:info@malosa.com
www.malosa.com

Carl Zeiss Meditec Vertriebsgesellschaft mbH

Rudolf-Eber-Straße 11
73447 Oberkochen
Germany
www.zeiss.com

Part III
Glaucoma: Canaloplasty

In 2015 the German patient glaucoma association declared canaloplasty as the new gold standard in glaucoma surgery, as this operation combines good results with a low risk profile. Prof. Scharioth from Gelsenkirchen, Germany, will demonstrate a novel technique for canaloplasty using a special suture from Onatec (Onalene, Germany). Prof. Körber from Cologne, Germany, is a pioneer in the surgery of canaloplasty. During this surgery, an illuminated microcatheter is introduced in Schlemm's canal and the canal is then widened through injection of viscoelastics.

Canaloplasty

5

Gabor B. Scharioth

Abstract

First successful antiglaucomatous surgery was performed by the German ophthalmologist Albrecht von Graefe in 1852. The described technique did work only in acute angle closure glaucoma. In the following 100 years various surgical techniques addressed open angle glaucoma problematic. Since early 1970th trabeculectomy became the standard of care in open-angle glaucoma surgery. This widely used procedure involves a surgically formed pathway for aqueous humour between the anterior chamber and the subconjunctival space to lower intraocular pressure (IOP) in treatment of glaucoma. Main goal is the formation of a conjunctival filtering bleb. This is a relatively unphysiological approach and scleral as well as conjunctival scarring led to introduction of antimetabolites as adjunctive for filtering bleb depending glaucoma surgeries. Numerous intraoperative and postoperative complications have been cited (Jones et al. in Curr Opin Ophthalmol 16:107–113, 2005; Mac and Soltau in Curr Opin Ophthalmol 14:91–94, 2003; Borisuth et al. in Curr Opin Ophthalmol 10:112–116, 1999; Ophir in Eye 6:348–352, 1992; Gedde et al. in Am J Ophthalmol 143:23–31, 2007). These include hypotony, maculopathy, blebitis/endophthlamitis, hyphema, suprachoroidal hemorrhage or effusions, encapsulation of the bleb with resultant IOP elevation, loss of visual acuity, and increased risk for cataract formation. In addition, intensive postoperative care, including bleb massage, laser suturolysis, release of releasable sutures, needling, or 5-fluorouracil injections, may be needed to achieve primary success. Recently several authors reported relatively high failure rate of trabeculectomy after long term follow-up (Jones et al. in Curr Opin Ophthalmol 16:107–113, 2005).

Keywords

Anterior chamber · Trabecular meshwork · Polypropylene suture · Anterior chamber angle · Scleral flap

Supplementary Information The online version contains supplementary material available at https://doi.org/10.1007/978-3-031-84204-7_5.

G. B. Scharioth (✉)
Aurelios Augenzentrum, Recklinghausen, Germany
e-mail: gabor.scharioth@augenzentrum.org

G. B. Scharioth
Department of Ophthalmology, Faculty of Medicine, University of Szeged, Szeged, Hungary

U. Spandau and G. B. Scharioth (eds.), *Cutting Edge of Ophthalmic Surgery*,
https://doi.org/10.1007/978-3-031-84204-7_5

First successful antiglaucomatous surgery was performed by the German ophthalmologist Albrecht von Graefe in 1852. The described technique did work only in acute angle closure glaucoma. In the following 100 years various surgical techniques addressed open angle glaucoma problematic. Since early 1970th trabeculectomy became the standard of care in open-angle glaucoma surgery. This widely used procedure involves a surgically formed pathway for aqueous humour between the anterior chamber and the subconjunctival space to lower intraocular pressure (IOP) in treatment of glaucoma. Main goal is the formation of a conjunctival filtering bleb. This is a relatively unphysiological approach and scleral as well as conjunctival scarring led to introduction of antimetabolites as adjunctive for filtering bleb depending glaucoma surgeries. Numerous intraoperative and postoperative complications have been cited [1–5]. These include hypotony, maculopathy, blebitis/endophthlamitis, hyphema, suprachoroidal hemorrhage or effusions, encapsulation of the bleb with resultant IOP elevation, loss of visual acuity, and increased risk for cataract formation. In addition, intensive postoperative care, including bleb massage, laser suturolysis, release of releasable sutures, needling, or 5-fluorouracil injections, may be needed to achieve primary success. Recently several authors reported relatively high failure rate of trabeculectomy after long term follow-up [1].

All this led surgeons to search for a more physiological and bleb independent surgical approach in IOP lowering glaucoma surgery. Surgical treatment of the natural aqueous outflow system, including Schlemm's canal, to restore normal function and IOP control without penetration of the intraocular space has long been the interest in the study of open-angle glaucoma as an alternative to penetrating and bleb depending methods [6, 7]. In the late 1950s [8] and early 1960s [9], surgical procedures, often described as sinusotomy, were introduced to expose Schlemm's canal and induce aqueous outflow without intraocular penetration. Further development of non-penetrating approaches included the use of a guarded scleral flap and creation of a descemetic window in the 1980s (deep sclerectomy) [10–12], dilatation of the surgical ostia of Schlemm's canal with viscoelastic substance in the late 1990s (viscocanalostomy) [13], and the use of implants at the surgical site in the late 1990s and early 2000s [14–16]. These implants were either resorbable (i.e. SK Gel, AquaFlow) or non-resorbable (T-Flux). Most surgeons preferred to close the scleral flap loose to induce subconjunctival filtration in contrast to a watertight closure in viscocanalostomy, which could be named the first bleb independent non-penetrating glaucoma surgery. Although these non-penetrating surgical procedures for glaucoma effectively reduced IOP and lowered the incidence of postoperative complications compared with penetrating procedures such as trabeculectomy, comparative clinical studies indicates that IOP decreases more significantly with trabeculectomy, especially when used in conjunction with antimetabolites [17–23].

Cannulation of Schlemm's canal with a silk suture was described in 1960 for partial trabeculotomy [24]. A modified technique using a 6 × 0 polypropylene suture was later used for 360° trabeculotomy for treatment of congenital glaucoma [25]. All previous non-penetrating glaucoma surgeries were able to reach two to three clock hours of Schlemm's canal while a procedure treating the entire canal should be theoretically more effective. We reported a technique using the 6 × 0 polypropylene suture for catheterization of the entire Schlemm's canal and while withdrawing the suture a 10 × 0 polypropylene suture is installed in the canal and finally knotted under tension [26]. Postoperative intraocular pressure after 1 year was 12.4 mmHg and medication was 0.3 IOP lowering drugs. This is a very difficult and time consuming technique with a relatively high risk of mispassage of the 6 × 0 polypropylene suture into the anterior chamber or suprachoroidal space. Recent advances in technology have allowed surgeons to use a flexible microcatheter to access the entire length of Schlemm's canal more atraumatically. This technique is called canaloplasty (Fig.

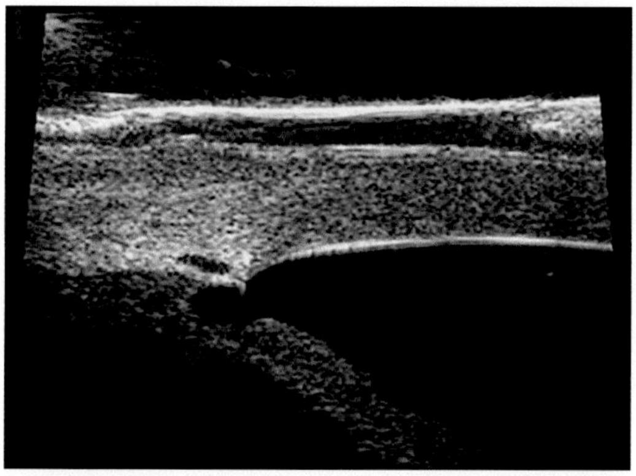

Fig. 5.1 UBM image after canaloplasty. *Note* Schlemm's canal clearly visible, gut distension of trabecular meshwork

5.1, Videos 5.1 and 5.2) and seems to be the logical evolution to viscocanalostomy [27, 28].

This procedure is intended to overcome some of the problems of the previous procedures with deep sclerectomy.

The idea of implanting a fine tensioning suture into the Schlemm's canal to enlarge the entire 360° of Schlemm's canal [29, 30] should theoretically.

- widen the intertrabecular spaces,
- preventing collapse of the canal, the surgical ostia and the descemetic window and herniation of the inner wall into the ostia of collector channels,
- keep the entire Schlemm's canal open and
- make collector channels away from the surgical site available for drainage.

First commercially available microcatheter for this technique was iTrack (Ellex, Australia, initially marketed from iScience Interventional, USA). This microcatheter has a 200 µm diameter shaft with an atraumatic distal tip approximately 250 µm in diameter. The device incorporates an optical fiber to provide an illuminated beacon tip to assist in surgical guidance. The illuminated tip is visible transsclerally during catheterization of Schlemm's canal to identify the location of the distal tip of the microcatheter. The iTrack is connected to an external light source (iLumin, Ellex, Australia). The microcatheter has a lumen of about 70 µm with a proximal Luer lock connector through which an OVD (e.g. Healon GV or Healon 5) or dye (e.g. trypane blue, indocyanin green, fluorescein) could be delivered. The procedure is called viscocanaloplasty if OVD is injected to further stretch and enlarge the Schlemm's canal. A dye could be used intraoperatively to control outflow system [31]. Later we developed a microcatheter (Glaucolight, DORC, The Netherlands) without lumen but reduced outer diameter for canaloplasty [32]. This device was directly connected to a sterile light source and less expensive. Currently Glaucolight is not commercially available. Recently a twisted polypropylene suture (Onalene for canaloplasty, Onatec, Germany) was marketed. The tip is atraumatic and catheterization seems to have a high success rate (personal experience). As it is not illuminated the advancement of the suture during catheterization cannot be controlled.

Surgical Technique (Videos 5.1 and 5.2)

1. **Preparation of a superficial scleral flap**

The conjunctiva may be opened either at the fornix or at the limbus. A 5×5 mm rectangular or parabolic shaped scleral flap (scleral flap marqueur) is performed (Fig. 5.2) including one-third of the scleral thickness (about 300 µm, depending on the total scleral thickness in the particular case) (Fig. 5.1). To be able to reach the Descemet's membrane later during the dissection of the deeper scleral flap, the superficial scleral flap has to be prepared 1–1.5 mm anteriorly into the perilimbal clear cornea (Fig. 5.3). The initial incision is made with a no.11 stainless steel blade (i.e. 15° slit knife for paracentesis) or a diamond knife. The flap dissection is made with a ruby blade or a bevel-up delicate crescent knife (i.e. 1 mm ultrasharp minidisc knife, Grieshaber Alcon, USA) (Fig. 5.4). Diathermy of episcleral vessels is prevented or reduced to a minimum. The episcleral vessels

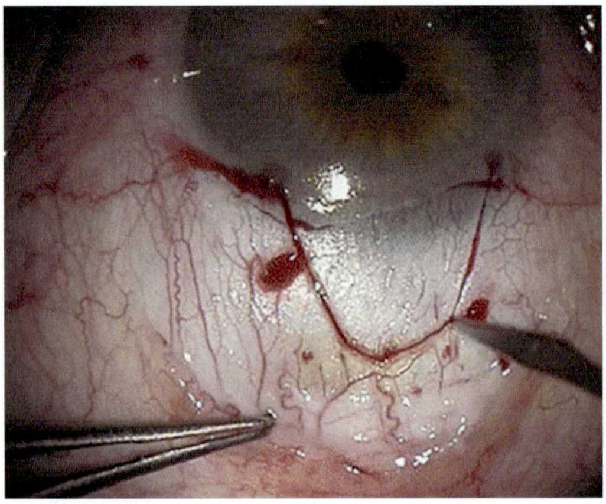

Fig. 5.2 Superficial scleral flap, note no diathermy of episcleral vessels is performed

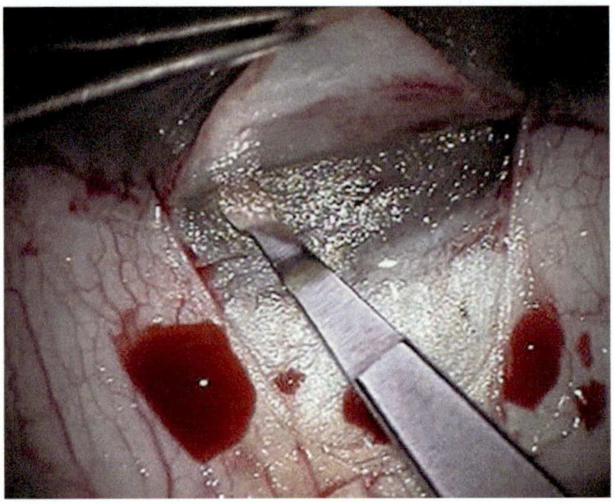

Fig. 5.4 Dissecting the superficial scleral flap into the clear cornea

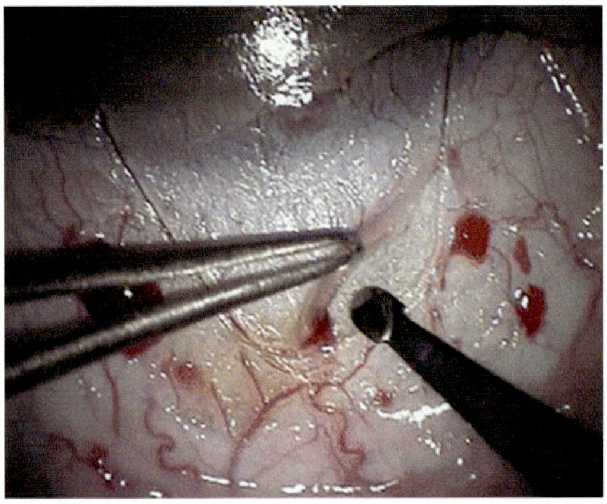

Fig. 5.3 Preparation of the superficial scleral flap with a mini crescent knife

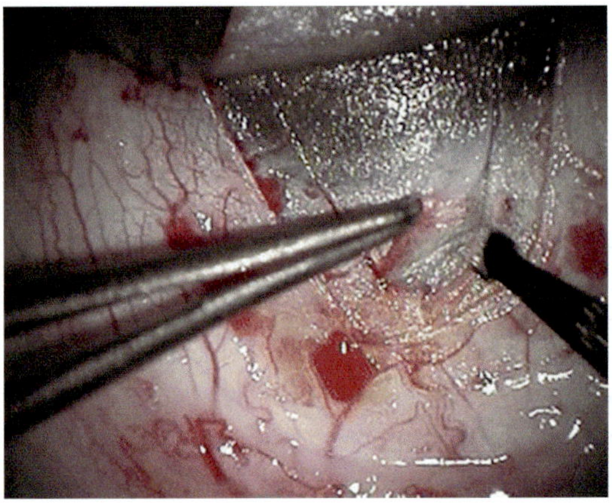

Fig. 5.5 Preparation of the deeper scleral flap using a mini crescent knife, note the smaller size of the deeper scleral flap

are part of the draining system and needed for successful canaloplasty. In case of excessive bleeding we use a delicate diathermy probe (25G endodiathermy probe) to perform focal diathermy.

2. **Preparation of a deep scleral flap**

Next deep sclerokeratectomy is performed by making a slightly smaller second flap then the superficial one, leaving a step of sclera at the sides allowing for a tighter closure of the superficial flap in case of an intraoperative perforation of the trabeculo-Descemet's-membrane or intended watertight closure for viscocanalostomy/canaloplasty. Then the deep scleral flap is dissected towards the cornea using ruby knife or delicate crescent stainless steel knife (Fig. 5.5). This dissection has to be made down to a depth very close to the choroids/ciliary body and carefully carried anteriorly keeping the level of dissection as constant as possible. In case of opening of the suprachoroidal space dissection is continued just a few scleral fibers above. The change of the direction of the scleral fibers to a limbusparallel bundle indicates the scleral spur (Fig. 5.6). Just behind this the Schlemm's canal is opened and unroofed. Care is taken to dissect the ostia of Schlemm's

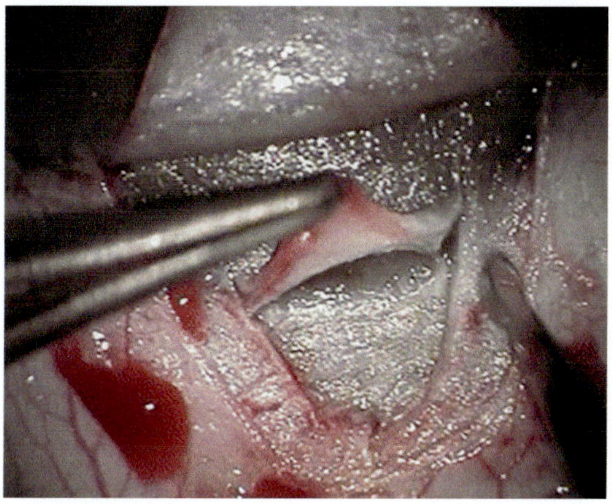

Fig. 5.6 Opening of the Schlemm's canal, note the colour difference in the scleral bed indicating the right depth of preparation

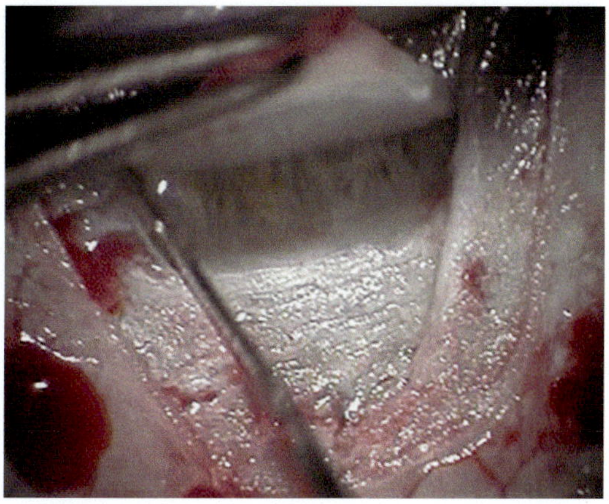

Fig. 5.7 Enlarging the descemetic window for optimal exposure of the trabeculo-descemetic membrane, note the percolation of aqueous humour without perforation of the membrane, iris is visible through the intact membrane

canal clearly, because it is believed that this reduces the risk of collapse and scarring of these surgical ostia. Also entering the Schlemm's canal with the microcatheter or a cannula is easier if the ostia can be identified clearly.

3. **Reduction of IOP**

A paracentesis/side port incision, which should be performed latest now is used to reduce intraocular pressure to very low level. This manoeuvre reduces the risk of perforation of the trabeculo-Descemet's-membrane. Also it is necessary to control later IOP or inject air in the anterior chamber.

4. **Creating a trabeculo-descemetic window**

The dissection is then carried forward to expose a small segment of the Descemet's membrane, creating a trabeculo-descemetic window of about 1–1.5 mm (Fig. 5.7). The corneal stroma can be blunt separated from the Descemet's membrane i.e. with a sponge while the edges of the deep scleral flap are cut towards the cornea with the knife. In some cases the adhesion of Descemet's membrane to the stroma is tighter. In these cases a blunt spatula or the mini crescent knife could be used with sweeping like limbusparallel motion to release these adhesions. This part of the surgery is quite challenging because there is a high risk of perforation of the anterior chamber. The deep sclerocorneal flap is then removed by cutting in the clear corneal part with a delicate small and very sharp scissor (i.e. Vannas or Galand scissor) (Fig. 5.8).

5. **Insertion of the microcatheter**

Now the ostia of Schlemm's canal are gently enlarged by injecting a high viscosity OVD with the help of a special 31G cannula (Fig. 5.9). This will also help to reduce reflux bleeding into the surgical field. As the IOP starts to drop this occurs frequently at this stage of surgery. A specially designed forceps (Glaucolight

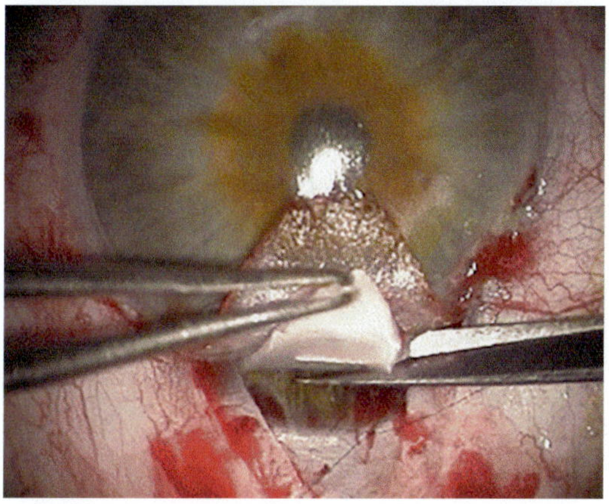

Fig. 5.8 Deep sclerectomy—dissection of the deeper scleral flap with Vannas scissors

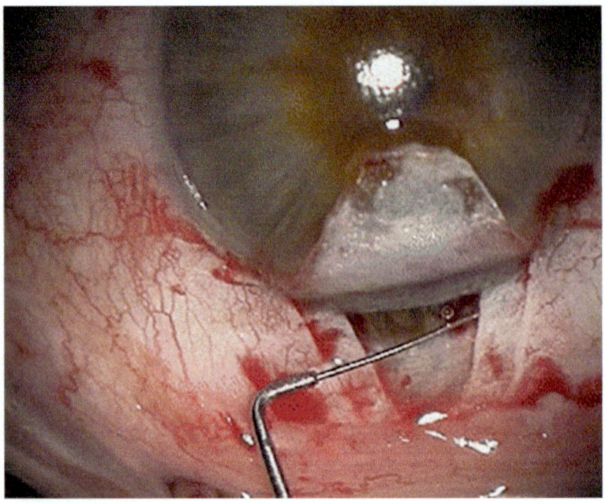

Fig. 5.9 Viscocanalostomy with injection of OVD into the ostia of Schlemm's canal with a special cannula

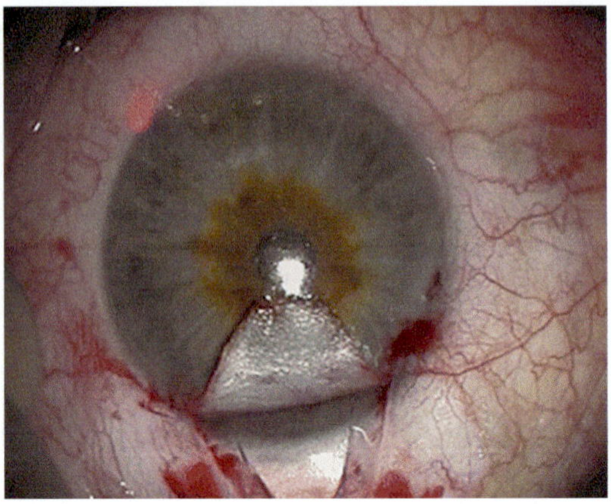

Fig. 5.11 Red spot indicating the position of the microcatheter at 5 o'clock position in the Schlemm's canal

forceps, DORC, The Netherlands) or a tying forceps is used to manipulate the microcatheter and place the tip into the surgically created ostia of Schlemm's canal (Fig. 5.10). The microcatheter is advanced 12 clock h within the canal while the surgeon observes the location of the beacon tip through the sclera (Figs. 5.11, 5.12 and 5.13). After the catheterization of the entire canal length with the microcatheter and with the distal tip exposed at the surgical site, a 10×0 polypropylene suture is tied to the distal tip and the microcatheter withdrawn, pulling the suture into the canal (Fig. 5.14). To enhance the effect of canaloplasty an OVD can be injected while the iTrack microcatheter is retracted. If this additional injection of OVD into the entire canal is necessary, is unclear, while we could prove that the procedure did work without the use of iTrack catheter and circumferential injection of OVD **33**.

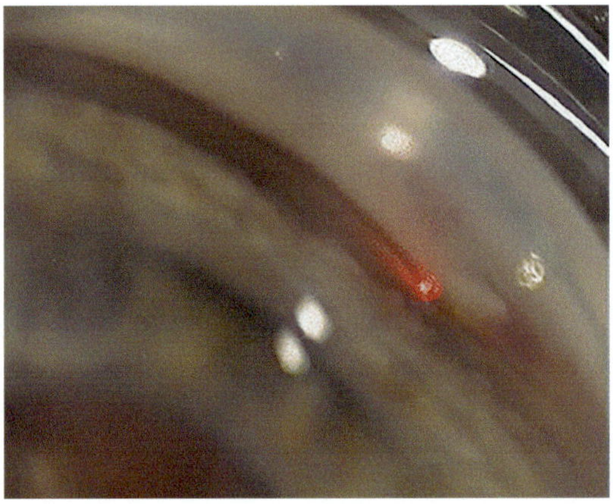

Fig. 5.12 Intraoperative gonioscopic few with illuminated tip of the microcatheter (red dot) in the Schlemm's canal, note the heavily pigmented trabecular meshwork in this eye

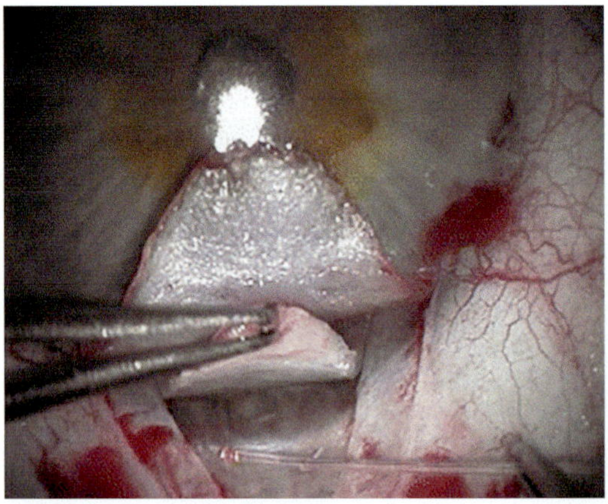

Fig. 5.10 Microcatheter before insertion into the Schlemm's canal

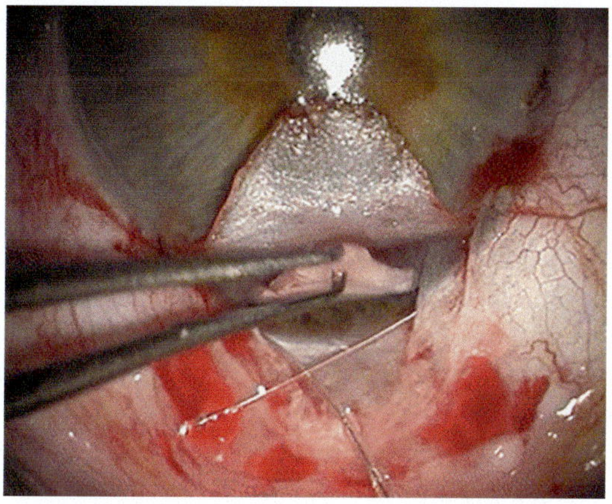

Fig. 5.13 After complete 360° cannulation of the Schlemm's canal

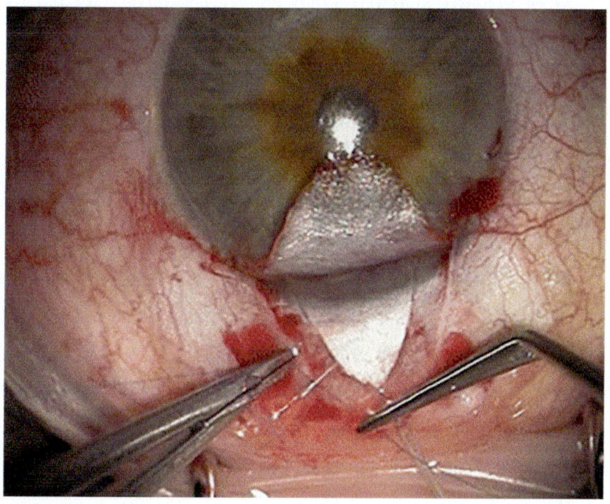

Fig. 5.14 10×0 Prolene tensioning suture is fixed to the microcatheter

6. **Insertion of a 10×0 polypropylene suture**

After the microcatheter is removed from Schlemm's canal the suture is cut from the microcatheter and then tied in a loop, encircling the inner wall of the canal using a slip knot or a locked four throw knot (Fig. 5.15). To reduce risk of rupture of descemetic membrane and to facilitate a more effective tensioning of the 10×0 polypropylene suture the IOP was previously lowered through a paracentesis.

7. **Check for perculation of aqueous**

At this stage of the procedure, there should be perculation of aqueous through the remaining

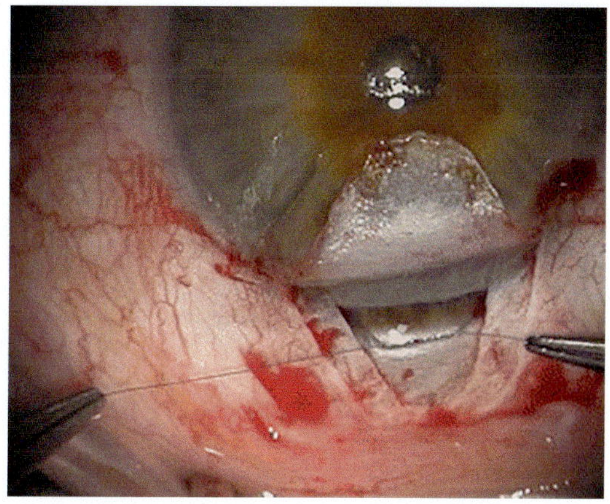

Fig. 5.15 After withdrawing of the microcatheter the suture is cut off and knotted under tension to pull the inner wall of Schlemm's canal and the descemetic window towards the anterior chamber to prevent failure of the surgery due to collapse of these structures

membrane evident. This can be checked also by applicating fluorescein to the surgical area (s.c. Rentsch-Seidel test). The amount of perculation is checked while drying the surgical area with a sponge. To increase the outflow facility, we peel partially the inner wall of the Schlemm's canal, including the endothelium and the juxtacanalicular trabecular meshwork. A special designed forceps or an ordinary capsulorhexis forceps could be used. Occasional the inner wall of the Schlemm's canal is fibrosed and an initial radial cut is necessary to be able to start the peeling. The next step of the surgery ophthalmic viscosurgical device (OVD) is injected in the surgical ostia of Schlemm's canal.

8. **Suturing of superficial scleral flap**

The superficial scleral flap is repositioned and tightly closed with five to seven single absorbable sutures (i.e. 10×0 Vicryl, Ethicon). The superficial scleral flap is sutured as watertight as possible for forcing internal filtration into the Schlemm's canal and then into the collector channels (Fig. 5.16). Now OVD is gently injected under the scleral flap to reduce the risk of bleeding into the sclerectomy site and to prevent scarring in this area. This will preserve the scleral lake. Anterior chamber is refilled with balanced salt solution to normal or slightly

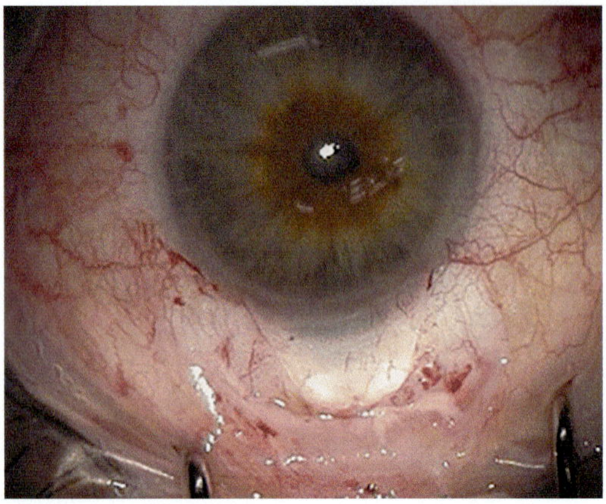

Fig. 5.16 Watertight closure of the superficial scleral flap with 5–7 interrupted sutures (9/0 absorbable suture), same suture is used to close conjunctiva

elevated IOP. In case of perforation or unstable anterior chamber alternatively air could be injected. Conjunctiva is repositioned and fixed with two to four single absorbable sutures.

Canaloplasty could be performed in combination with phacoemulsification. In contrast to phacotrabeculectomy results of phacocanaloplasty is not negatively affected by cataract surgery. It seems that the non perforating character of canaloplasty and the postoperative stable anterior chamber are important factors for the favourable outcome. There is no evidence that separate or shared incision is better. If separate incision is planned first a clear cornea microincisional cataract surgery is performed. This is then followed by deep sclerectomy and canaloplasty as described. We favour a shared incision. Preparation of deep sclerectomy is carried out until the Schlemm's canal is opened. Then the phacoincision is placed between the superficial and deep scleral flap and a standard MICS is performed with injector assisted IOL implantation. OVD is left in the anterior chamber and canaloplasty is performed. After superficial flap is sutured the OVD is removed with bimanual irrigation-aspiration.

Complications

Only very limited data are available about complications in canaloplasty. Intraoperative complications should be separately discussed from those occurring in the postoperative period. Most intraoperative complications are related to difficulties during the deep sclerectomy and are not specially caused by the catheterization of Schlemm's canal and the placement of a tensioning suture.

Typical intraoperative complications of deep sclerectomy are:

- Superficial preparation of the scleral flaps
  This will cause either a button holing in the superficial scleral flap or difficulties to localize and open Schlemm's canal during preparation of deep scleral flap. The superficial flap should be about one third scleral thickness. This is needed to leave enough scleral tissue for deeper scleral flap and to facilitate surgical manipulations. Deep scleral flap should be almost opening the suprachoroidal space. As scleral thickness is variable a preset knife is not recommended. We have performed deep sclerectomy in patients with very thin sclera of less then 400 μm. Here only surgeons experience can help to create the correct scleral flaps.
- Deep preparation of scleral flaps
  Opening the suprachoroidal space usually is not causing severe complication. After the surgeon has realized this problem preparation can be continue a few microns more superficial. And if then this level is kept during preparation this will guide to anatomical landmark scleral spur and finally to Schlemm's canal.
- Perforation of Descemet's membrane
  Most frequent complication in deep sclerectomy is a perforation of the Descemet's membrane (Figs. 5.17, 5.18 and 5.19). As a standard in all non-penetrating procedures a

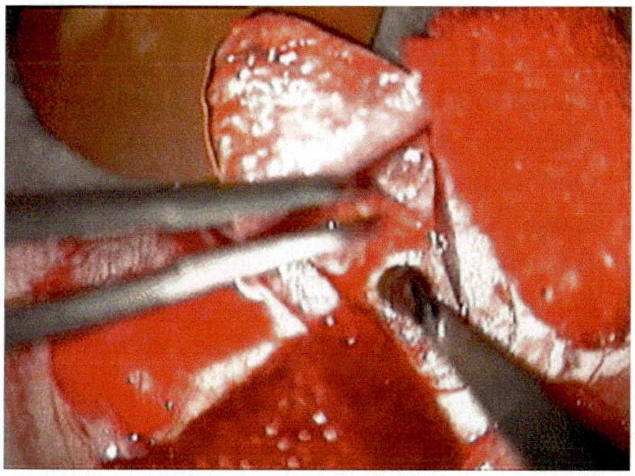

Fig. 5.17 Radial opening of suprachoroidal space during preparation of deep scleral flap. *Note* Minimal prolapse of ciliary body, no bleeding, and canaloplasty was completed without any further complication

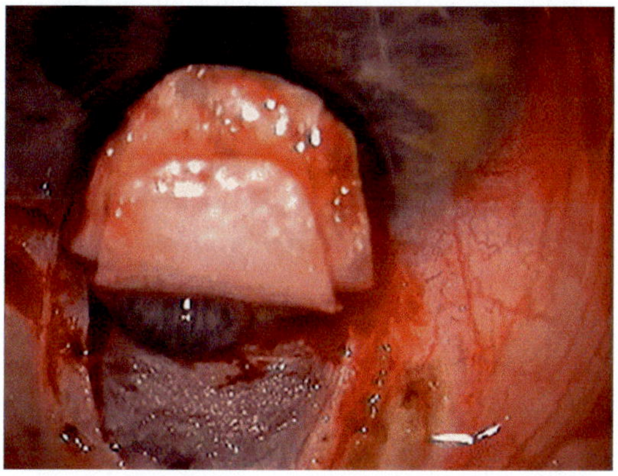

Fig. 5.18 Intraoperative iris prolapse through Descemet's membrane during preparation of deep scleral flap

paracentesis should be performed latest when Schlemm's canal is reached. This will allow control of intraocular pressure, as experience has shown, that lowering the IOP will reduce stress to Descemet's membrane and reduce risk for perforation. In case of perforation further strategy will depend on size of perforation and appearance of iris prolapse. If the perforation is minimal surgery can be continued. Anterior chamber might be refilled with balanced salt solution or even better with air (higher surface tension) to form the eye. Miochol could be gently injected to bring the pupil down and to pull the iris root away from the perforation side. If a larger perforation with iris prolapse occurs surgery usually needs to be converted into a "modified" trabeculectomy. Iridectomy is performed and superficial flap is closed.

Typical intraoperative complications of canaloplasty:

- Difficult catheterization
  The most frequent complication is an unsuccessful catheterization (Fig. 5.20). In the literature it is reported in up to 30% of cases. This could be caused by a non-perfect deep sclerectomy resulting in difficulties to find the surgically created ostia of Schlemm's canal. But more frequent in difficulties

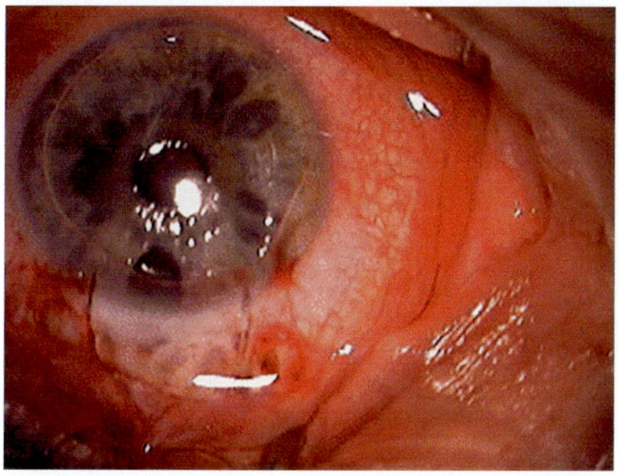

Fig. 5.19 Same eye after deep sclerectomy, peripheral iridectomy and air injection in anterior chamber

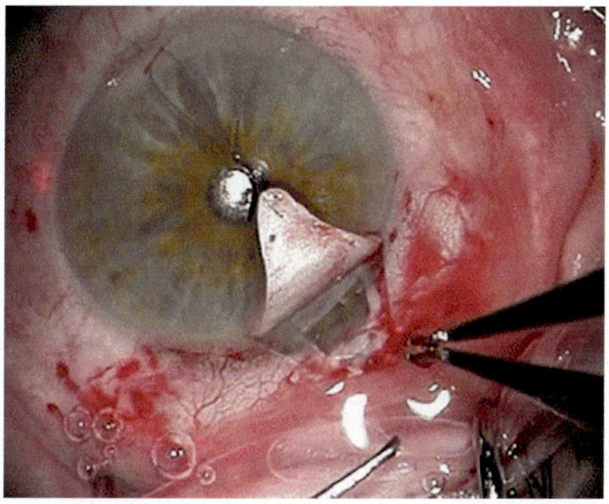

Fig. 5.20 Illuminated tip of microcatheter is indicating correct position in the Schlemm's canal

during 360° catheterization. The microcatheter could stop at any point during passage. This is mostly caused by larger ostia of collector channels in the outer wall of Schlemm's canal. Gently massage ab externo in this area might help sometimes to overcome this problem. If this does not help the microcatheter is withdrawn and the tip is bended a little. Then the microcatheter is again inserted. The bended tip should be directed towards the trabecular meshwork to reduce the risk for mispassage into an ostia of a collector channel. If this will not overcome the problem the microcatheter is again withdrawn and introduced in the opposite ostia of Schlemm's canal. In almost all cases this will lead to a successful passage.

- Mispassage
  The tip of the microcatheter could perforate the wall of Schlemm's canal and become located suprachoroidal or in the anterior chamber. If the microcatheter will perforate into the anterior chamber usually it will be advanced in the anterior chamber angle. First sign could be a reduced distance to the limbus. This will be usually followed by little iris movement. In most cases this will not cause any severe complications and catheterization could be performed successfully in the opposite direction. But in some cases the tip can damage the peripheral iris vessels and cause anterior chamber bleeding. Also the tip can penetrate the anterior chamber angle and appears in the suprachoroidal space. The illuminated tip will indicate if the microcatheter enters the suprachoroidal space. Distance to the limbus will increase and finally the tip will move posteriorly. Microcatheter should be removed. Depending on surgeons experience catheterization could be repeated. Most cases passage will be possible in the opposite direction. Special care should be taken that the tip of the microcatheter is correctly introduced in the ostia of Schlemm's canal.
- Suture related problems
  Placement of the polypropylene suture into the Schlemm's canal is the next step during canaloplasty (Fig. 5.21). The suture is knotted to the microcatheter. If this knot is loose the suture could be lost and the catheterization has to be repeated. A larger knot could stop at the ostium of Schlemm's canal. One should not pull to strong as this could cause perforation of trabecular meshwork or Descemet's membrane. The knot should be turned towards the trabecular meshwork.
  Tightening the polypropylene suture is the major step in canaloplasty. This will prevent collapse of Schlemm's canal and will overcome some problems of other non-penetrating procedures. There are different techniques how to create a tensioned suture (e.g. slippage knot and four throw blocked knot). Correct tension should be checked by pulling the suture before cutting the loose ends. If the knot cannot be moved over the scleral spur and the surgeons feels some tension from the suture it is believed to be the right tension. To verify the so called distension and status of Schlemm's canal an intraoperative ultrasound biomicroscopy or optical coherence tomography could be performed. If the suture is loose and cannot be tightened more a new suture should be placed into Schlemm's canal (Fig. 5.21).

Rarely a too tight suture could cause cheese wiring of trabecular meshwork (Fig. 5.22). This is usually related to a more complicated surgery and/or unexperienced surgeon. If the suture is

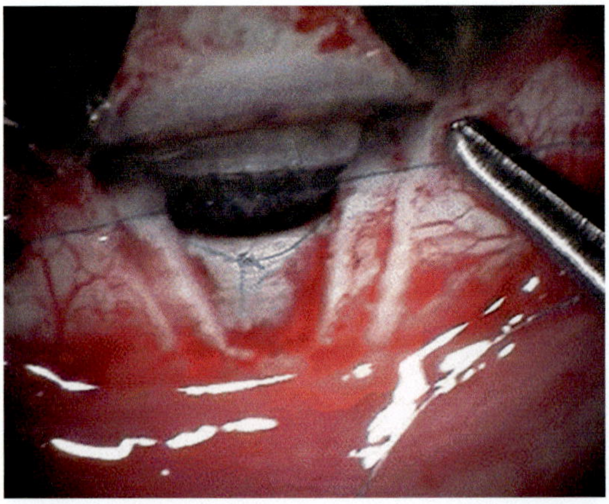

Fig. 5.21 Placement of a second tighter tensioning suture. *Note* First suture became very loose after tightening the second suture

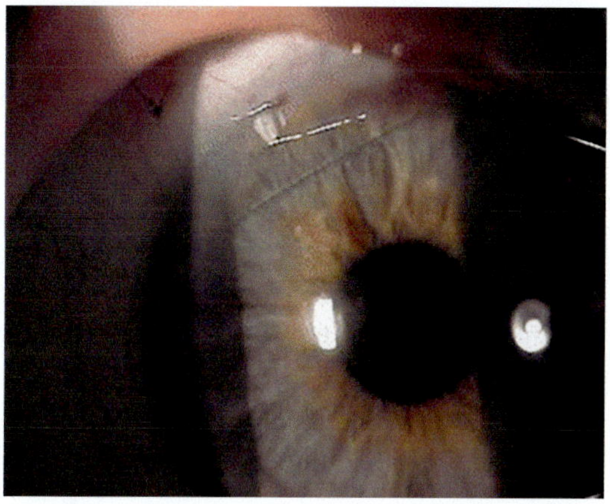

Fig. 5.22 Tensioning suture in the superior nasal quadrant of anterior chamber after complicated canaloplasty. *Note* No pupil distortion, no inflammation, IOP 13 mmHg

only in the peripheral anterior chamber visible it could be left. In our experience this will not cause further complications. If the suture is in the pupillary area or has contact to iris surface it is recommended to remove it. There are only very few cases reported on this complication. Some were recognized only later postoperative and thought to be caused by the permanent tension of the suture. But we believe they where always caused intraoperative. The tension of the 10/0 polypropylene suture is minimal and if accidentally cut during NdYAG goniopuncture procedure the loose ends will move only one or maximum 2 mm.

- Descemet's membrane detachment
  In viscocanaloplasty vasodilatation of Schlemm's canal is intended. A special syringe is used with iTrack® to inject viscoelastic device through the microcatheter. Originally this was used for 360° viscocanalostomy, but this procedure did not prove to be more effective then standard viscocanalostomy. The effect of viscoinjection in the more or less closed system is not predictable. The same amount of viscoelastic device may cause only dilatation of Schlemm's canal, microrupture of trabecular meshwork, Descemet's membrane detachment or even viscodetachment into suprachoroidal space [33]. There are several reports on hemorrhagic Descemet's membrane detachment in the literature (Figs. 5.23 and 5.24). Spontaneous resorption will take up to 1 year. But if central cornea is not affected vision is stable and cornea stroma remains clear. An immediate surgical intervention with lavage of the hemorrhagic Descemet's membrane detachment could be indicated if the visual axis is affected [34]. Because of this complication we have abandoned vasodilatation and have not found any difference with regards to postoperative intraocular pressure.
- Bleeding from anterior chamber angle
  Even in uncomplicated canaloplasty intraoperative bleeding from anterior chamber angle might occur. This is related to a reflux bleeding from episcleral vessels into Schlemm's canal caused by low intraocular pressure. If trabecular meshwork is permeable the blood might appear in the anterior chamber angle and is not a sign of a complication. Early postoperative it might be followed by hyphaema. Resorption will take a few days and only very rarely anterior chamber lavage is needed.

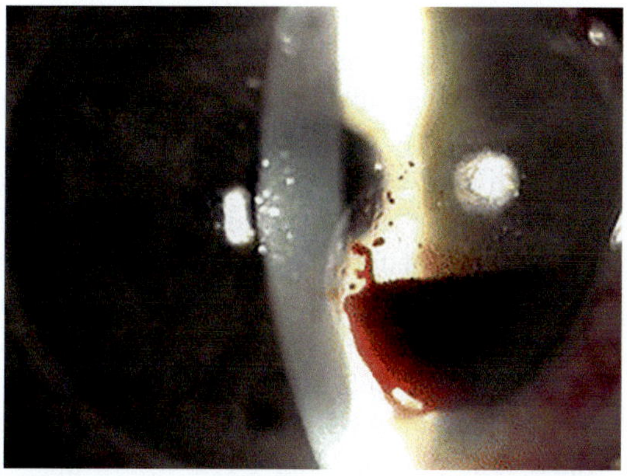

Fig. 5.23 Hemorrhagic Descemet's membrane detachment after viscocanaloplasty with iTrack® bleb is filled with blood and viscoelastic device

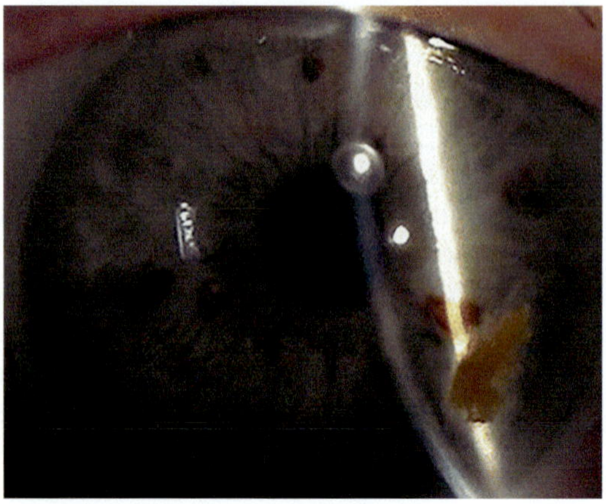

Fig. 5.24 Same eye 10 months postoperative, visual acuity remained 20/20, IOP 13 mmHg

Typical postoperative complications of canaloplasty:

- Early postoperative hyphaema
  If intraocular pressure early postoperative is lower then episcleral vein pressure a reflux bleeding via collector channels, Schlemm's canal and trabecular meshwork might cause intracameral hemorrhage. This could result in a microhyphaema (frequent postoperative appearance) or even a excessive hyphaema of up to 4–5 mm. Reduced visual acuity stresses patients and the surgeon but spontaneous resorption should be awaited at least for one week. In case of missing resorption or intraocular pressure rise the anterior chamber could be lavaged with bimanual irrigation/aspiration.
  As a minor anterior chamber bleeding is very common and does not affect the final outcome it should not be considered a complication. Some surgeons consider it as a positive prognostic sign and have found a positive correlation between early postoperative microhyphaema and lower postoperative intraocular pressure after 1 year follow up.
- Transient decreased visual acuity
  Even in case of clear optical media in some patients visual acuity is decreased for some weeks or even months postoperatively. Beside surgically induced astigmatism no specific reason was found and in almost all cases visual acuity recovered spontaneously.
- Steroid induced elevation of intraocular pressure
  As canaloplasty is a non-penetrating procedure in up to thirty percent of cases steroid response is possible. Most surgeons are using prednisolone acetate or dexamethasone eye drops as standard postoperative care. If two weeks postoperatively the intraocular pressure rises and gonioscopy does not show any abnormality this might be caused by steroid response and therapy should be changed to NSAID. In most cases intraocular pressure will drop again after one to two weeks.
- Postoperative hypotonia
  Sometimes postoperative intraocular pressure is below 6 mmHg. This might be caused by some subconjunctival filtration. After uncomplicated canaloplasty anterior chamber is formed even in this cases and choroidal detachment is very rare. Interruption of postoperative antiphlogistic therapy for 1 or 2 days is usually enough to induce healing processes at the scleral flap and to stop subconjunctival filtration. After increase of intraocular pressure steroid eye drops should be continued for about 4 weeks. If this does not help reintervention with placement of additional sutures to scleral flap might be indicated. In case of flat anterior chamber injection of air is very helpful.
- Postoperative pressure rise
  Other causes for postoperative uncontrolled intraocular pressure could be increased outflow resistance in trabecular pressure or gonosynechiae in the area of deep sclerectomy / Descemet's window. Usually NdYAG laser synechiolysis and/or goniopuncture are very effective (Fig. 5.25). Special care should be taken, that the tensioning suture is not cut by the laser.
- Iris prolapse
  There is an increased risk for iris prolapse through descemetic window into the sclerectomy area (scleral lake) after complicated surgery or blunt trauma. This is a rare complication and if intraocular pressure remains

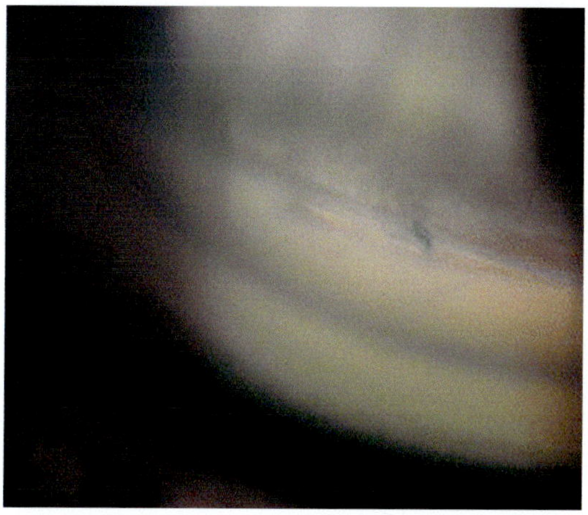

Fig. 5.25 Gonioscopic view after NDYAG goniopuncture. *Note* Defects in descemetic window, tensioning suture intact, scleral lake open

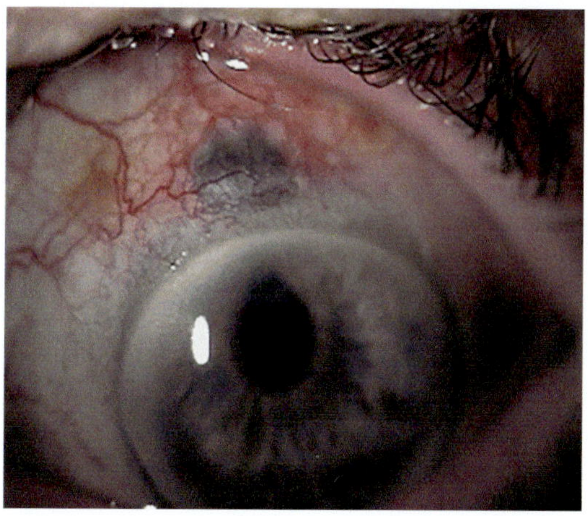

Fig. 5.26 Late postoperative iris prolapse after blunt trauma

low and optical axis is not affected from pupil distortion no intervention is required. If needed iris prolapse could be repositioned ab interno in early phase. Miochol and air is injected into the anterior chamber. Additionally a peripheral iridectomy could be performed with a vitrectome. Later a revision ab externo is preferable. After conjunctival peritomy superficial scleral flap is lifted and prolapsed iris dissected (Fig. 5.26).

- Expulsive intraocular haemorrhage
  One of the worst complication of a surgical intervention in a seeing eye is an expulsive suprachoroidal haemorrhage. This is usually caused by very low intraocular pressure in the early postoperative phase, fragile choroidal vessels, sudden elevation of cranial blood pressure (e.g. forward bending or pressing) and anticoagulation. There is no report of such an event in the literature. We have had two cases with expulsive suprachoroidal haemorrhage in canaloplasty. Both eyes where high myopic and vitrectomized. Early postoperative pressure was very low. In the first patient the complication occurred during the first night whereas in the second patient it occurs at third postoperative morning during tooth brushing. One should wait 7–10 days before intervention. We favour pars plana vitrectomy, suprachoroidal lavage via sclerotomy and silicone oil tamponade.
- Endophthalmitis
  There is no endophthalmitis reported after canaloplasty. In the last 15 years we have performed more then 3000 non-penetrating glaucoma surgeries without any endophthalmitis. If endophthalmitis occur one should take same considerations like for a case of endophthalmitis after phacoemulsification.

Postoperative Treatment

In routine canaloplasty only minimal postoperative care is needed. The anterior chamber is deep and the IOP in the first postoperative days is around 10 mmHg. As described hyphaema might be present, but is usually absorbed within 2–3 days spontaneously.

We refer for local steroid therapy with five times daily prednisolone 1% eye drops. This therapy is continued for 5–6 weeks.

IOP fluctuations within the first few weeks might be present. We use gonioscopy to differentiate between steroid response, iris adhesion, bleeding into scleral lake, early excessive

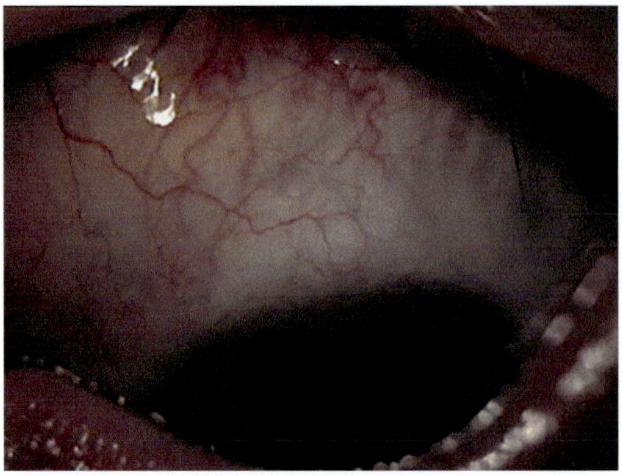

Fig. 5.27 Status 4 years post canaloplasty, IOP 13 mmHG, no antiglaucomatous medication. *Note* No bleb formation or sign of subconjunctival filtration

scaring of scleral lake etc. Intervention is adapted to the cause of IOP rise.

Canaloplasty is a highly effective non-perforating bleb independent glaucoma surgery (Fig. 5.27). The postoperative IOP is usually in the low tens and comparable to the results of trabeculectomy. But there is a much lower complication rate reported. It has the potential to re-establish the natural pathway of aqueous humour outflow in patients with open angle glaucoma.

Material and Companies Address

Ellex

Ellex Medical Lasers Ltd.
82 Gilbert Street,
Adelaide, SA 5000 Australia
Phone + 61 8 8104 5200.
http://www.ellex.com/.

Geuder

Hertzstr. 4
69126 Heidelberg
Germany
Tel: 06,221/3066
Fax: 06,221/303,122
info@geuder.de
www.geuder.de.

Electronic Supplementary Material

Below is the link to the electronic supplementary material.Video 5.1Canaloplasty (MPG 104696 kb)Video 5.2Canaloplasty with Onalene (MPG 177941 kb)

References

1. Jones E, Clarke J, Khaw PT. Recent advances in trabeculectomy technique. Curr Opin Ophthalmol. 2005;16:107–13.
2. Mac I, Soltau JB. Glaucoma-filtering bleb infections. Curr Opin Ophthalmol. 2003;14:91–4.
3. Borisuth NSC, Phillips B, Krupin T. The risk of glaucoma filtration surgery. Curr Opin Ophthalmol. 1999;10:112–6.
4. Ophir A. Encapsulated filtering bleb; a selective review—new deductions. Eye. 1992;6:348–52.
5. Gedde SJ, Herndon LW, Brandt JD, et al. Surgical complications in the tube versus trabeculectomy study during the first year of follow-up. Am J Ophthalmol. 2007;143:23–31.
6. Ellingsen BA, Grant WM. Trabeculotomy and sinusotomy in enucleated human eyes. Investig Ophthalmol. 1972;11:21–8.
7. Johnstone MA, Grant WM. Microsurgery of Schlemm's canal and the human aqueous outflow systeme. Am J Ophthalmol. 1973;76:906–17.
8. Epstein E. Fibrosing response to aqueous; its relation to glaucoma. Br J Ophthalmol. 1959;43:641–7.
9. Krasnov MM. Externalization of Schlemm's canal (sinusotomy) in glaucoma. Br J Ophthalmol. 1968;52:157–61.
10. Koslov VI, Bagrov SN, Anisimova SY, et al. (Nonpentrating deep sclerectomy with collagen) Russian. Oftalmokhirurgiia. 1990;3:44–6.
11. Fyodorov SN, Ioffe DI, Ronkina TI. Deep sclerectomy: technique and mechanism of a new antiglaucomatous procedure. Glaucoma. 1984;6:183–281.
12. Zimmerman TJ, Kooner KS, Ford VJ, et al. Trabeculectomy vs. nonpenetrating trabeculectomy: a retrospective study of two procedures in phakic patients with glaucoma. Ophthalmic Surg. 1984;15:734–40.
13. Stegmann R, Pinenaar A, Miller D. Viscocanalostomy for open-angle glaucoma in

black African patients. J Cataract Refract Surg. 1999;25:316–22.
14. Sourdille P, Santiago P-Y, Villain F, et al. Reticulated hyaluronic acid implant in nonperforating trabecular surgery. J Cataract Refract Surg. 1999;25:332–9.
15. Ambresin A, Shaarawy T, Mermoud A. Deep sclerectomy with collagen implant in one eye compared with trabeculectomy in the other eye of the same patient. J Glaucoma. 2002;11:214–20.
16. Sanchez E, Schnyder CC, Sickenberg M, et al. Deep sclerectomy: results with and without collagen implant. Int Ophthalmol. 1996/97;20:157–62.
17. Wiermann A, Zeitz O, Jochim E, Matthiessen ET, Wagenfeld L, Galambos P, Scharioth G, Matthiesen N, Klemm M. A comparision between absorbable and non-absorbable scleral implants in deep sclerectomy (T-Flux and SK-Gel). Ophthalmologe. 2007;104(5):409–14.
18. Schreyger F, Scharioth GB, Baatz H. SKGEL implant versus T-Flux implant in the contralateral eye in deep sclerectomy with phacoemulsification: long-term follow-up. Open Ophthalmol J. 2008;2:57–61.
19. O'Bart DPS, Shiew M, Edmunds B. A randomized, prospective study comparing trabeculectomy with viscocanalostomy with adjunctive antimetabolite usage for the management of open angle glaucoma uncontrolled by medical therapy. Br J Ophthalmol. 2004;88:1012–7.
20. Yalvac IS, Sahin M, Eksioglu U. Primary viscocanalostomy versus trabeculectomy for primary open-angle glaucoma; three years prospective randomized clinical trial. J Cataract Refract Surg. 2004;30:2050–7.
21. Carassa RG, Bettin P, Fiori M, Brancato R. Viscocanaolostomy versus trabeculectomy in white adults affected by open-angle glaucoma; a 2-year randomized, controlled trial. Ophthalmology. 2003;110:882–7.
22. Kobayashi H, Kobayashi K, Okinami S. A comparision of the intraocular pressure-lowering effect and safety of viscocanalostomy and trabeculectomy with mitomycin C in bilateral open-angle glaucoma. Graefes Arch Clin Exp Ophthalmol. 2003;241:359–66.
23. Cillino S, Di Pace F, Casuccio A, Lodato G. Deep sclerectomy versus punch trabeculectomy: effect of low dose mitomycin C. Ophthalmologica. 2005;219:281–6.
24. Lüke C, Dietlein TS, Jacobi PC, et al. A prospective ranndomized trial of viscocanalostomy versus trabeculectomy in open-angle glaucoma: a 1-year follow-up study. J Glaucoma. 2002;11:294–9.
25. Goldsmith JA, Ahmed IK, Cradall AS. Nonpenetrating glaucoma surgery. Ophthalmol Clin N Am. 2005;18(3):443–60.
26. Smith R. A new technique for opening the canal of Schlemm. Br J Ophthalmol. 1960;44:370–3.
27. Beck AD, Lynch MG. 360° trabeculotomy for primary congenital glaucoma. Arch Ophthalmol. 1995;113:1200–2.
28. Scharioth GB. Cartheterless Viscocanaloplasty, 6th congress of Romanian society of ophthalmology. In: 3rd international meeting on innovative glaucoma surgery, Recklinghausen, Germany; 2007; Sinaia, Romania
29. Lewis RA, von Wolff K, Tetz M, et al. Canaloplasty: circumferential viscodilation and tensioning of Schlemm's canal using a flexible microcatheter for the treatment of open-angle glaucoma in adults: interim clinical study analysis. J Cataract Refract Surg. 2007;33:1217–26.
30. Lewis RA, von Wolff K, Tetz M, et al. Canaloplasty: circumferential viscodilation and tensioning of Schlemm's canal using a flexible microcatheter for the treatment of open-angle glaucoma in adults: two-year interim clinical study results. J Cataract Refract Surg. 2009;35:814–23
31. Grieshaber MC. Channelography and mechanism of action in canaloplasty. Ophthalmologe. 2015;112(4):319–24.
32. Scharioth GB. Glaucolight assisted Canaloplasty. Highlights Ophthalmol. 2012;40(6):2–7.
33. Scharioth GB. Risk of circumferential viscodilatation in viscocanalostomy. J Cataract Refract Surg. 2015;41(5):1122–3.
34. Rękas M, Petz K, Wierzbowska J, Byszewska A, Jünemann A. Evacuating a pre-Descemet hematoma through a clear corneal incision during acanaloplasty procedure. J Cataract Refract Surg. 2014;40(12):1953–7.

Canaloplasty with iTrack

6

Norbert Körber

Abstract

In black patients all fistularising procedures tend to heal aggressively and thereby the success rate is low, even with the use of mitomycin.

Keywords

Black patient · Trabecular meshwork · Vicryl suture · Senile cataract · International multicenter study

In 2015, the German glaucoma patient association declared *canaloplasty* as the new gold standard in glaucoma surgery, as this operation combines good results with a low risk profile. Prof. Körber from Cologne, Germany, is a pioneer in the surgery of canaloplasty. During this surgery, an illuminated microcatheter is introduced in Schlemm's canal and the canal is then widened through injection of viscoelastics.

Supplementary Information The online version contains supplementary material available at https://doi.org/10.1007/978-3-031-84204-7_6.

N. Körber (✉)
Augencentrum Köln, Köln, Germany
e-mail: n.koerber@gmx.de

In black patients all fistularising procedures tend to heal aggressively and thereby the success rate is low, even with the use of mitomycin.

Robert Stegmann worked very early with Healon for various indications as ocular trauma, pediatric and senile cataract surgery and glaucoma.

His first studies involved visco-trabeculotomy, which was disappointing as there was scarring of the trabecular meshwork in the trabeculotomy segments and also descemet's membrane dissection occurred frequently.

Thus, he developed viscocanalostomy and later canaloplasty as a logical step to improve the results.

Viscocanalostomy showed good long term results in a long term follow up study for black as well as for Caucasian patients.

Canaloplasty is effective on a long term base as well, as the international multicenter study could show.

In Europe, canaloplasty was performed for the first time in 2005 in three surgical centers in Germany (v. Wolff and Bull; Tetz; Koerber) and one in the UK (C. Peckar).

Since then, canaloplasty has been adopted by numerous surgeons in Europe. In Germany, it is coded in the DRG system and in the public health system. Thus, we can state, that this operation has been accepted officially. This year, a patient association named canaloplasty as the

U. Spandau and G. B. Scharioth (eds.), *Cutting Edge of Ophthalmic Surgery*,
https://doi.org/10.1007/978-3-031-84204-7_6

new gold standard in glaucoma surgery, as this operation offers good results with a low risk profile.

Viscocanalostomy

The Surgery Step-by-Step

Viscocanalostomy is performed according to Stegmann's technique, with the creation of a parabolic 5 × 5 mm limbal-based one-third scleral thickness flap (Figs. 6.1 and 6.2). With the goal of achieving a watertight closure, cautery is avoided and 1:10,000 epinephrine is applied using a Weck-cel sponge to achieve hemostasis (Fig. 6.3). A deep scleral flap is created 0.5 mm inside the superficial flap, dissecting down until the choroid is just visible. Schlemm's canal is unroofed and a membrane is cleaved from the cornea, creating a Descemetic window through which aqueous can permeate (Fig. 6.4). The inner, deep scleral flap is then excised, forming the scleral lake (Fig. 6.5). The two surgically created ostia of Schlemm's canal are injected six times with Healon™ GV (Abbott Medical Optics, Santa Ana, California) using a 150 μm cannula (ViscoCanalostomy Cannula, Grieshaber, Schaffhausen, Switzerland) (Fig. 6.6).

The superficial flap is sutured tight to achieve internal drainage and prevent bleb formation (Fig. 6.7).

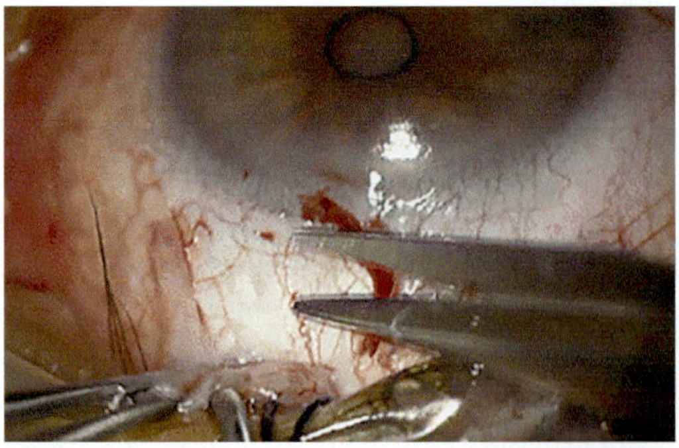

Fig. 6.1 Opening of the conjunctiva

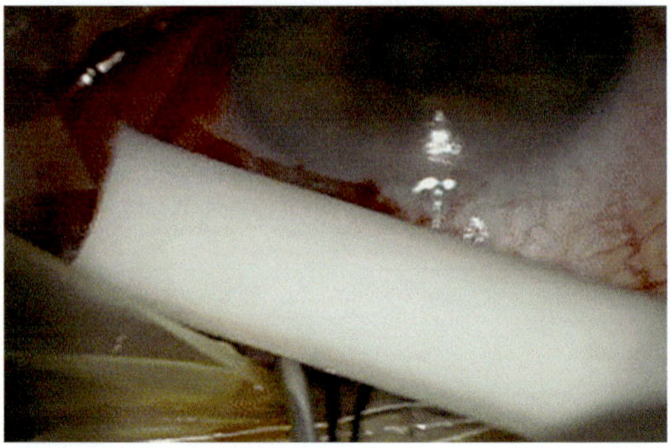

Fig. 6.2 Compression of sclera with suprarenine

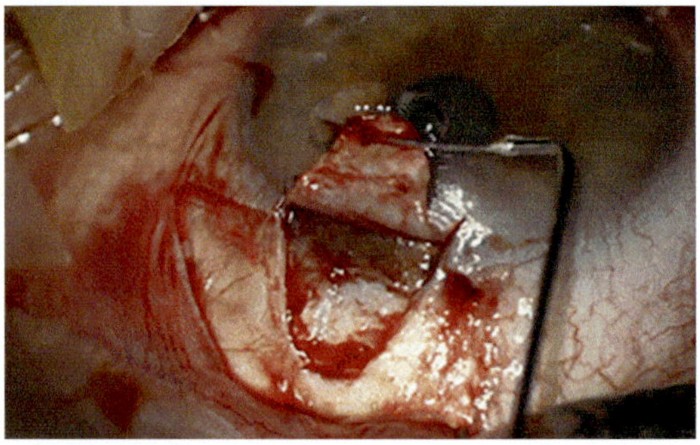

Fig. 6.3 First flap

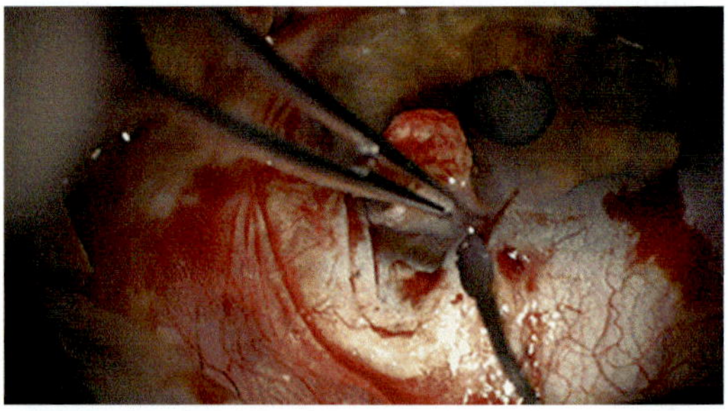

Fig. 6.4 Preparation of the inner flap—descemet window

Canaloplasty (Videos 6.1, 6.2, and 6.3)

The Surgery Step-by-Step

Canaloplasty essentially uses the same non-penetrating surgical technique discussed for viscocanalostomy and has been described in detail in previous reports. After exposing Schlemm's

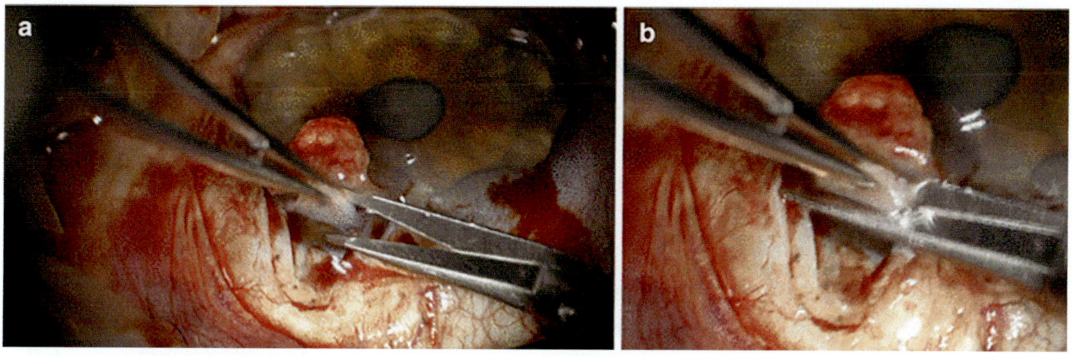

Fig. 6.5 (**a**) Deep sclerectomy bei CP. (**b**) Excision of the inner flap

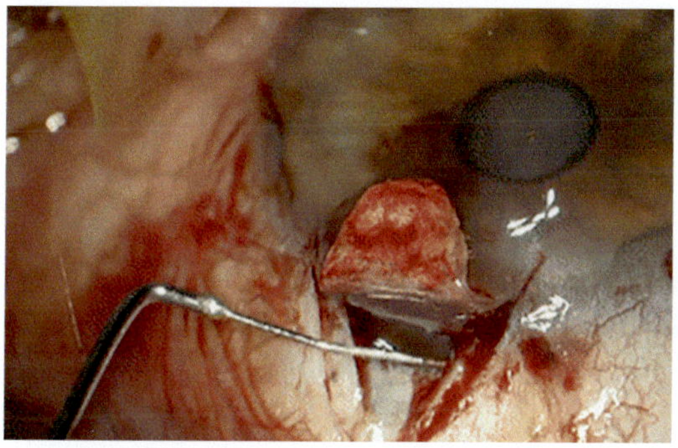

Fig. 6.6 Dilation of Schlemm's canal ostium

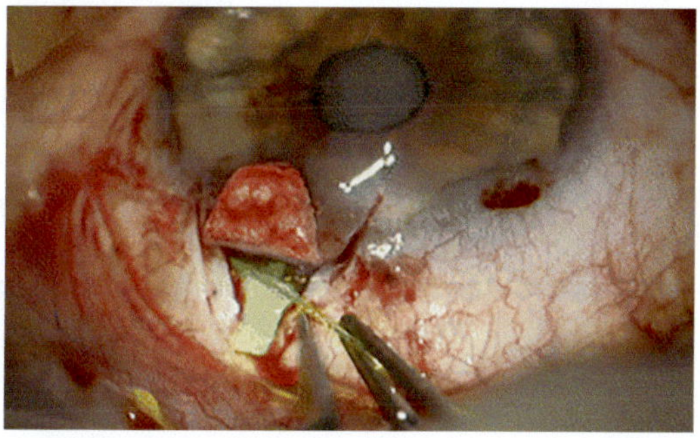

Fig. 6.8 iTrack entering Schlemm's canal

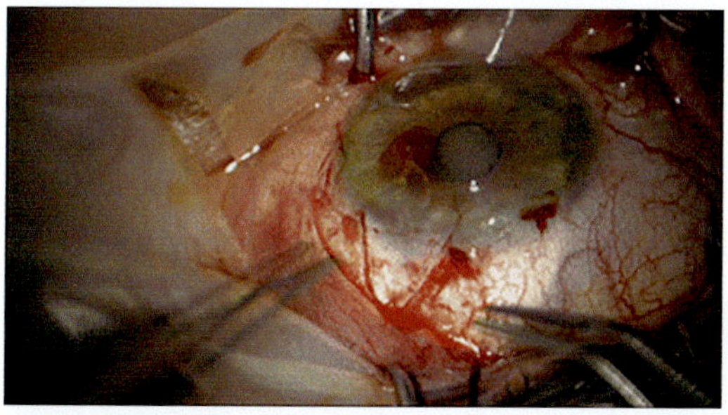

Fig. 6.7 Suturing the outer flap

canal, a flexible microcatheter (iTrack™ 250A Canaloplasty Microcatheter, Nova Eye Medical,Kent Town, Australia) is used to dilate the full circumference of the canal by injecting Healon GV during catheterization (Fig. 6.8). The microcatheter has a 200 micron diameter shaft with an atraumatic distal tip of approximately 250 microns in diameter (Figs. 6.9 and 6.10). The device, which has a lumen through which the viscoelastics is delivered, has an illuminated tip so that the surgeon can observe the location of the beacon tip trans-sclerally (Fig. 6.11). A 10-0 prolene suture (Ethicon Inc., Somerville, New Jersey) is tied to the distal tip (Fig. 6.12) and the microcatheter is withdrawn slowly, pulling the suture into the canal. After tying the suture in a loop encircling the inner wall of the canal, the suture loop is tightened to distend the trabecular meshwork inwards placing the tissues in tension and then locking knots are added (Fig. 6.13).

The scleral lake and the ostia of Schlemm's canal are filled with Healon GV (Fig. 6.14) and the superficial flap is closed with typically 7 10-0 vicryl sutures. The conjunctiva is reattached with one 10-0 vicryl suture with an inverted knot to prevent foreign body sensation during the first days.

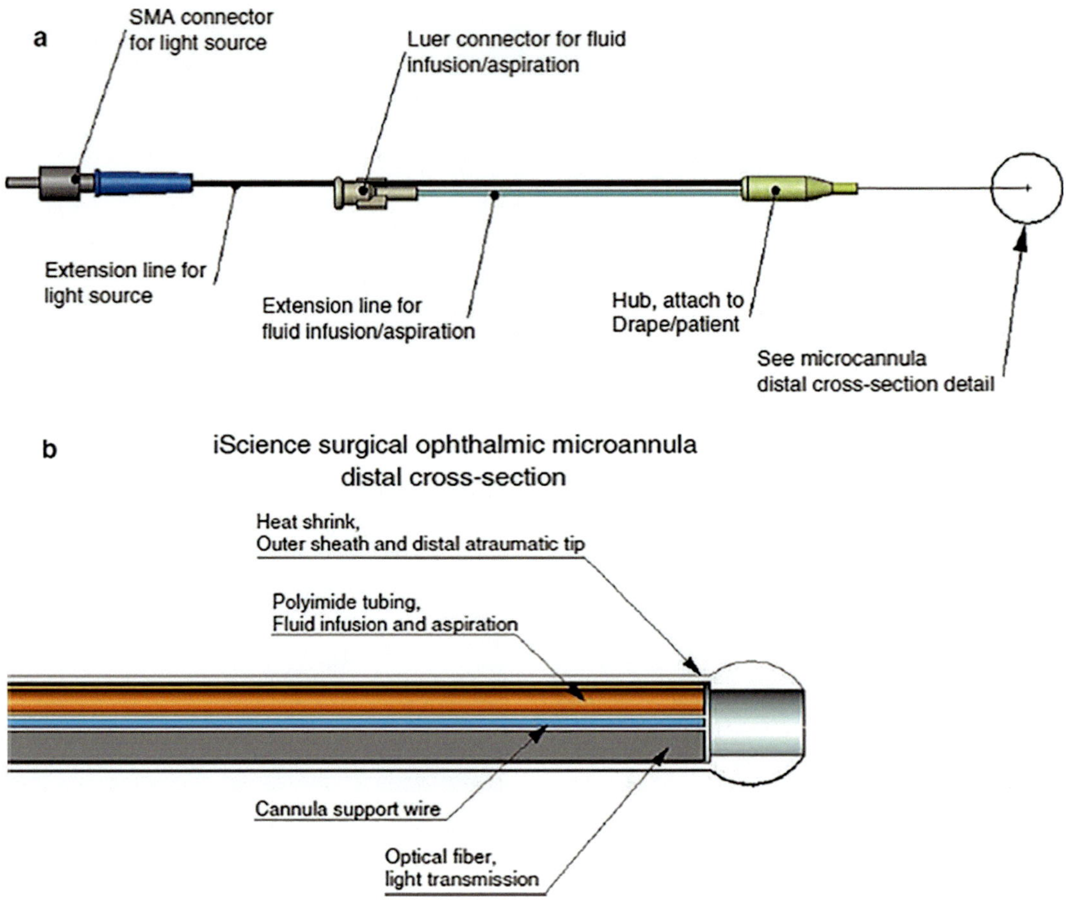

Fig. 6.9 The images show the complete catheter design (**a**). In detail (**b**) we can see a cross-section of the tip depicting the size of the inner structure. We can imagine, that passing a high viscositiy OVD like Healon GV creates an enormous pressure inside the inner tubing, which is made from polyimide

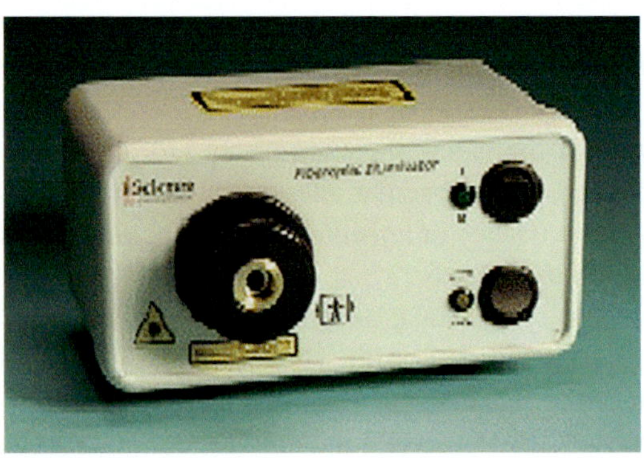

Fig. 6.10 The light source (iLumin II). The light fiber connection is on the left side. On the right side is the on-off switch and a selection button for continuous or intermittent light

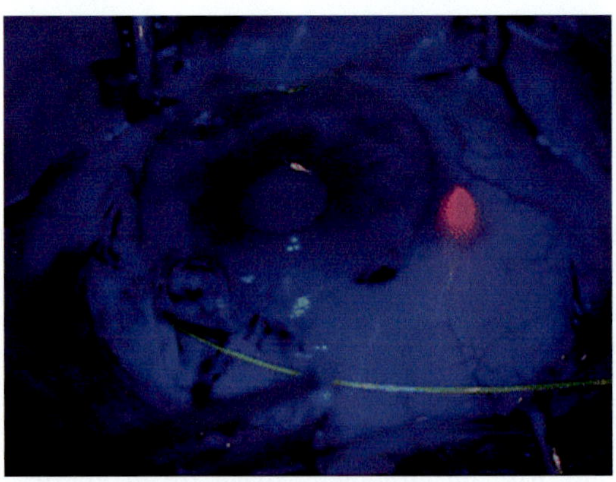

Fig. 6.11 Tip of catheter visible by red dot and visible outflow vessels

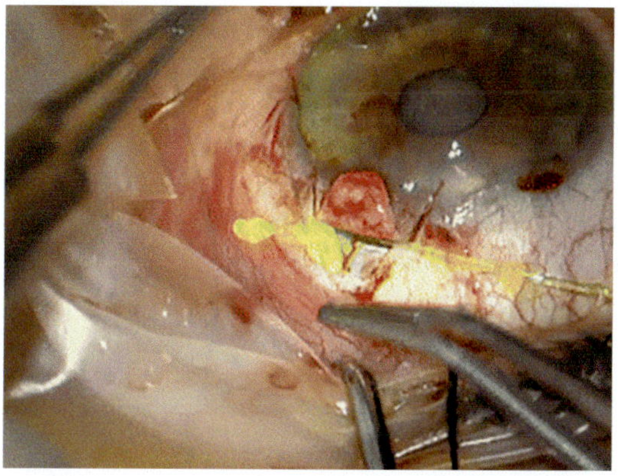

Fig. 6.12 iTrack after 360° dilation, fixation of the 10-0 prolene

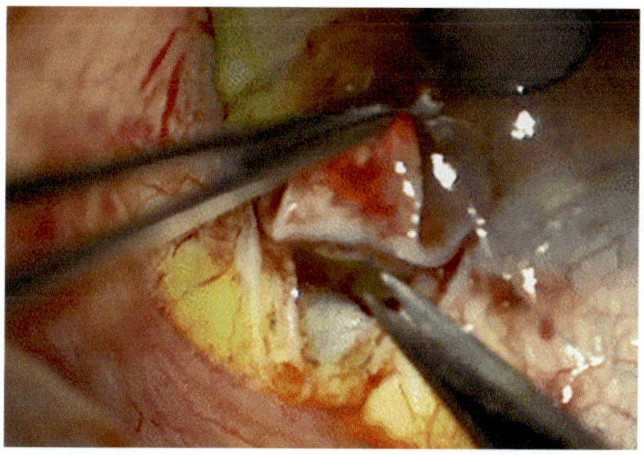

Fig. 6.13 Prolene suture in place, cutting of the end

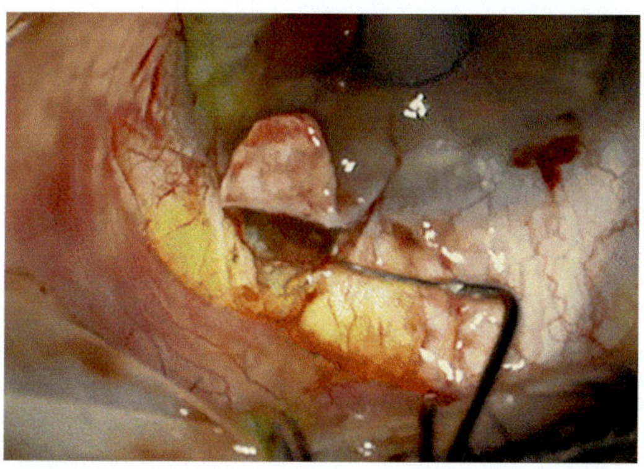

Fig. 6.14 Filling of the lake with Healon GV before suturing the flap

Complications

The complication profile of viscocanalostomy and canaloplasty is not much different, so we will describe both in one chapter.

Ocular-related surgical and post-surgical complications (3 year study Europe)	
Surgical/early postoperative complications (≤ 90 days post-op)	n (%)
Microhyphema: < 1.0 mm layered blood	14 (12.8%)
Hyphema: ≥ 1.0 mm layered blood	6 (5.5%)
Elevated intraocular pressure	6 (5.5%)
Descemet's membrane detachment	4 (3.7%)
Hypotony: IOP ≤ 5 mm Hg with shallow anterior chamber	0
Flat/shallow anterior chamber	0

n sample size, *mm* millimeter

Management of Complications

Hyphema and microhyphema usually do not make an intervention necessary. They resolve in a few days up to 1 week.

Post-op pressure rises during the first days are rare and the reason is still unknown. A local and systemic therapy is sufficient—a surgical intervention/revision is not indicated. Exception: trauma with subsequent incarceration of iris to the scleral lake.

After 2–3 weeks steroid-induced pressure rises are not uncommon. Local therapy and change of steroid (from pred forte to fluorometholone) or stop of steroids and therapy with NSAID's alone is usually sufficient and effective.

Descemet detachment occurs intraoperatively, when a local "overdose" of Healon GV is injected into the canal while being dilated. Most of the detachments are only peripheral and resolve spontaneously after some weeks. If blood enters the detachment space and the visual axis is close or covered, intraoperative aspiration by a paracentesis and air tamponade of the anterior chamber is indicated.

If during the preparation of the Descemet window a Descemet's rupture (parallel to the trabecular meshwork) occurs, it is necessary to perform a small iridotomy to prevent an iris adhesion or prolapse into the scleral lake post-op. Usually the canaloplasty or viscocanalostomy can be continued successfully, as it is still possible to enter the ostia of Schlemm's canal.

Material and Companies Address

Nova Eye Medical

107 Rundle Street,
Kent Town, 5067, Australia,
http://www.nova-eye.com.

Part IV
Iris: Iris Surgery

Iris surgery has made a huge leap forward with the advent of a foldable iris prosthesis from Human Optics, Germany, and new iris instruments from Geuder, Germany. The iris prosthesis enables the treatment of aniridia with a 2.5 mm incision, and the new instruments allow a simple surgery for traumatic mydriasis. Asst. Prof. Spandau will demonstrate the surgical techniques step by step and show several videos.

Iris Surgery

7

Ulrich Spandau

Abstract

An iridoplasty has become surgically much easier with the introduction of a foldable iris prosthesis from Human Optics (Germany) and of novel iris instruments and suture from Geuder (Germany).

Keywords

Anterior chamber · Purse string suture · Lens capsule · Iris instrument · Main incision

Iris surgery has made a huge leap forward with the advent of a foldable iris prosthesis from Human Optics, Germany, and new iris instruments from Geuder, Germany. The iris prosthesis enables the treatment of aniridia with a 2.5 mm incision and the new instruments allow a simple surgery for traumatic mydriasis. Asst. Prof. Spandau will demonstrate the surgical techniques step by step and show several videos.

Supplementary Information The online version contains supplementary material available at https://doi.org/10.1007/978-3-031-84204-7_7.

U. Spandau (✉)
Stockholm University Hospital, Stockholm, Sweden
e-mail: ulrich_spandau@yahoo.de

An iridoplasty has become surgically much easier with the introduction of a foldable iris prosthesis from Human Optics (Germany) and of novel iris instruments and suture from Geuder (Germany).

There are two surgical options for iris surgery. The first one is an iris prosthesis (Figs. 7.1 and 7.2) and the second is an iris suture (Fig. 7.3). An iris suture is more preferable than an iris prosthesis because it causes less anterior chamber irritation. The iridoplasty with an iris suture has been made possible for VR surgeons through the advent of novel iris instruments (Fig. 7.3, Geuder, Germany) and a suture with a short needle (Onatec, Germany) (Fig. 7.4). A traumatic mydriasis can be operated easily and a video for this technique is presented.

<u>There are several important features which determine the surgical planning</u>:

- (Partial) iris defect (Figs. 7.5 and 7.6)?
- Old traumatic mydriasis (Figs. 7.7 and 7.8)?
- Aniridia and aphakia (Figs. 7.9, 7.10 and 7.11)?
- Recent traumatic mydriasis (Figs. 7.12 and 7.13)?

Eyes with aniridia and aphakia secondary to trauma can be provided with an iris prosthesis and with/without an IOL prosthesis. The company Human Optics (Germany) produces a

U. Spandau and G. B. Scharioth (eds.), *Cutting Edge of Ophthalmic Surgery*,
https://doi.org/10.1007/978-3-031-84204-7_7

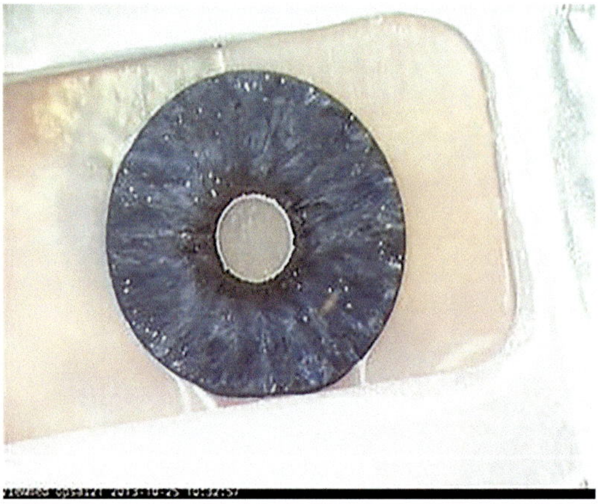

Fig. 7.1 A foldable and hand painted iris prosthesis from Human Optics (Germany). The material is Goretex. The body is 12 mm in diameter

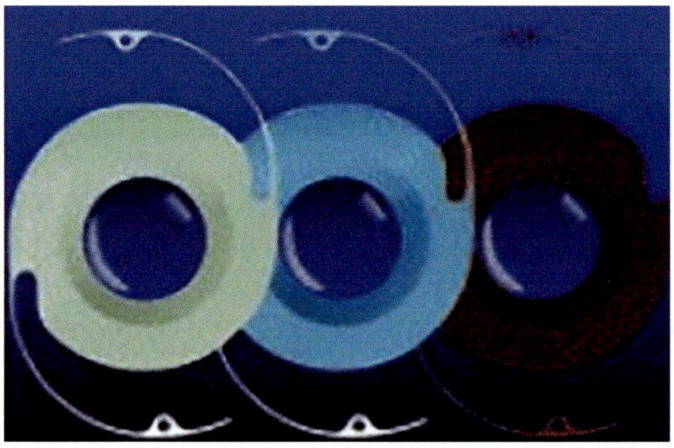

Fig. 7.2 A non foldable and not hand painted iris + IOL prosthesis from Ophtec (Netherlands). The material is PMMA. The body is 12 mm in diameter

foldable iris prosthesis, which is hand painted (Fig. 7.1). It has a diameter of 12 mm and needs to be customized to the eye with a trephine (Opthec).

<u>Prosthesis size for Human optic iris prosthesis:</u>

- Sulcus implantation: 10.0 mm
- In the bag implantation: 9.0 mm

The companies Morcher (Germany) and Ophtec (The Netherlands) offer a combined iris and IOL prosthesis made from PMMA and are therefore not foldable (Fig. 7.11). Whereas Morcher produces a hand painted iris prosthesis offers Ophtec a range of four colours. The Morcher and Ophtec iris—IOL prosthesis require a 10.0 mm broad main incision.

The foldable iris prosthesis from Human Optics can be implanted with an IOL injector into the sulcus (Figs. 7.14, 7.15, 7.16, 7.17, 7.18, 7.19, and 7.20). For eyes with aniridia and aphakia the iris prosthesis from Human Optics can be combined with a 3-piece IOL: The iris prosthesis is fixated into the haptics of a 3-piece IOL (MA60AC, Alcon). I call this a combo iris and IOL prosthesis. It is implanted through a 2.4 mm main incision with an IOL injector (Alcon).

<u>Our surgical management is as follows:</u>

In case of an aniridia and an old traumatic mydriasis we prefer the foldable iris prosthesis (Human Optics®). You can check if a traumatic mydriasis is feasible for surgery by pulling on the old iris with an intravitreal forceps. If it bleeds and cannot be constricted then a prosthesis is the only option.

In case of a fresh traumatic mydriasis, I recommend an iridoplasty with iris instruments from Geuder (Germany) and a special suture from Onatec®, Germany (Figs. 7.3 and 7.4). If an aphakia is also present I would perform an iridoplasty and implant at the same time a retropupillar iris claw-IOL (Figs. 7.21, 7.22, 7.23, and 7.24).

In case of an aniridia with aphakia, I prefer a combined iris and IOL prosthesis (Figs. 7.14, 7.15, 7.16, 7.17, 7.18, 7.19, and 7.20). The foldable iris prosthesis is implanted together with a 3-piece IOL (Alcon, AMO). In case of aniridia with a phakic lens, I would implant the foldable iris with the IOL inside the bag.

<u>Implantation site:</u>

The Ophtec iris-IOL can be scleral fixated with a 9-0 polypropylene suture.

The artificial iris (Human Optics) can be implanted into the lens capsule or in the sulcus. The combo IOL-iris prosthesis can be implanted in the bag and be scleral fixated with 10-0 polypropylene suture. An alternative is a Scharioth intrascleral fixation with the 3-piece IOL.

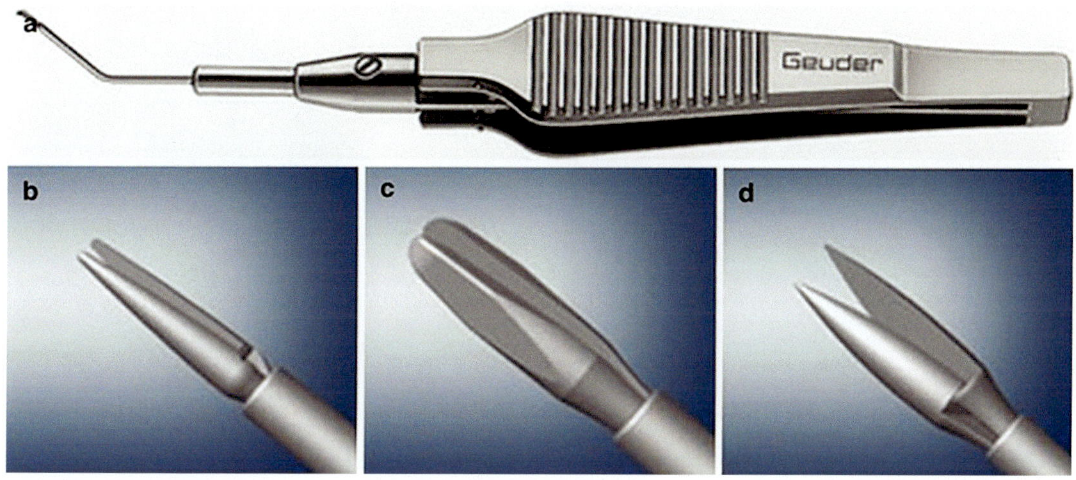

Fig. 7.3 (**a–d**) Hattenbach iris instruments from Geuder (Germany) (**a**). It includes a needle holder (**b**), an iris holder (**c**) and scissors (**d**). The instruments are very easy to use

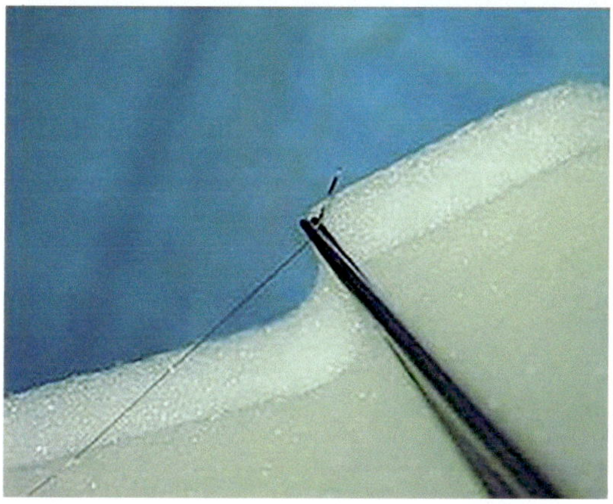

Fig. 7.4 A special suture with short needle for iris sutures (Onatec, Geuder, Germany)

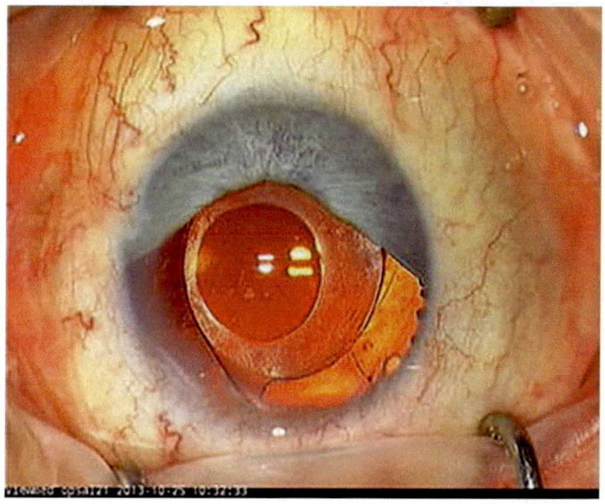

Fig. 7.5 A sector iris defect after complicated phacoemulsification

Complications of the above mentioned surgical methods:

- Iridoplasty for traumatic mydriasis: No complications.
- Iridoplasty for sector defects: May cause an anterior chamber inflammation. A perioperative subconjunctival triamcinolone injection is recommended.
- The foldable iris prosthesis in the sulcus position may cause a low grade chronic inflammation and discomfort if the diameter is too large. A diameter of 10 mm and a trephine (Opthec) is recommended.

Implantation of a Foldable Iris Prosthesis (Human Optics®)

Video 7.1: Foldable iris and IOL prosthesis (very short version).

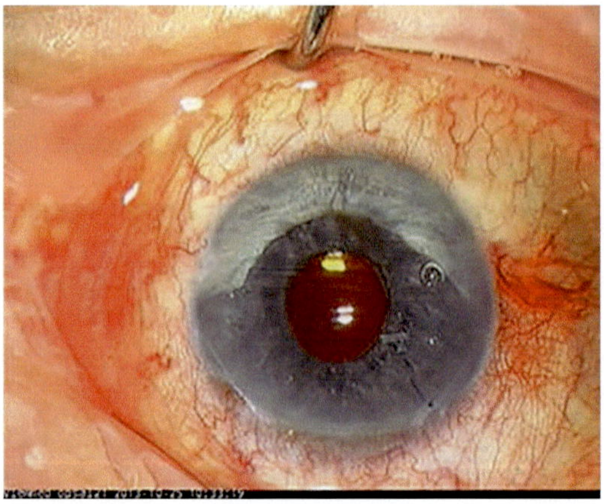

Fig. 7.6 After implantation of a hand painted Human Optics iris prosthesis into the sulcus

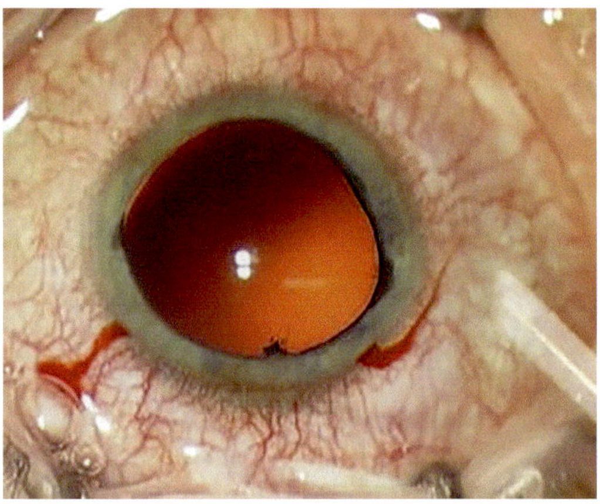

Fig. 7.7 An eye with an old traumatic mydriasis and natural lens

Video 7.2: Combo IOL-iris prosthesis (long version).

Video 7.3: Combo IOL iris prosthesis in lens capsule (short version).

Instruments

- 10 mm corneal trephine (Opthec)
- 23G or 25G endgripping forceps
- IOL injector

Material

- Iris prosthesis (Human Optics)
- MA60AC IOL (Alcon)

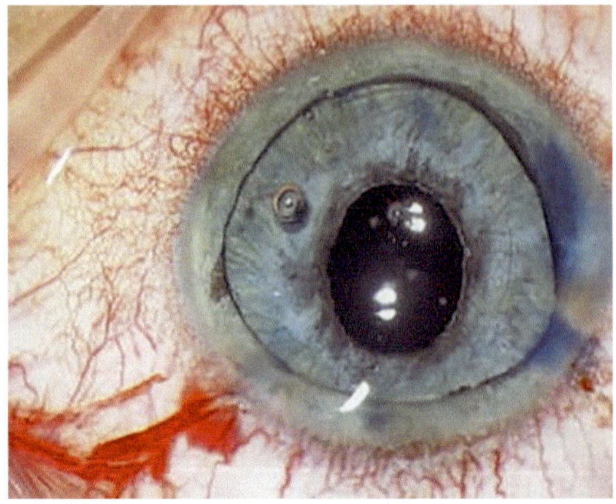

Fig. 7.8 After implantation of a hand painted Human Optics iris prosthesis together with a 3-piece IOL into the lens capsule

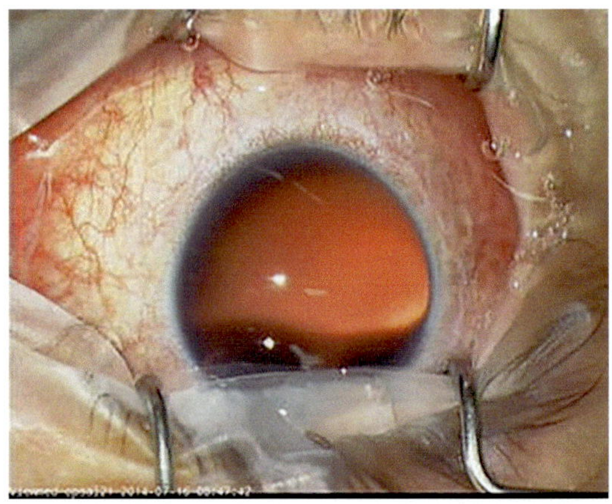

Fig. 7.9 An aniridia and aphakia after a blunt perforation with an i-pad

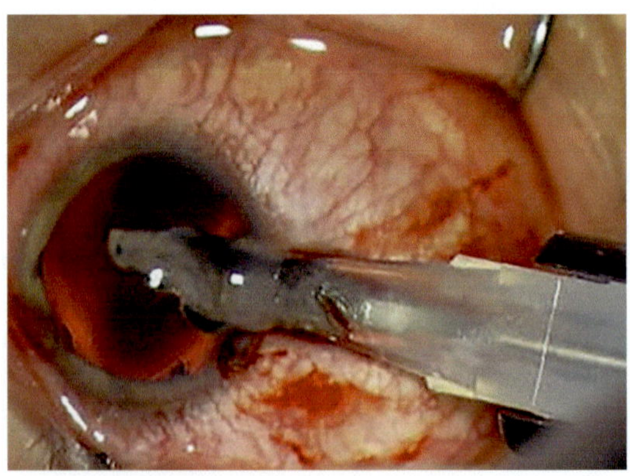

Fig. 7.10 Scleral fixation of a combined Human Optics iris prosthesis + 3-piece IOL

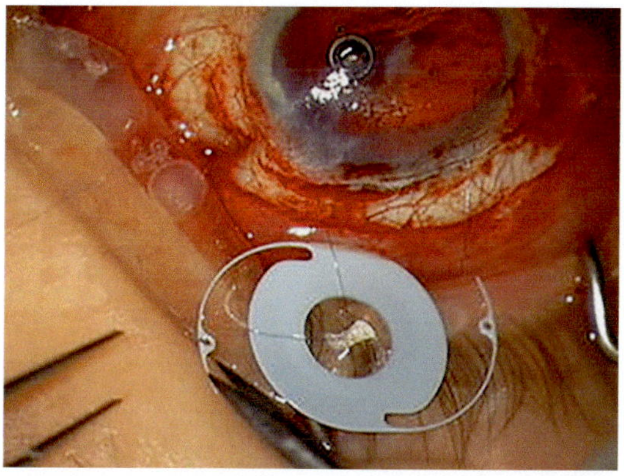

Fig. 7.11 Scleral fixation of a hard Opthec iris-IOL prosthesis (12 mm diameter)

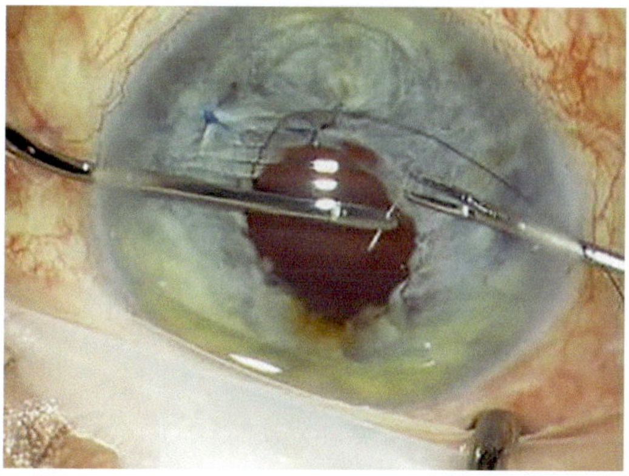

Fig. 7.12 Intraoperative view on an eye with a recent traumatic mydriasis and aphakia after blunt trauma. The Hattenbach iris instruments in action

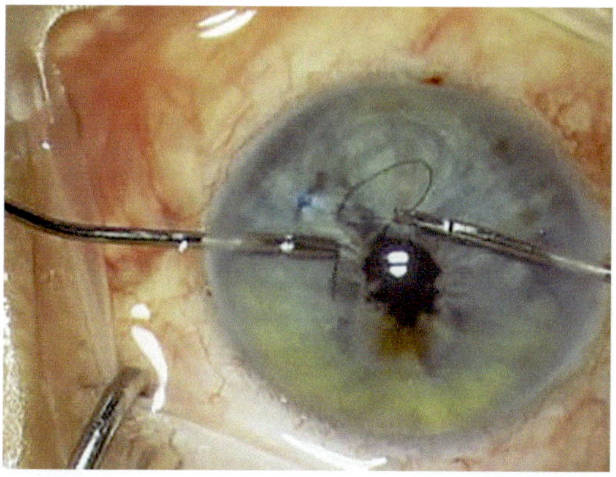

Fig. 7.13 After performing a purse string suture a retropupillar iris-claw IOL is implanted. Postoperative VA = 1.0

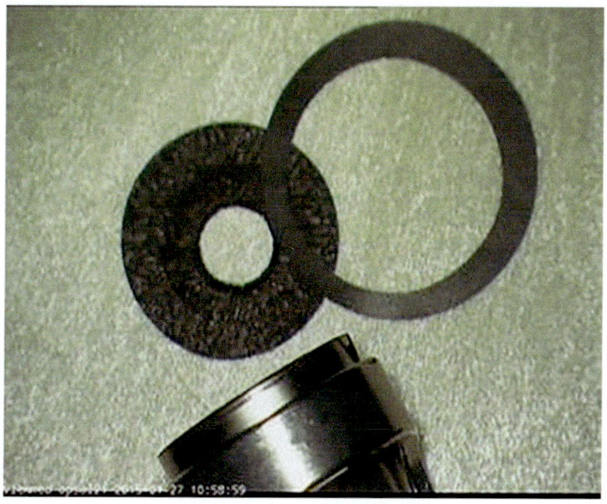

Fig. 7.14 Cutting the Human Optics iris prosthesis (12 mm body) with a 10 mm trephine for sulcus implantation

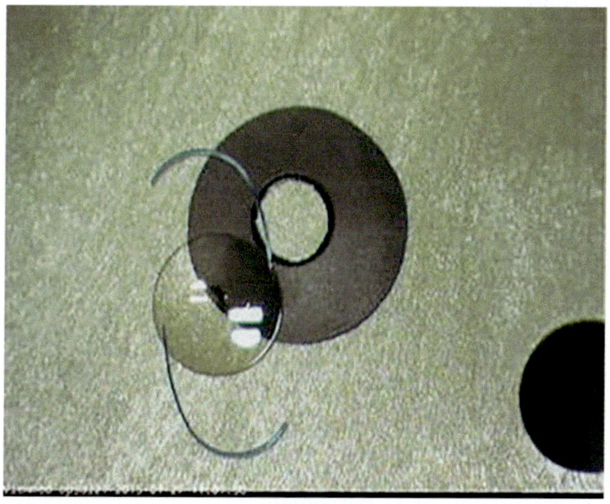

Fig. 7.15 A 3-piece IOL (Alcon, AMO) will be combined with the foldable prosthesis

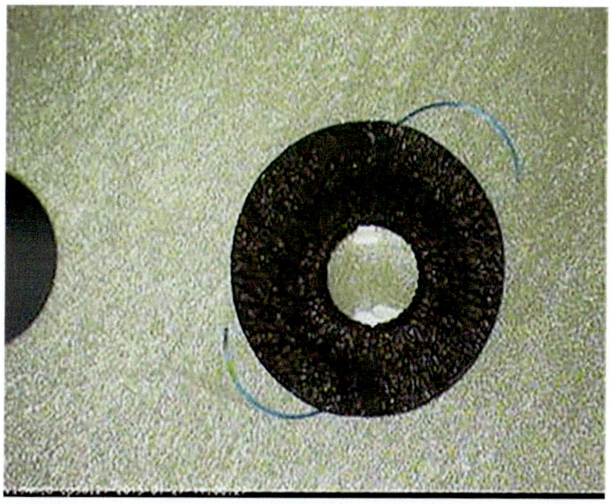

Fig. 7.16 The haptics of the 3-piece IOL were inserted into the iris prosthesis

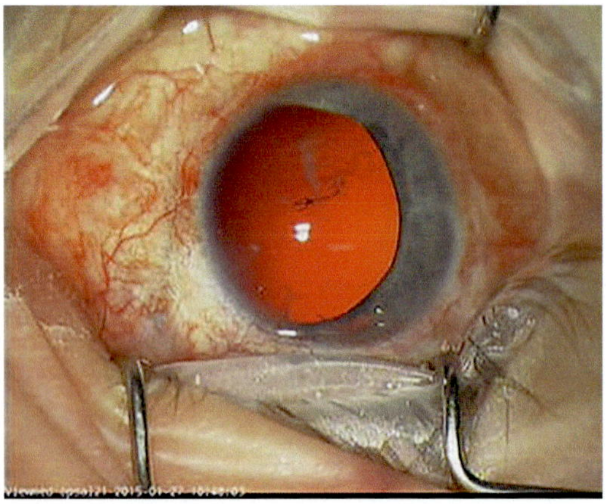

Fig. 7.17 The preoperative status after an explosive trauma. A healed corneal perforation, partial aniridia and aphakia

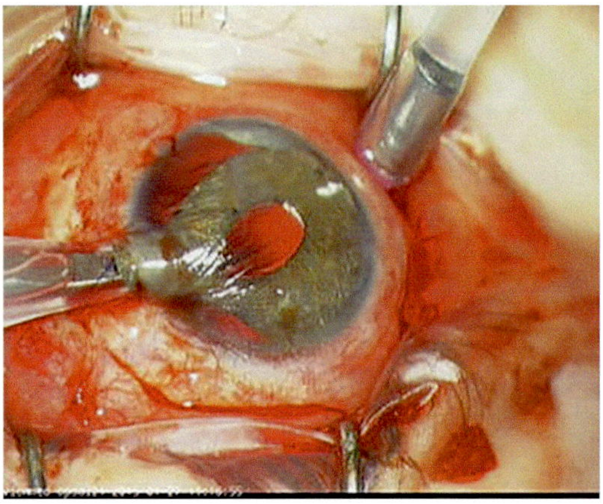

Fig. 7.18 Implantation of the combined iris prosthesis with 3-piece IOL with a regular IOL injector

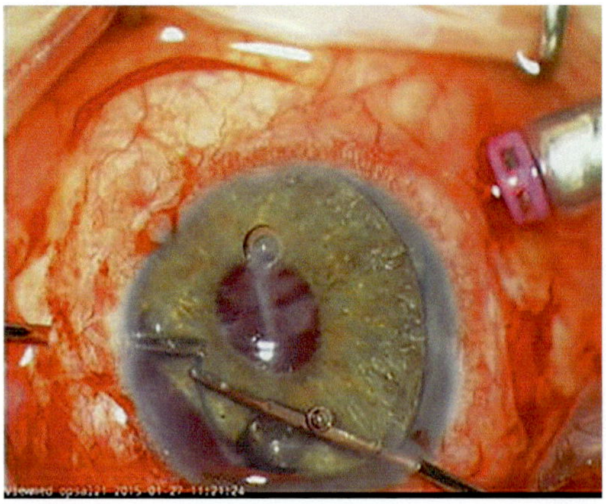

Fig. 7.19 Scleral fixation of the IOL

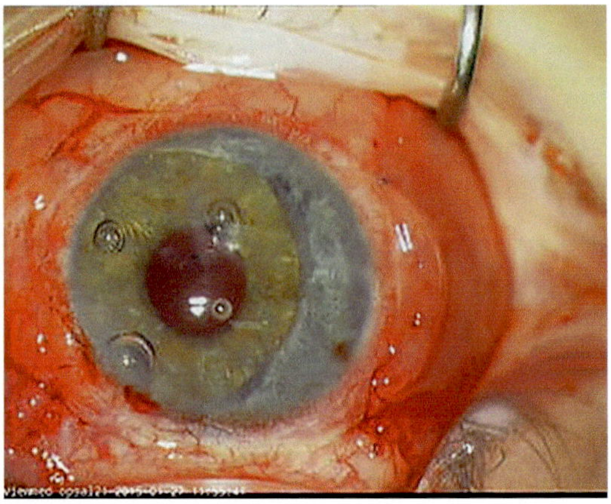

Fig. 7.20 Immediate postoperative status. The 3-month postoperative VA = 0.4

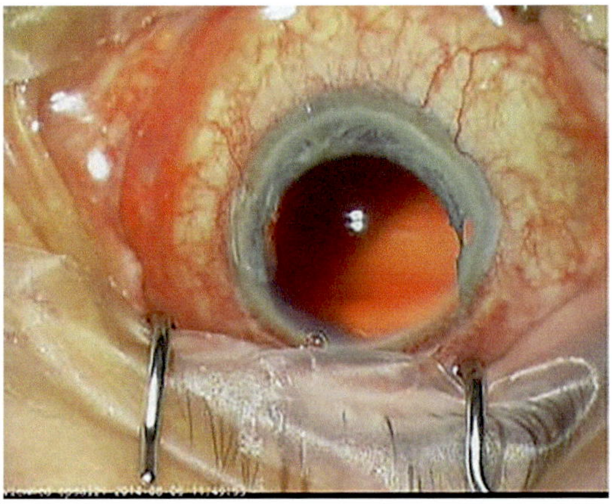

Fig. 7.21 A recent traumatic mydriasis and aphakia after a blunt trauma with a plastic ball

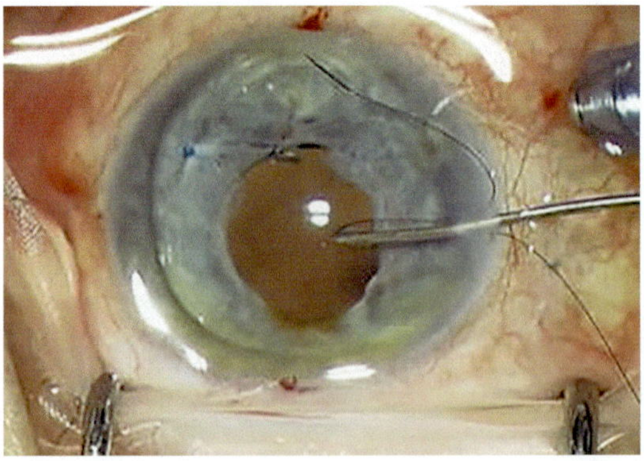

Fig. 7.22 Insert the suture into the anterior chamber with a Sinskey hook

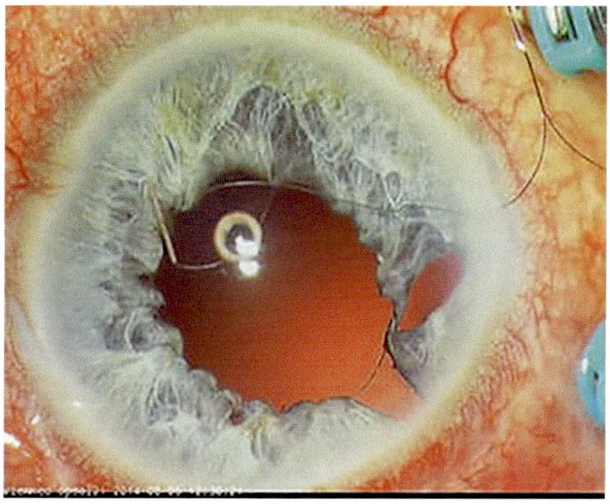

Fig. 7.23 Purse string suture with Hattenbach iris instruments

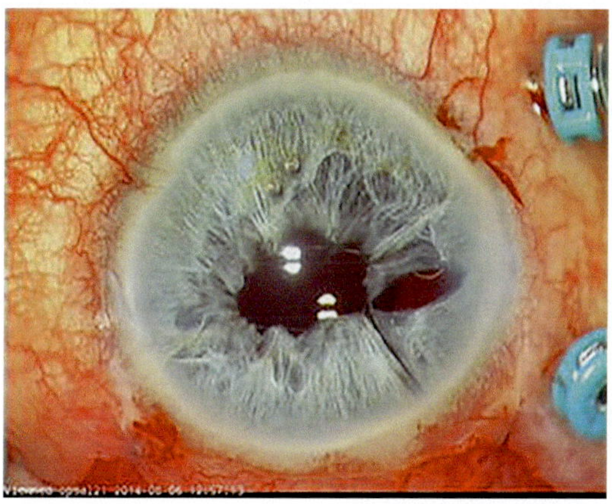

Fig. 7.24 After implantation of an Artisan IOL and closing the knot of the purse string suture. The 1-week postoperative VA = 0.9

<u>**Individual steps**</u>

- **Preparation of an iris-IOL prosthesis**
- **Insertion of iris-IOL prosthesis into a cartridge**
- **Implantation of iris-IOL prosthesis**
- **Fixation of iris prosthesis**

The surgery step-by-step: Figs. 7.14, 7.15, 7.16, 7.17, 7.18, 7.19, and 7.20

- **Preparation of an iris-IOL prosthesis**

The size of the iris prosthesis depends on an implantation in the sulcus or in the capsular bag. In case of a capsular bag implantation we use a 9.0 mm corneal trephine. In case of a sulcus implantation we use a 10.0 mm corneal trephine (Fig. 7.14). Place the 3-piece IOL on the backside of the foldable iris and place two incisions at each haptic with a 15 deg. knife (Alcon). Tunnel the 25G endgripping forceps through the two incisions, grab an end of a haptic and pull the haptic through the incisions (Figs. 7.15 and 7.16). Repeat the manoeuvre with the other haptic.

2. Insertion of iris-IOL prosthesis into a cartridge
3. Implantation of iris-IOL prosthesis

Fold or roll the combo prosthesis and insert it into an IOL cartridge (Alcon) and finally into an injector. Continue with a 2.4 mm main incision and implant then the combo iris-prosthesis into the anterior chamber (Fig. 7.18).

4. Fixation of iris prosthesis

Rotate the combo iris-IOL prosthesis into the lens capsule. If a lens capsule is not present a scleral fixation has to be performed: (1) Intrascleral Scharioth method or (2) scleral fixation with sutures (Figs. 7.19 and 7.20). For details read the book "Complications during and after cataract surgery" from Ulrich Spandau and Gabor Scharioth.

Iridoplasty and Iris-Claw IOL Implantation

Video 7.4: Iridoplasty for traumatic mydriasis.
Video 7.5: Iridoplasty for traumatic mydriasis + iris claw IOL.

<u>**Instruments**</u>

- Iris instruments (Geuder)
- 23G or 25G intravitreal scissors

Material

- Onalene suture (Geuder)

Individual steps

1. **Anterior chamber maintainer or pars plana infusion**
2. **Four paracentesis at 12, 3, 6 and 9 o'clock**
3. **Insert the Onalene suture into the anterior chamber with a Sinskey hook**
4. **Perform a 360° suture around the pupillary margin (purse string suture)**
5. **Retropupillary implantation of the iris-claw IOL**
6. **Tying of the Onalene suture**

The surgery step-by-step: Figs. 7.21, 7.22, 7.23 and 7.24.

1. Anterior chamber maintainer or pars plana infusion

Eyes with aphakia tend to be hypotony under surgery because the lens-iris diaphragma is impaired. In order to avoid intraoperative hypotony I recommend the use of an anterior chamber maintainer or even better a pars plana infusion. The anterior chamber maintainer may disturb the suturing within the anterior chamber.

2. Four paracentesis at 12, 3, 6 and 9 o'clock
3. Insert the Onalene suture into the anterior chamber

Perform a paracentesis at 12, 3, 6 and 9 o'clock. Then push the suture with a Sinskey hook (push–pull instrument) into the anterior chamber (Fig. 7.22).

4. Perform a 360° suture around the pupillary margin (purse string suture)

Place the needle behind the iris, pierce the tissue at the pupillary margin, grasp the needle with the second forceps and pull the needle completely through. Continue 360°. Before tying the suture we must implant the IOL (Fig. 7.23). Alternatively you could tie the suture now and implant the iris-claw IOL antepupillary.

5. Retropupillary implantation of the iris-claw IOL
6. Tying of the Onalene suture

Perform a 6 mm broad incision at the limbus or at the sclera. Place the IOL on the iris and rotate the claws at the 3 and 9 o'clock position. Hold the IOL in an upside-down position with the IOL forceps (AMO), place the IOL behind the iris. Now the assistant must pull on both ends of the purse string suture so that the pupil is constricted. Using an iris spatula from Sekundo (Geuder) enclavate the iris tissue within the iris claws. Tie finally the purse string suture (Fig. 7.24).

Material and Companies Address

Opthec BV

- Schweitzerlaan 15
- 9728 NR Groningen
- Netherlands
- Phone: +31 050 5,251,944
- www.opthec.com

Human Optics

- Dr. Schmidt Intraocularlinsen GmbH
- Westerwaldstraße 11–13
- 53,757 Sankt Augustin
- Germany
- e-mail: iris@humanoptics.com
- http://www.artificial-iris.com

Geuder

- Hertzstr. 4
- 69,126 Heidelberg
- Germany
- Tel: 06,221/3066
- Fax: 06,221/303122
- info@geuder.de
- www.geuder.de

Part V
Cataract: Femto-Cataract, Laser Phaco, Congenital Cataract

The most exciting development in cataract surgery is surely the advent of the laser. Prof. Nagy from Budapest, Hungary, is the developer of the femto cataract. He will present his technique step-by-step and show the pros and cons of this exciting new surgery. Dr. Sauder from Stuttgart, Germany, will demonstrate a novel phaco handpiece which removes the nucleus with laser instead of ultrasound. And finally will Dr. Nyström from Gothenburg, Sweden, demonstrate congenital cataract surgery with implantation of a Tassignon IOL.

Femtosecond Laser Assisted Cataract Surgery: Principles and Results

8

Zoltan Z. Nagy

Abstract

Ophthalmology always had a pioneer role in use of lasers (Light Amplification by Stimulated Emission of Radiation). A great variety of lasers have been employed since the first laser appeared within the ophthalmic armamentarium for more than 50 years. The German ophthalmologist Meyer-Schwickerath applied the first laser for photocoagulation in the retina in 1949 (Meyer-Schwickerath in Ber Dtsch Ophthalmol Ges. 55:256–9, 1949). A laser is a special surgical device which emits specific electromagnetic light via stimulated emission. Ophthalmic lasers operate at one specific fixed wavelength, pulse pattern, energy, duration, repetition rate, spot size and causing most of the time thermal effects, but photocoagulation, evaporation and non-thermal effects also important, regarding laser-tissue interaction.

Keywords

Optical coherence tomography · Femtosecond laser · Cataract surgery · Crystalline lens · Corneal incision

Ophthalmology always had a pioneer role in use of lasers (Light Amplification by Stimulated Emission of Radiation). A great variety of lasers have been employed since the first laser appeared within the ophthalmic armamentarium for more than 50 years. The German ophthalmologist Meyer-Schwickerath applied the first laser for photocoagulation in the retina in 1949 [1]. A laser is a special surgical device which emits specific electromagnetic light via stimulated emission. Ophthalmic lasers operate at one specific fixed wavelength, pulse pattern, energy, duration, repetition rate, spot size and causing most of the time thermal effects, but photocoagulation, evaporation and non-thermal effects also important, regarding laser-tissue interaction.

Femtosecond lasers (Fig. 8.1) first applied in refractive surgery to replace mechanical and blade-operated microkeratomes to create

The most exciting development in cataract surgery is surely the advent of the laser. Prof. Nagy from Budapest, Hungary, is a developer of femtosecond cataract surgery. He will present his technique step by step and show the pros and cons of this exciting new surgery.

Supplementary Information The online version contains supplementary material available at https://doi.org/10.1007/978-3-031-84204-7_8.

Z. Z. Nagy (✉)
Director of Department of Ophthalmology, Semmelweis University, Budapest, Hungary
e-mail: zoltan.nagy100@gmail.com

U. Spandau and G. B. Scharioth (eds.), *Cutting Edge of Ophthalmic Surgery*,
https://doi.org/10.1007/978-3-031-84204-7_8

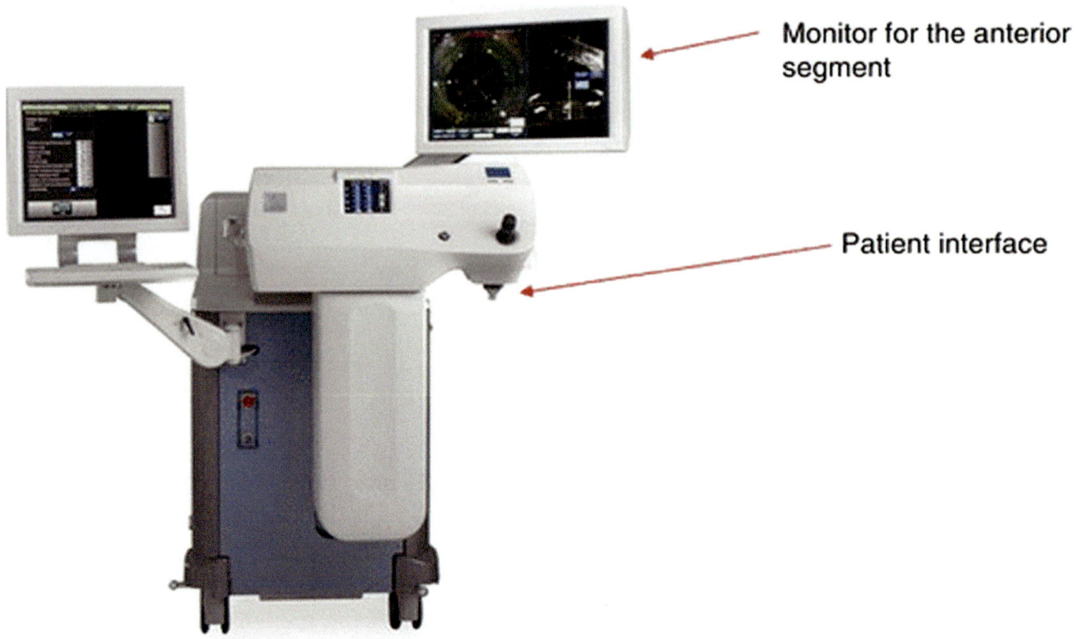

Fig. 8.1 The Alcon-LenSx femtolaser. The left monitor is for to set the treatment parameters, the right LCD monitor helps the surgeon throughout the femtolaser treatment, underneath the patient interface (PI) which comes into contact with the treated eye

corneal flaps during laser in situ keratomileusis (LASIK) [2]. Thereafter the indication has changed and widened to all types of lamellar and penetrating keratoplasties, ring-segment implantation in keratoconus and presbyopia inlay pocket creation [3, 4].

The femtosecond laser beam is sharply focused and generates plasma within the affected corneal tissue. This plasma rapidly expands causing an acoustic shock wave and by this way displacing the surrounding tissue, cavitation bubbles and a cut plane are formed. At tissue level, photodisruption occurs exactly at the laser's focal point without any thermal effect or collateral tissue damage. Due to the photodisruptive effect, the femtolasers are capable of creating very precise cuts within the cornea, lens capsule and crystalline lens (Fig. 8.2) by the principle of tissue separation [5].

The repetition rate of femtosecond lasers has doubled recently from 30 to 60 kHz and recently a 160 kHz femtosecond laser has also became available, which is able to create a corneal flap within 10–12 s. The higher the repetition rate, the less energy is needed to achieve the same tissue effect. Femtosecond lasers used in laser assisted cataract surgery perform with a pulse duration of 400–800 femtosecond (fs) and the energy range is in micro Joules ($10–^{6}$ J). During the surgery of the crystalline lens of the eye, the femtosecond laser energy is usually increased to 8–15 μJ.

The femtosecond laser generated plasma rapidly expands causing an acoustic shock wave which displacing the surrounding tissue. When the plasma cools, cavitation bubbles are being formed [2, 3, 5]. At tissue level, photodisruption occurs without any thermal effect of the collateral tissue.

Cataract surgery at the moment is the most commonly performed ocular implantation procedure not only within ophthalmology, but within medicine worldwide [6]. It is estimated that approximately 32 million cataract operations will be performed globally by 2020 with a gradual increase year by year, due to aging population, demographic changes, and the change in indications for surgery [9]. Cataract

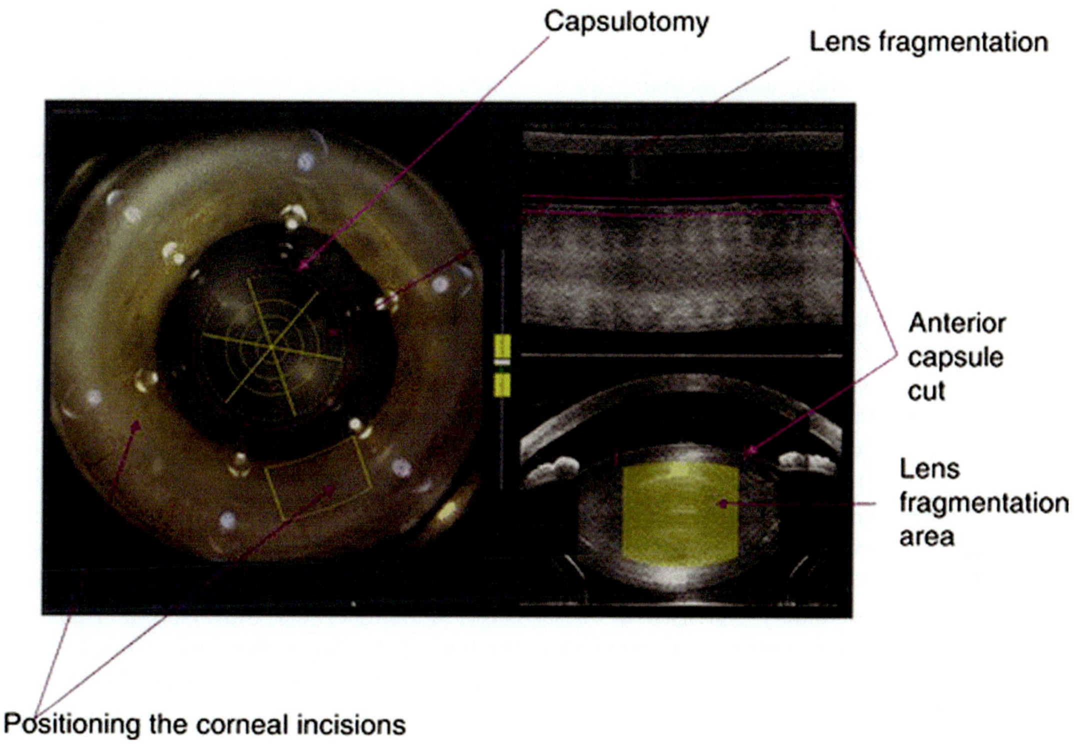

Fig. 8.2 Screen of the Alcon-LenSx femtolaser

surgery and refractive surgery are being merged, so cataract surgery is not only a purely vision restoration entity, regarding the clarity of the optic media, but became a refractive procedure as well. Ophthalmic surgeons now also change the refractive power of the eye, compensate for astigmatism, spherical and other higher order aberrations of the eye. Further, the restoration of near vision has also become possible with the use of premium artificial lenses, such as multifocal or accommodating intraocular lenses [7, 8].

Patient expectation has also risen, doctors need to take longer chair time with patients explaining the benefits and drawbacks of different surgical approaches and using different intraocular lenses. [10]. To avoid refractive surprises possible solutions include better intraocular lens calculation using more precise formulas and performing a better and more thorough preoperative assessment, especially when the patient had refractive surgery before [11]. Now more consistent surgical results came in the focus of ophthalmic community which is no longer depending on the dexterity of the surgeon. In this field, femtolasers offer new possibilities and potential for surgeons and patients alike. Regarding the new trends in ophthalmology, compound and coupled diagnostic and surgical tools helping surgeons to achieve the final goal: the postoperative refraction should be within ± 0.5 Dpt to ± 0.25 Dpt as was achieved already in refractive surgery.

The Surgical Technique (Videos 8.1 and 8.2)

Docking Maneuver

The first and one of the most important steps of femtosecond laser assisted cataract surgery is the docking procedure with any types of femtosecond lasers. The Alcon-LenSx femtosecond laser (Fig. 8.1) operates with a curved soft contact lens which is integrated with a sterile limbal suction ring (SoftFit Patient Interface = PI). The tubing uses vacuum with a 16–20 mm Hg suction force to fixate the treated eye. The patient interface should be docked centrally then the rest of the procedure seems easier [12]. In case of decentered docking, incisions might be incomplete, due to paralaxis and geometrically attenuated femtolaser beam. Otherwise it is simple to dock and it provides a large viewing for the surgeon, which allows performing the peripheral corneal incisions and arcuate keratotomy incisions. Due to the low suction force, ocular perfusion and visual perception is usually not disturbed during the femtolaser pretreatment. With the new PI and soft contact lens use, there are no corneal folds, which allows using lower energy and the rate of free floating capsulotomy increased to 98% [12]. Other femtosecond lasers also operate with a special PI, some of them using coupling fluid to avoid corneal folds. All femtosecond lasers at the moment using moderate suction force to stabilize the eye during femtolaser pretreatment.

The femtolaser has an in-built HD (high definition) optical coherence tomography (HD-OCT) system and a live video with a separate screen to assist the surgeon and to provide total control for the surgeon during the docking procedure and surgical pattern determination [12]. The OCT uses the same optical path as the laser beam. Therefore the surgeon knows by micrometer precision where the laser beam will incise within the ophthalmic tissues. The high-definition OCT (HD-OCT) covers the complete anterior segment of the eye up to the posterior capsule with dilated pupil and is also able to assess the clinical density of the crystalline lens. The surgical pattern is offered automatically and performed by the LenSx femtosecond laser. However, the surgeon should check and alter treatment parameters if necessary prior starting the treatment. The femtosecond laser produces approximately a 100 μm acoustic shock wave (very small); therefore a minimum of 500 μm safety distance from the posterior capsule is recommended (Fig. 8.2).

Due to the technical development a new preoperative assessment tool has been created, which is called the Verion system. It allows a complete preoperative assessment and post-operative follow-ups as well. Meanwhile with data transfer it helps the surgeon in the OR to perform the surgery with the greatest exactness. The Verion pre-operative assessment system identifies the conjunctival, scleral vessels and iris characteristics. In the OR all structures are recognized automatically and information is provided where to perform corneal incisions, shows the diameter and localization of the capsulotomy and helps implanting the intraocular lenses in the best available position, which is especially useful during toric lens implantation.

The first human femtolaser assisted cataract surgery was performed in 2008 by Zoltan Z. Nagy at Semmelweis University in Budapest, Hungary [5]. Since then the United States Food and Drug Administration (FDA) has granted approval and the European Conformité Européene (CE) mark has granted for femtosecond lasers, and femtolasers became available for the public. There are currently four international companies producing and providing this new technology for cataract surgery. The number of peer-reviewed publications is increasing on femtosecond laser assisted cataract surgery and it is foreseen that within a decade the method could be spread generally in the largest ophthalmic centers in the world.

Indications

The main indications of the femtolaser during cataract surgery are:

- Anterior capsulotomy (4.5–7.0 mm) (Fig. 8.3.)
- Laser fragmentation and liquefaction of hard and soft lenses respectively, hybrid pattern: central liquefaction and fragmentation using a cake or cross pattern (six cuts at least)
- Single plane or multiplane corneal incisions with any geometry

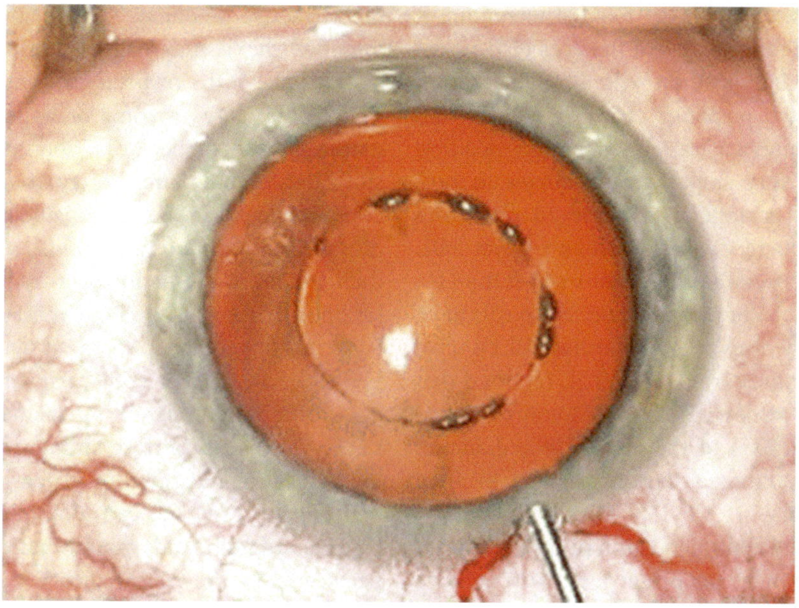

Fig. 8.3 Femto-capsulotomy sharp edge incision performed by the femtosecond laser before phacoemulsification

- Arcuate corneal incisions to control pre-operative corneal astigmatism

Contraindications

- Small, non-dilating pupil (the only and relative contraindication)

The small, non-dilating pupil less than 6 mm in diameter is recognized as a relative contraindication to femtolaser cataract surgery (lens fragmentation). If the laser beam hits the iris it may cause more miosis and freeing inflammatory mediators within the iris. It is possible to perform an anterior capsulotomy with a 5.0 mm pupil, but there is a high risk of iris injury. Malyugin rings or iris hooks offer a good solution in such cases [13, 14].

The order of the three main steps of femtosecond laser assisted cataract surgery is as follows: first the anterior capsulotomy should be created, secondly the lens fragmentation and or liquefaction and thirdly the corneal incisions. The anterior capsulotomy is performed before the lens fragmentation/liquefaction because the lens fragmentation/liquefaction may create a gas bubble, which may elevate the anterior capsule. In that case the laser beam will not cut in the same plane as it was planned during the preoperative OCT assessment. The corneal incisions are performed lastly and they are performed from the inside to outside. Conjunctiva should be avoided. In the latter case the penetration with a special spatula can be quite difficult if not impossible.

Clinical Results

Capsulotomy Studies

During the first study the accuracy of the diameter of the anterior capsulotomies have been evaluated and compared to standard manual capsulotomies targeting also the same diameter of 5 mm and found that using the manual technique the diameter was 5.88 ($\pm$0.73) but it was 5.02 ($\pm$0.04) mm using the Alcon LenSx femtosecond laser. During the surgery of human crystalline lenses, the Alcon LenSx FSL was able to perform all capsulotomies within $\pm$0.25 mm accuracy, whereas with the manual technique it was only achieved in 10% of the eyes [15].

The in-the bag position with an 0.25–0.5 mm coverage of the posterior chamber lens by the anterior capsule, so the effective lens position (ELPo) is a very important parameter in predictability of postoperative achieved refraction against the planned one. Therefore exact IOL calculation especially with multifocal IOLs [10, 21] and the accuracy of the size and position of rhexis is very important regarding ELPo [14, 15] A recent study by Packer et al. reported that planning and achieving the capsulotomy centred on the optical axis of the lens with a diameter of 5.25 mm optimizes the consistency of final ELPo-s [20].

The size and central location of capsulorhexis is one of the most important factors to achieve the targeted accurate final post-operative refraction (Figs. 8.3 and 8.4). In the literature there not too much about the accuracy of the standard manual technique because for more than two decades it has been the only method available, little attention has been paid to the effect of capsulotomy diameter and localization on the refractive outcome. A larger or smaller than intended rhexis may cause anterior or posterior shift of the IOL, respectively or IOL tilt [15–17]. In that cases myopic or hyperopic shift or increase in the higher order aberrations and possibly in the final ocular astigmatism may be the consequences. Irregular capsulotomies cannot provide enough defence against remaining epithelial cells so the incidence of posterior capsular opacification also may increase.

In a study of our team, it was found that Femto Second Laser (FSL) capsulotomies were not stronger compared to manual capsulotomies, but due to perfect circularity and central location, the predictability of tearing was much better than in manual capsulotomies [18, 19]. A capsule strength study found that capsulotomies performed by the OptiMedica FSL required two to three times more force to tear compared with the manual capsulotomies [17, 20].

So the real strength of FSL created capsulotomies is still debated in the literature and it is depending what method was used for force testing, but it is questionable that a less regular edge capsulotomy tested by the electron microscopy

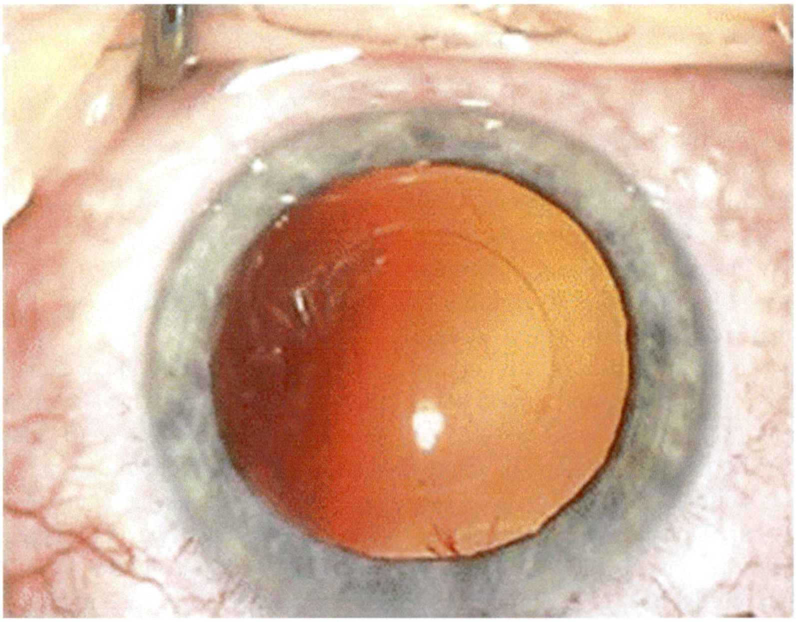

Fig. 8.4 Femto-capsulotomy after removal of the crystalline lens and before implantation of the posterior chamber lens

would be 3 times stronger than manual ones. Femtosecond laser creates small circular shape irregularities ("saw teeth shape") within the capsule, the lower the energy, the more regular is the edge of the capsulotomies and the stronger the capsule against tearing forces [18].

Circularity of the Anterior Capsulotomy and PCL Centration

Authors performed two studies at Semmelweis University in Budapest in an assessed the accuracy of the circularity of the femtosecond laser created rhexis with the Alcon LenSx and the effect on IOL centration postoperatively. They found that the LenSx performed anterior capsulotomy was more regular and circular shaped and provided better centration and capsule/IOL overlap compared with the manual capsulorhexis. Vertical and horizontal IOL decentration following the standard manually created rhexis was found to be statistically higher than the LenSx [15] even if capsulorhexis was performed by the same experienced surgeon.

In another anterior comparative study, anterior capsulotomy was created by the Alcon LenSx femtosecond laser (Figs. 8.3 and 8.4). The circularity was statistically significantly better in the FSL group ($p=0.032$) and there was significantly less incomplete overlap of capsulotomies with the manual rhexis (28% of eyes versus 11%; $p=0.033$). In highly myopic eyes the capsulotomy tended to be larger in the manual group than in normal eyes. The possible cause is the larger size of myopic eyes, the larger dilated pupil, which may deceive the surgeon assessing the relation to anatomy [16]. The letter one is very important in ELPo and predictability, so in high myopic eyes the size and centration of capsulotomies have a higher importance than in eyes with normal axial length and less or no preoperative refractive error.

Lens Fragmentation and Phacoemulsification Energy Studies

The various femtosecond laser platforms offer different types of lens fragmentation. With soft lenses, LOCS grading less than 2.0, a central 0.25 mm central liquefaction is typically used. This technique is especially important in clear lens extraction, in patients with high myopia or high hyperopia or in presbyopic subjects who are seeking a refractive solution for the refractive error and not for cataract. During lens liquefaction concentric rings (cylindrical pattern) are created within the nucleus of the crystalline lens, rings elevate from the bottom toward the anterior part of the crystalline lens. With LOCS grading greater than 2.0, lens fragmentation is typically recommended and used. This can be a cross pattern (two perpendicular incisions within the lens), or can be customized with an increased number of cuts. Typically six cuts are performed and called "cake" or "pizza" pattern by the surgeons on the LenSx platform. The surgeon might decide to choose a hybrid pattern which means a central 3.0 mm diameter of liquefaction and a six lines fragmentation especially at the peripheral part of the crystalline lens [6]. This allows a quick nuclear removal and a help to fragment the remaining part of the crystalline lens. The final aim is to increase the safety of the method. The fragmentation length area should not be greater than 1–2.0 mm of the capsulorhexis diameter, due to the concave shape of the back of the lens surface. With longer fragmentation lines, the risk of trauma to the posterior capsule might be above acceptable risks.

Cubicle pattern was introduced first by another platform (Catalys), by now it is available in most types of the femtosecond lasers. The author found that using the cubicle pattern, two main planes are still required in order to chop the crystalline lens and to avoid the epinuclear 'bowl' phenomenon that can make the rest of the surgery really difficult to remove due to limited accessibility either to phaco or to irrigation-aspiration hand-pieces [13].

The use of the cross pattern and 'quick chop' surgical technique with the LenSx femtosecond laser compared to standard phacoemulsification resulted in a 43% reduction in cumulative dissipative energy (CDE) and a 51% reduction in effective phacoemulsification time (EPT) using the Infiniti (Alcon, Forth Worth, Texas, USA) phacoemulsification device already at the early phase of femtosecond laser use [5]. Since a decrease of more than 90% is reported in the literature using FSL technology. Of course this result is depending what type of cataract is being pre-treated by the FSL.

Corneal and Limbal Incisions

Manually created incisions with a blade usually require stromal hydration at the conclusion of cataract surgery due to irregular, sometimes imprecise tunnel structure. If the wound is smaller than required a tear during phacoemulsification or lens implantation might be the consequence, therefore wound hydration is a must. If wound leaks during the postoperative period a lower intraocular pressure might cause the manual wound to open with free entering of bacteria from the conjunctival sac, leading possibly to endophthalmitis [22]. Precise wound position, geometry and architecture are very important in controlling postoperative infection and also to minimize surgically induced astigmatism (SIA) [22, 23]. FSL offers a new horizon due to precise wound geometry and architecture resulting in a better wound closure and no need for stromal hydration at the end of the surgery [22]. The consistency of wound structure is of utmost importance also important, especially implanting toric and multifocal IOLs [22]. Femtosecond laser created corneal incisions should be as peripheral as possible. Conjunctiva must be avoided, because if laser incision hits the conjunctiva the wound usually cannot be opened with the special blunt spatula. The reason is different laser absorption in conjunctiva and possible hemorrhage from peripheral conjunctival vessels may cause loss of laser absorption. In order to control preoperative corneal astigmatism corneal incisions can be arcuate or limbal relaxing and case reports with the LenSx and Catalys OptiMedica FSLs indicate successful correction of large amounts of corneal astigmatism [24].

The LenSx uses an image-guided capability enabling the control of corneal thickness, incision length, width, depth shape, and location. The surgeon may determine preoperatively the depth up to 90% of thickness, the length and position of the corneal arcuate incisions. After planning the procedure is completely computer-controlled, precise and predictable. It is possible to open the incision immediately following the FSL pre-treatment or the surgeon can wait until the next post-operative day. With topography control, opening of the incisions might be customized at the slit lamp. This allows a better control of decreasing preoperative corneal astigmatism, according to the real need, which in turn increases predictability [22].

Refractive Outcomes, Fine Vision Tuning

A study from Semmelweis University, Budapest, compared internal aberrations and quality of vision in eyes treated with the LenSx FSL and standard manual phacoemulsification. The study was performed by the Nidek Optical Path Difference (OPD) scanner (NIDEK Inc., Japan) [8]. It was revealed that the anterior capsulotomy with the LenSx induced significantly less internal aberrations. Other outcome comparisons included: post-operative visual acuity (uncorrected and best corrected spectacle), residual refraction, ocular and internal aberrations, Strehl ratio and the modulation transfer function (MTF). No statistically significant differences were found between the post-operative refraction, and distant visual acuity (uncorrected and corrected), regarding standard manual phacoemulsification and femtosecond laser assisted cataract surgery (FLACS). On the other hand, the femtosecond treated eyes had lower values of intraocular vertical tilt (Z_1^{-1}) and coma aberrations (Z_3-^1), higher Strehl ratios and higher MTF values at all measured cycles per degree ($p<0.05$) [8]. Other studies in the literature have reported no difference in post-operative refractive error between FSL and standard cataract surgery [25, 26].

Szigeti and colleagues found less IOL tilt and decentration with a FSL created anterior capsulorhexis of 5.5 mm compared with 6 mm [7] in case of implanting accommodative type of lenses (Crystalens). In this type of lens, the capsulotomy diameter should be above 5.0 mm in order to allow anterior and posterior movement of the implanted posterior chamber lenses. Subjective comparative studies on outcomes between FSL cataract surgery and standard manual cataract surgery regarding quality of vision and quality of life [10] are still scarce and welcomed.

Safety Issues

Effects on the Corneal Endothelium

It is estimated that there is 8.5% endothelial loss with standard cataract surgery [27]. Abell and colleagues found no difference in endothelial cell loss between the Catalys OptiMedica FSL and standard cataract surgery 3 weeks post-operatively. Abell performed femtosecond laser assisted cataract surgery in a group of 405 eyes; among them 118 had automated laser corneal incisions and 287 had manual corneal incisions. Interestingly, endothelial cell loss was significantly less in eyes with manually created corneal incisions [28].

Takács and colleagues compared the corneal thickness, corneal volume stress index, and endothelial density following FSL with the LenSx and standard cataract surgery. They reported better outcomes with the LenSx in the early post-operative period in terms of significantly lower corneal thickness compared to the manual group; and the difference disappeared by the second postoperative week and 1 month. Presumed causes for this finding account for the less phacoemulsification time and corneal edema associated with the FSL technique [27]. Therefore FSL assisted cataract surgery might be an option in eyes with reduced endothelial number, e.g.: Fuchs disease, previous ocular surgery, glaucoma, etc.

Effects on the Macula

In the most recent studies macular problems following FSL surgery seem no safety issue. In a study comparing changes in macular thickness following FSL with the LenSx versus standard cataract surgery, there was less gain in macular thickness in the FSL group at 1 week post-operatively and there was no difference after 1 month [29]. Nagy et al. also compared thickness changes in the retinal layers in the macula with optical coherence tomography (OCT) after femtosecond laser-assisted phacoemulsification (study group) and conventional manual phacoemulsification (control group). After cataract surgery, macular edema was detectable mainly in the outer nuclear layer in both groups but was significantly less using the femtosecond laser technology, presumably due to shorter phacoemulsification time and less ultrasound energy. Uveitis patients may therefore also benefit from FSL cataract surgery. Less cystoid macular edema (CME) might be expected due to above mentioned facts [30]. Levitz et al. reported also no difference in macular edema between groups of patients having FSL cataract surgery compared to standard manual phacoemulsification [31].

Complications

Complications are rare with the FSL. The most common issues encountered are:

Pupillary Constriction

Pupillary dilation is an important issue during preoperative care in FSL surgery. The pupil diameter should be at least 6 mm to avoid iris injury. In case of poorly dilated pupil, bleeding and inadvertent miosis may occur. At the early stage authors experienced miosis in 1/3 of the femtosecond laser pretreated eyes, the reason behind was the elevation of prostaglandin (PG) level in the anterior chamber (within the aqueous). By now it is cleared based on lab test and peer-reviewed literature data, that the PG level might elevate de novo during FSL surgery [13, 32]. Preoperatively additional dilating drops and non-steroidal anti-inflammatory drugs (NSAIDS) should be used to prevent disabling miosis [32]. In case of small, non- dilating or adhered pupil, Malyugin ring or iris hooks offer a good solution [13, 14].

Capsular Blockage Syndrome

Roberts and colleagues were the first to report capsular block syndrome, occurring during the first cases of FSL surgery [33]. A capsular block syndrome usually occurs during hydrodissection if the fluid is injected with high volume and speed under the anterior capsule and intranuclear/−lenticular gas bubbles are pressed towards the posterior capsule. The gas bubbles may rupture the posterior capsule followed subsequently by drop of the nucleus into the vitreous cavity. The 'rock and roll' technique described by Nagy reduces the risk of this possible complication [13]. The technique involves slow and titred injection of hydrodissection fluid and careful moving of the nucleus which helps to release intra-lenticular gas bubbles. By this way the intralenticular gas leaves the eye toward the anterior chamber and then through the corneal wound. The rock refers to gentle down and upward force to the lens and the roll refers to the gentle moving around of the crystalline lens. This is the most important safety maneuver during the first part following femtosecond laser assisted pretreatment.

Corneal Incisions

With a thorough preoperative planning and the proper insertion of PI, the surgeon is able to ensure the optimal anatomical situation to perform a central and even free-floating capsulotomy, as peripheral as possible corneal wounds and a proper liquefaction/even fragmentation within the crystalline lens. Precise docking has a paramount importance avoiding lens tilt, centrally localized corneal wounds, creating higher surgically induced astigmatism which was expected and uneven cuts within the crystalline lens [22].

Other complications listed in the literature include anterior capsule tear and clinically significant increases in intraocular pressure (with the Victus platform) [34]. In a very large study by Abell et al. evaluating 4080 eyes, 1852 had FSL assisted cataract surgery with the Catalys Laser System, an incomplete capsulotomy was found to occur in 21 eyes. An anterior capsulotomy tag occurred in 30 eyes compared to one with non-FSL surgery ($P=0.001$). Posterior capsular tear occurred in eight eyes compared to four with non-FSL surgery, which was not statistically significant. Usually most of the complications occurred during the first 100 cases. Certainly there is a learning curve for surgeons. FSL technology is different from standard manual phacoemulsification. Surgeons should respect this fact and should start surgery with a slower technique compared to manual phacoemulsification. Corneal haze occurred in 12 eyes compared to one with non-FSL surgery ($P=0.0009$), the reason behind this is unknown. An unstable pupil was experienced by the surgeons in 30 eyes compared to 14 with non-FSL surgery ($P=0.003$) [26]. The latter is extremely important in eyes with floppy iris syndrome.

More pupil dilation and preoperative non-steroid anti-inflammatory drops one day earlier may help to avoid unwanted pupillary constriction during surgery.

Special Indications

FSL cataract surgery has been successfully used in ocular trauma [35], phacomorphic glaucoma [14], following penetrating keratoplasty [36], keratoconus, Marfan syndrome [37], in a nanophthalmic eye [38], in Alport syndrome [39] and pediatric cataract surgery [40], white intumescent cataract. The indications of FSL assisted cataract surgery still widens and more indications are to be expected in the future [41]. Special focus should be placed on the pediatric cataract. The anterior and posterior capsulotomies are prone to have a larger diameter than planned due to the elastic lens capsule. FSL helps avoiding inadvertently larger capsulotomies in infants and young children. There should be a solution to avoid the need to use double PI-s with unnecessary doubled costs in pediatric cases.

Conclusion

The FSL at present is utilized in four main areas: corneal incisions, anterior capsulotomy, lens fragmentation and arcuate corneal incisions to control preoperative corneal astigmatism. Customized corneal wounds with any geometry, size and location, desired centration of capsulotomy, guaranteed size of capsulotomy diameter, pre-fragmented or liquefied lens nucleus offers increased precision and predictability and higher consistency in postoperative refractive results. FSL technology is still an expensive technology with additional costs compared to standard phacoemulsification. Peer-reviewed studies are still needed, with more realistic pricing and then a quicker spread of this technology is expected.

Material and Companies Adress

Alcon

- Alcon Laboratories (UK) Ltd.
- Pentagon Park
- Boundary Way
- Hemel Hempstead
- Herts HP2 7UD, England
- Phone: 44+1442.341.234
- www.alcon.com
- https://www.myalcon.com/products/surgical/lensx-laser/index.shtml

References

1. G Meyer-Schwickerath 1949 Koagulation der Netzhaut mit Sonnenlicht Ber Dtsch Ophthalmol Ges. 55 256 9
2. RM Kurtz C Horvath HH Liu RR Krueger T Juhasz 1998 Lamellar refractive surgery with scanned intrastromal picosecond and femtosecond laser pulses in animal eyes J Refract Surg 14 541 8
3. P Kim GL Sutton DS Rootman 2011 Applications of the femtosecond laser in corneal refractive surgery Curr Opin Ophthalmol 22 238 44
4. J Marshall 1988 Lasers in ophthalmology: the basic principles Eye 2 Suppl S98 112
5. Z Nagy A Takacs T Filkorn M Sarayba 2009 Initial clinical evaluation of an intraocular femtosecond laser in cataract surgery J Refract Surg 25 1053 60
6. ZZ Nagy 2014 New technology update: femtosecond laser in cataract surgery Clin Ophthalmol 8 1157 67
7. Szigeti A, Kranitz K, Takacs AI, Mihaltz K, Knorz MC, Nagy ZZ. Comparison of long-term visual outcome and IOL position with a single-optic accommodating IOL After 5.5- or 6.0-mm Femtosecond laser capsulotomy. J Refract Surg. 2012;28:609–13
8. K Mihaltz MC Knorz JL Alio AI Takacs K Kranitz I Kovacs ZZ Nagy 2011 Internal aberrations and optical quality after femtosecond laser anterior capsulotomy in cataract surgery J Refract Surg 27 711 6
9. C McAlinden M Jonsson M Kugelberg M Lundstrom J Khadka K Pesudovs 2012 Establishing levels of indications for cataract surgery: combining clinical and questionnaire data into a measure of cataract impact Invest Ophthalmol Vis Sci 53 1095 101
10. C McAlinden K Pesudovs JE Moore 2010 The development of an instrument to measure quality of vision: the Quality of Vision (QoV) questionnaire Invest Ophthalmol Vis Sci 51 5537 45

11. C Hodge C McAlinden M Lawless C Chan G Sutton A Martin 2015 Intraocular lens power calculation following laser refractive surgery Eye Vision 2 7
12. Nagy ZZ, Kiss HJ, Takacs AI, Kranitz K, Czako C, Filkorn T, Dunai A, Sandor GL, Kovacs I. Results of femtosecond laser-assisted cataract surgery using the new 2.16 software and the SoftFit(R) patient interface. Orv Hetil. 2015;156:221–5
13. ZZ Nagy AI Takacs T Filkorn K Kranitz A Gyenes E Juhasz GL Sandor I Kovacs T Juhasz S Slade 2014 Complications of femtosecond laser-assisted cataract surgery J Cataract Refract Surg 40 20 8
14. K Kranitz AI Takacs A Gyenes T Filkorn R Gergely I Kovacs ZZ Nagy 2013 Femtosecond laser-assisted cataract surgery in management of phacomorphic glaucoma J Refract Surg 29 645 8
15. ZZ Nagy K Kranitz AI Takacs K Mihaltz I Kovacs MC Knorz 2011 Comparison of intraocular lens decentration parameters after femtosecond and manual capsulotomies J Refract Surg 27 564 9
16. K Kranitz K Mihaltz GL Sandor A Takacs MC Knorz ZZ Nagy 2012 Intraocular lens tilt and decentration measured by Scheimpflug camera following manual or femtosecond laser-created continuous circular capsulotomy J Refract Surg 28 259 63
17. NJ Friedman DV Palanker G Schuele D Andersen G Marcellino BS Seibel J Batlle R Feliz JH Talamo MS Blumenkranz WW Culbertson 2011 Femtosecond laser capsulotomy J Cataract Refract Surg 37 1189 98
18. GL Sándor Z Kiss ZI Bocskai K Kolev ÁI Takács É Juhász K Kránitz G Tóth A Gyenes I Bojtár T Juhász ZZ Nagy 2015 Evaluation of the mechanical properties of the anterior lens capsule following femtosecond laser capsulotomy at different pulse energy settings J Refract Surg 31 153 7
19. GL Sándor Z Kiss ZI Bocskai K Kolev AI Takács E Juhász K Kránitz G Tóth A Gyenes I Bojtár T Juhász ZZ Nagy 2014 Comparison of the mechanical properties of the anterior lens capsule following manual capsulorhexis and femtosecond laser capsulotomy J Refract Surg 30 660 4
20. M Packer EV Teuma A Glasser S Bott 2015 Defining the ideal femtosecond laser capsulotomy Br J Ophthalmol 99 1137 42
21. T Filkorn I Kovacs A Takacs E Horvath MC Knorz ZZ Nagy 2012 Comparison of IOL power calculation and refractive outcome after laser refractive cataract surgery with a femtosecond laser versus conventional phacoemulsification J Refract Surg 28 540 4
22. ZZ Nagy A Dunai K Kránitz AI Takács GL Sándor R Hécz MC Knorz 2014 Evaluation of femtosecond laser-assisted and manual clear corneal incisions and their effect on surgically induced astigmatism and higher-order aberrations J Refract Surg 30 522 5
23. Hu YJ, Hou P, WQ C. Factors affecting stromal hydration of clear corneal incision architecture. J Cataract Refract Surg. 2010;36:528
24. D Viswanathan NL Kumar 2013 Bilateral femtosecond laser-enabled intrastromal astigmatic keratotomy to correct high post-penetrating keratoplasty astigmatism J Cataract Refract Surg 39 1916 20
25. TV Roberts M Lawless SJ Bali C Hodge G Sutton 2013 Surgical outcome and safety of femtosecond laser cataract surgery: a prospective study of 1500 consecutive cases Ophthalmology 120 227 33
26. RG Abell E Darian-Smith JB Kan PL Allen SY Ewe BJ Vote 2015 Femtosecond laser-assisted cataract surgery versus standard phacoemulsification cataract surgery: outcomes and safety in more than 4000 cases at a single center J Cataract Refract Surg 41 47 52
27. AI Takács I Kovacs K Mihaltz T Filkorn MC Knorz ZZ Nagy 2012 Central corneal volume and endothelial cell count following femtosecond laser-assisted refractive cataract surgery compared to conventional phacoemulsification J Refract Surg 28 387 91
28. RG Abell NM Kerr AR Howie MA Mustaffa Kamal FL Allen BJ Vote 2014 Effects of femtosecond laser assisted cataract surgery on the corneal endothelium JCRS. 40 1777 83
29. M Ecsedy K Mihaltz I Kovacs A Takacs T Filkorn ZZ Nagy 2011 Effect of femtosecond laser cataract surgery on the macula J Refract Surg 27 717 22
30. ZZ Nagy M Ecsedy I Kovacs A Takacs E Tatrai GM Somfai DD Cabrera 2012 Macular morphology assessed by optical coherence tomography image segmentation after femtosecond laser-assisted and standard cataract surgery J Cataract Refract Surg 38 941 6
31. L Levitz J Reich TV Roberts M Lawless 2015 Incidence of cystoid macular edema: femtosecond laser-assisted cataract surgery versus manual cataract surgery J Cataract Refract Surg 41 683 6
32. HJ Kiss AI Takacs K Kranitz GL Sandor G Gabor Toth B Beatrix Gilanyi ZZ Nagy 2015 One-day use of preoperative topical non-steroidal anti-inflammatory drug prevents intraoperative prostaglandin level elevation during femtosecond laser-assisted cataract surgery Curr Eye Res 17 1 4
33. TV Roberts G Sutton MA Lawless S Jindal-Bali C Hodge 2011 Capsular block syndrome associated with femtosecond laser-assisted cataract surgery J Cataract Refract Surg 37 2068 70
34. NB Baig GP Cheng JK Lam V Jhanji KK Chong VC Woo CC Tham 2014 Intraocular pressure profiles during femtosecond laser-assisted cataract surgery J Cataract Refract Surg 40 1784 9
35. ZZ Nagy K Kranitz A Takacs T Filkorn R Gergely MC Knorz 2012 Intraocular femtosecond laser use in traumatic cataracts following penetrating and blunt trauma J Refract Surg 28 151 3
36. ZZ Nagy AI Takacs T Filkorn E Juhasz G Sandor A Szigeti MC Knorz 2013 Laser refractive cataract surgery with a femtosecond laser after penetrating keratoplasty: case report J Refract Surg 29 8

37. T Schultz E Ezeanosike HB Dick 2013 Femtosecond laser-assisted cataract surgery in pediatric Marfan syndrome J Refract Surg 29 650 2
38. AI Martin P Hughes C Hodge 2014 First report of femtosecond laser cataract surgery in a nanophthalmic eye Clin Exp Ophthalmol 42 501 2
39. Ecsedy M, Sándor GL, Takács ÁI, Kránitz K, Kiss Z, Kolev K, Nagy ZZ. Femtosecond laser-assisted cataract surgery in Alport syndrome with anterior lenticonus. Eur J Ophthalmol. 2015;25:507–11. https://doi.org/10.5301/ejo.5000603 [Epub ahead of print]
40. HB Dick T Schultz 2013 Femtosecond laser-assisted cataract surgery in infants J Cataract Refract Surg 39 665 8
41. M Lawless SJ Bali C Hodge TV Roberts C Chan G Sutton 2012 Outcomes of femtosecond laser cataract surgery with a diffractive multifocal intraocular lens J Refract Surg 28 859 64

Nano Laser Photofragmentation

9

S. Mödl, E. Ruf, and Gangolf Sauder

Abstract

The use of lasers for the fragmentation of the lens in cataract surgery is an interesting alternative to traditional ultrasonic phacoemulsification. Since the beginning of phacoemulsification it has been a constant ambition to reduce the operative trauma and collateral damage of intraocular tissue during phacoemulsification. Parameters to be changed are operating time, total intraocular energy used, incision size, tissue heating, corneal endothelial cell loss and induced corneal astigmatism. During the last years different laser systems have been developed to minimize thermal and mechanical damage of the intraocular tissue (Alzner and Grabner in J Cataract Refract Surg 25:800–3, 1999; Dodick JM, Christiansen J. Experimental studies on the development and propagation of shock waves created by the interaction of short Nd: YAG laser pulses with a titanium target. Possible implications for Nd: YAG laser phacolysis of the cataractous human lens. J Cataract Refract Surg. 1991;17:794–4;Dodick et al. in Curr Opin Ophthalmol 4:107–9, 1993).

Keywords

Cataract surgery · Corneal endothelium · Operative trauma · Endothelial cell count · Lens tissue

The use of lasers for the fragmentation of the lens in cataract surgery is an interesting alternative to traditional ultrasonic phacoemulsification. Since the beginning of phacoemulsification it has been a constant ambition to reduce the operative trauma and collateral damage of intraocular tissue during phacoemulsification. Parameters to be changed are operating time, total intraocular energy used, incision size, tissue heating, corneal endothelial cell loss and induced corneal astigmatism. During the last years different laser systems have been developed to minimize thermal and mechanical damage of the intraocular tissue [1–3].

One possibility to replace phacoenergy by laser energy is the usage of Nd:YAG lasers. Laser technologies like the Nd:YAG laser have been studied for use in the removal of cataractous lens tissue for nearly two decades [4]. One disadvantage of this procedure was that laser

Supplementary Information The online version contains supplementary material available at https://doi.org/10.1007/978-3-031-84204-7_9.

S. Mödl (✉) · E. Ruf · G. Sauder
Charlottenklinik in Stuttgart, Stuttgart, Germany
e-mail: sarah.moedl@charlottenklinik.de

U. Spandau and G. B. Scharioth (eds.), *Cutting Edge of Ophthalmic Surgery*,
https://doi.org/10.1007/978-3-031-84204-7_9

energy could be used only partly for the disruption of the lens tissue and only very soft nuclei could be emulsified efficiently. This technique has been continuously improved. Studies have demonstrated the ability of a Nd:YAG laser system to safely and effectively emulsify the lens nucleus [5]. The cetus nano laser (A.R.C. Laser company) is a pulsed Nd:YAG laser with a wavelength of 1064 nm. The laser light is carried by a 300 μm fiber and hits a titanium target inside the tip, thus generating a plasma followed by a circumscript cavitation just around the opening (Fig. 9.1). The laser induced plasma and shock wave disrupt the nuclear material and thus induce a photofragmentation of the crystalline lens into particles, which then can be aspirated through the same needle. Similar to conventional phacoemulsification irrigation can be done via the same handpiece (Fig. 9.2).

Using this technique no laser light is being emitted into the eye because the lens material is emulsified indirectly. The nano laser is effective for lenses with grade 1–4 nuclear sclerosis (LOCS-classification).

Nano laser photofragmentation and ultrasonic phacoemulsification are two physically completely different techniques, resulting in different conditions during surgery.

The holdability of the lens particles in the phaco procedure is superior to the nano laser because the laser induced cavitation out of the port and the aspiration in the opposite direction are always competing with itself. The holdability has been improved by shortening the nano laser pulses. The deep impaling necessary for an efficient chopping technique is not possible because the laser handpiece is missing the phaco oscillations.

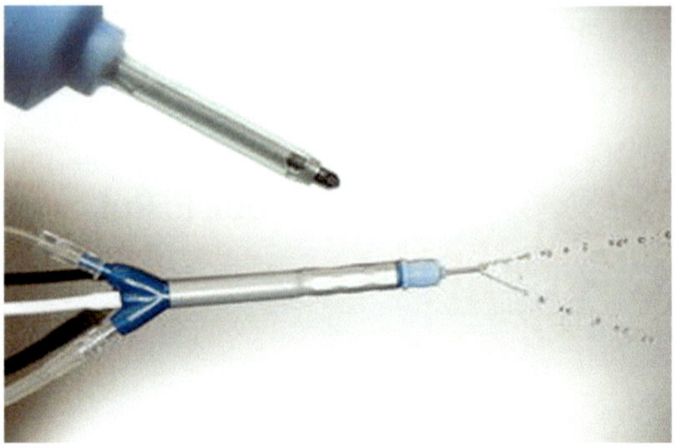

Fig. 9.2 Similar to phacoemulsification the irrigation is done with the same handpiece

In clinical practice two different techniques for the removal of lens tissue proved to be effective.

Softer nuclei (LOCS 1–2) can be removed with a so called bowling technique. The lens nucleus is photo fragmented by slightly rotating the tip down posteriorly from the middle of the surface. The tip is positioned with the port bevel down to protect the corneal endothelium. The epinucleus and cortex need to be untouched in order to protect the posterior capsule. For harder cataracts a lower frequency of laser pulses

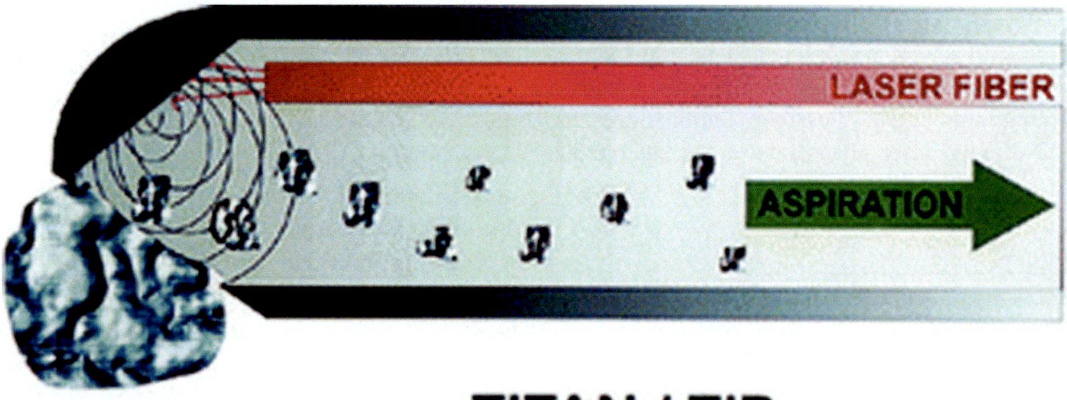

Fig. 9.1 The titan tip of a nano laser (ARC, Germany). The laser induces a plasma and shock wave and disrupts the nucleus. The nuclear material is aspirated through the same needle

Table 9.1 Technical settings of cetus nanolaser

Technical data	
	Nano Laser Cetus (A.R.C. Laser company)
Handpiece	Quartz fiber (300 μm)
Single pulse energy	0–10 mJ
Frequency	0–20 Hz
Single pulse duration	8 nsec
Vacuum	250–350 mm Hg

should be used. After the removal of the nucleus the epinucleus and cortex can be aspirated with the standard I/A Table 9.1.

Harder cataracts (LOCS 3–4) can be more efficiently emulsified by a "groove & crack" technique. Again with port bevel down a small hole or a little grove is created in the lens center up to approximately 50% of the lens thickness. Then the lens nucleus can be cracked with a second instrument, for example an iris hook or a Neuhann chopper. With aspiration half of the lens can be elevated in the iris level to fragment the half completely. If possible the same technique can be used to produce four quadrants. After removal of the nucleus the cortex and epinucleus are aspirated.

The complete nano laser cataract surgery is performed with single use instruments and thus features a very high hygienic standard.

The theoretically expectation and advantage of the laser photofragmentation over phacoemulsification are the lesser induction of shockwaves resulting in a gentler effect on corneal endothelium and intraocular tissue.

A major difference of the laser photofragmentation is the operation time which implies a higher consumption of jetting liquid and which would theoretically lead to a higher corneal endothelial cell loss.

First own investigations demonstrated a 20% higher fluid consumption with the laser procedure compared to conventional phacoemulsification and a longer effective laser – /phacotime. Concerning endothelial cell count and corneal thickness no significant differences were found. Intraocular energy release was significantly lower using the laser technology which might have a protective effect on the corneal endothelium. No differences could be shown for postoperative corrected visual acuity.

Conclusion

In addition to phacoemulsification as the gold standard nano laser photolysis is an efficient and safe procedure in cataract surgery. Main advantages are the lowest possible intraocular energy and heat release and minimal mechanical complications. A further advantage is that the complete cataract surgery is performed with single use instruments. Disadvantages are the longer operation time and the harder manipulation of the lens nucleus due to different physical characteristics of the laser photolysis compared to phacoemulsification.

Nano laser photofragmentation is a promising new procedure for cataractous lens removal. Further studies are required to see if this new technique is to be an improvement over current techniques.

FAQ

1. *What are the advantages of laser compared to ultrasound regarding phacoemulsification?*

The main advantages of the Nano laser compared to ultrasound are much lower required energy levels, no thermal or mechanical side effects and the possibility to perform the whole procedure with single use instrument

2. *How high is the risk of the input of laser energy for the eye?*

As no laser radiation is being emitted directly into the eye there is no risk of any laser induced damage to the intraocular tissue

3. *How long is the learning curve?*

The learning curve is short. An experienced phaco surgeon needs only a few weeks to adapt to this new technique.

4. *What are the main surgical differences when changing from phaco to laser?*

There are two major differences an experienced phaco surgeon has to adapt to when switching to Nano laser photo fragmentation. First the holdability of the lens particles is reduced using the laser technique compared to phacoemulsification. Second the deep impaling needed for an efficient chopping procedure is not possible with the Nano laser. Because of these different characteristics different surgical techniques as described above are required.

5. *How high is the risk to rupture the posterior capsule?*

The risk to rupture the posterior capsule is low due to the operating method of the laser. If the laser is pointed at the posterior capsule no rupture occurs unless the capsule is aspirated at the same time. In such a case a circular hole in the posterior capsule occurs similar to a posterior capsulorhexis.

6. *If we assume a surgical time of 10 min with phacoemulsification for a LOCS 3 nucleus; how long does it take with the laser handpiece?*

In our whole study group (30 nano laser patients and 30 phacoemulsification patients) a surgical time of 10 min was never needed.

Material and Companies Adress

A.R.C. Laser GmbH

- Bessemerstraße 14
- 90,411 Nürnberg
- Germany
- http://www.arclaser.de/en/

References

1. E Alzner G Grabner 1999 Dodick laser phacolysis: thermal effects J Cataract Refract Surg 25 800 3
2. Dodick JM, Christiansen J. Experimental studies on the development and propagation of shock waves created by the interaction of short Nd: YAG laser pulses with a titanium target. Possible implications for Nd: YAG laser phacolysis of the cataractous human lens. J Cataract Refract Surg. 1991;17:794–4
3. JM Dodick JM Lally LT Sperber 1993 Lasers in cataract surgery Curr Opin Ophthalmol 4 107 9
4. JM Dodick LTD Sperber JM Lally M Kazlas 1993 Neodymium-YAG laser phacolysis of the human cataractours lens (case report Arch Ophthalmol 111 903 4
5. Kanellopoulos AJ, Dodick JM, Brauweiler P, Alzner E. Dodick photolysis for cataract surgery. Early experience with the Q-switched Neodymium: YAG laser in 100 consecutive patients. Ophthalmology 1999;106:2197–202

Congenital Cataract Surgery

10

Alf Nyström and Lothar Schneider

Abstract

Dr. Nyström from Gothenburg, Sweden, has operated the most congenital cataracts in Scandinavia and implants always an IOL. He will demonstrate his technique and the implantation of a Tassignon IOL.

Keywords

Congenital cataract · Posterior capsular opacification · Corneal diameter · Anterior vitrectomy · Unilateral cataract

Indication for Surgery

To develop vision in an eye, a child must have an image on the retina. This can be checked with retinoscopy in a non-dilated child. Note that newborns often have very small pupils which are much bigger only a few weeks later.

A child with a non-dilated retinoscopy reflex has a good enough image which can be left without surgery regardless in which area the lens is opacified. If a child has a readable retinoscopy reflex then follow up with retinoscopy and a vision test (Fig. 10.1). If visual acuity under repeated examinations does not rise or even drops then the child should undergo surgery. Within the first 3 months of life at least two examinations should be performed, and then every second month within the first year and every third month within the second year of life.

If the child does not have a readable retinoscopy reflex and haze covers the pupil, the child should then undergo surgery; otherwise severe amblyopia will develop.

It is advantageous to carry out surgery after the age of 1 month in order to reduce the risk of secondary glaucoma and not later than 7–8 weeks to reduce the risk of grave amblyopia. After 3 months, the child often has a nystagmus if surgery has not been carried out, and reduces the chance of good visual acuity levels.

If the child does not have a readable retinoscopy reflex but the opacity does not completely cover the pupil, then the retinoscopy reflex is adjusted by adding different glasses. Not infrequently, cataract eyes are short and thus greatly hyperopic, but also grave myopia occurs due to a small anterior segment or spherical lens shape. It does not require so many diopters ametropia for the retinoscopy reflex to deteriorate.

Supplementary Information The online version contains supplementary material available at https://doi.org/10.1007/978-3-031-84204-7_10.

A. Nyström · L. Schneider (✉)
Sahlgrenska University Hospital Mölndal, Mölndal, Sweden
e-mail: lothar.schneider1@gmx.de

U. Spandau and G. B. Scharioth (eds.), *Cutting Edge of Ophthalmic Surgery*,
https://doi.org/10.1007/978-3-031-84204-7_10

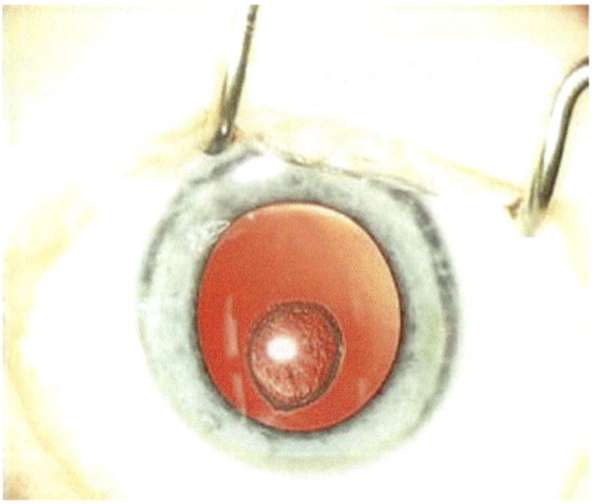

Fig. 10.1 A lens with inferior opacification and retinoscopy reflex

If you achieve a retinoscopy reflex with glass then you should refrain from surgery and following the above actions.

Why should you not operate a partial cataract?

The child's visual development is faster if it is phakic than if it is pseudophakic or aphakic (Fig. 10.2).

Unilateral cataracts should probably be operated slightly earlier. Unilateral cataracts are seldom caused by a syndrome and the risk for glaucoma is less (this does not apply for very small eyes).

Intraocular Lens

Video 10.1: 3D animation Bag in the lens

The Morcher 89 A IOL (Tassignon IOL, Fig. 10.3) is hydrophilic and called a BIL (Bag in the lens IOL) because the anterior and posterior lens capsules are clamped inside the IOL (Fig. 10.3). There are two sizes of IOL, one for adults and one for children. In the most cases an adult IOL (89 A) is used even in children eyes. In case of small eye and poorly dilated pupil the model 89D is preferred (Fig. 10.4).

The advantages of the Morcher 89 A IOL is that no posterior capsular opacification forms, the view to the fundus is excellent. The IOL causes much less inflammation than a usual three-piece IOL. Finally, in case of severe ametropia the IOL can be explanted against a new Tassignon IOL.

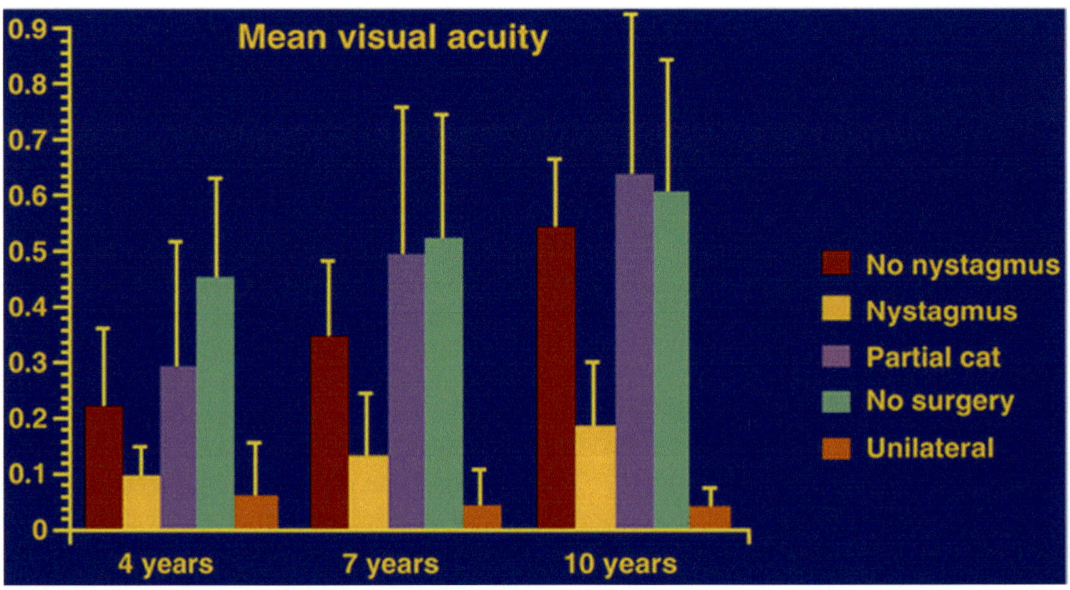

Fig. 10.2 Development of visual acuity of children with congenital cataract. Observe the poor VA for eyes with nystagmus and the increasing VA for eyes with no surgery

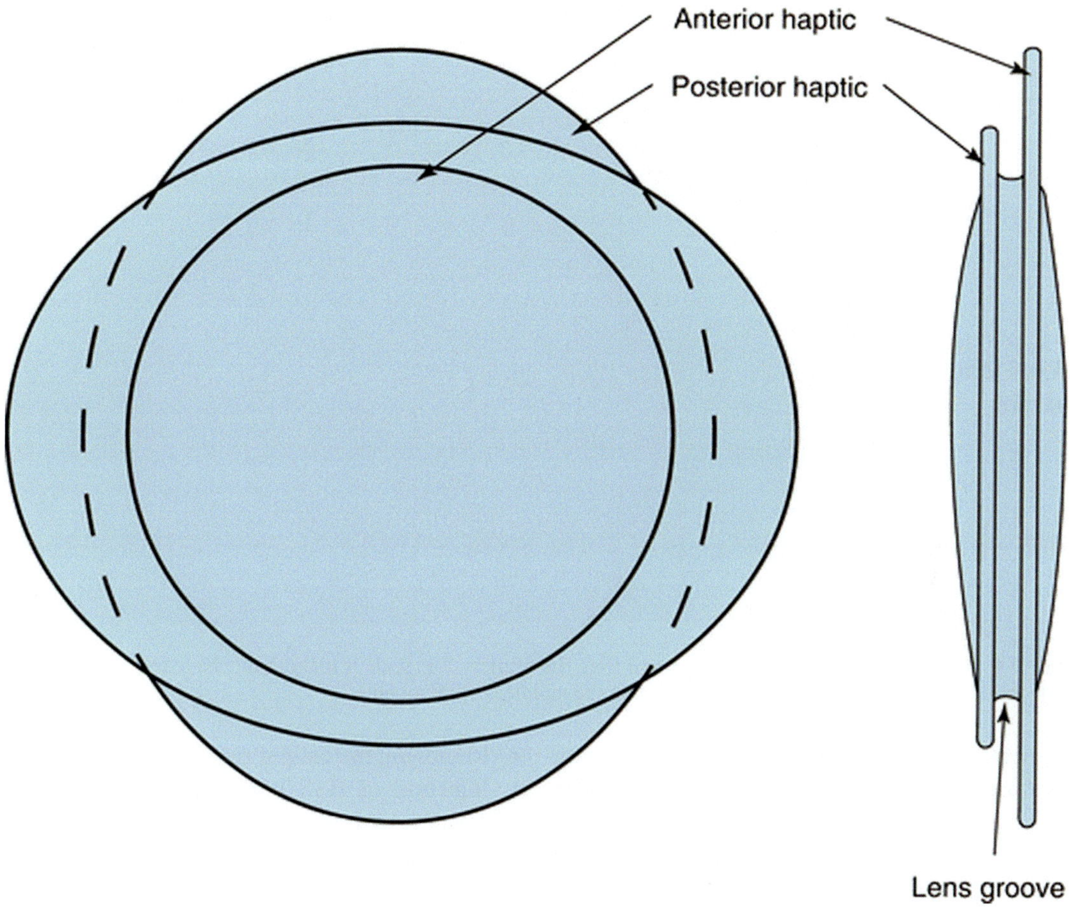

Fig. 10.3 The 89 A MORCHER hydrophilic IOL. The IOL has an anterior and posterior haptic and a groove between both haptics (Photocourtesy Morcher)

Morcher IOL type	Total diameter (mm)	Optic diameter (mm)
Type 89 A	7.5	5.0
Type 89D	6.5	4.5

Figure 10.4 there are two different sizes of "Tassignon" IOL.

Die IOL has an anterior and posterior haptic (Fig. 10.3). Between both haptics is a lens groove. Both rhexis sheets are located in this groove. Both haptics are located at a 90° angle to each other. The IOL is implanted so that the posterior haptic points towards 6 o'clock.

Target Refraction of IOL

In order to find out the target refraction the normal ocular axial growth curve from Sampaolesi is required (Fig. 10.4) [1]:

Example Congenital cataract in a 4 month old child, The AXL is measured with 20 mm. The Normal ocular axial growth curve from Sampaolesi (Fig. 10.4) shows now that the AXL will be 23 mm at the age of 80 months (6.5 years). The difference between 23 mm–20 mm = 3 mm. Three millimeter equals 9D (1 D = 3 mm). The target refraction is therefore + 9D.

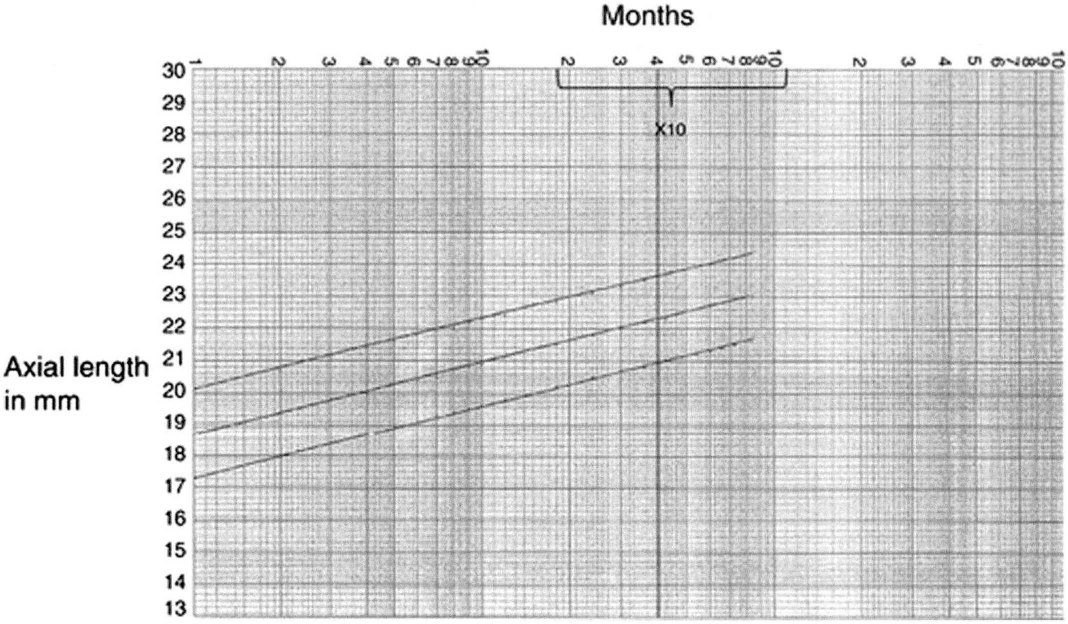

Fig. 10.4 The normal ocular axial growth curve from Sampaolesi. The scale is logarithmic. Note that on the months scale the months on the left are 2–10 months and in the middle 20–100 months

Remark Short eyes tend to grow less (require approximately 2D less target refraction); long eyes tend to grow more (approximately 2D more target refraction); Down syndrome eyes tend to grow significantly more (approximately 4D more target refraction) (unpublished results).

Surgical Protocol

Video 10.2: child's eye

Surgical protocol according to Prof Tassignon [2] **(Fig.** 10.5)

- Opening of the limbus with a knife 2.8 mm (eventually 2.5 mm) [1]
- Injection of 1.0 ml adrenalin solution (see procedure medication) [2]
- Injection of Healon GV for corneal protection [3]
- Insertion of the caliper ring type 5 NO Tassignon [4] using the ring caliper inserter (sk-7017 EyeTech) [5]
- Opening of the anterior capsule with the capsulorhexis forceps [6] (Ikeda 30° forceps) (Rr. 2268 EyeTech)
- Removing the caliper ring
- Injection of BSS between the lens and the capsule, hydrodissection [7]
- Phaco-emulsion of the lens content [8]
- Removing lens remnants with the I/A mode [9]
- Cleaning the capsule with BSS using the Helsinki needle (1273E Steriseal)
- Injection of Healon GV on top of the anterior capsule [3] (never fill the capsular bag!)
- Puncturing of the posterior capsule by using the tuberculin needle or 36G needle [10]
- Injection of Healon through the puncture hole within the space of Berger until the size of the blister is slightly larger than the anterior capsulorhexis [11]
- Attention not to overfill the space of Berger
- Performing the capsulorhexis with the Ikeda forceps [6]
- Insertion of the lens with the injector (Medicel Lp 604,410)
- Injection of miostat [12]
- Removing of the Healon with the I/A mode
- Refilling the anterior chamber with BSS and hydration of the corneal wound [9]
- Control of the water tightness of the wound
- Injection of zinacef solution (see procedure medication) [13].

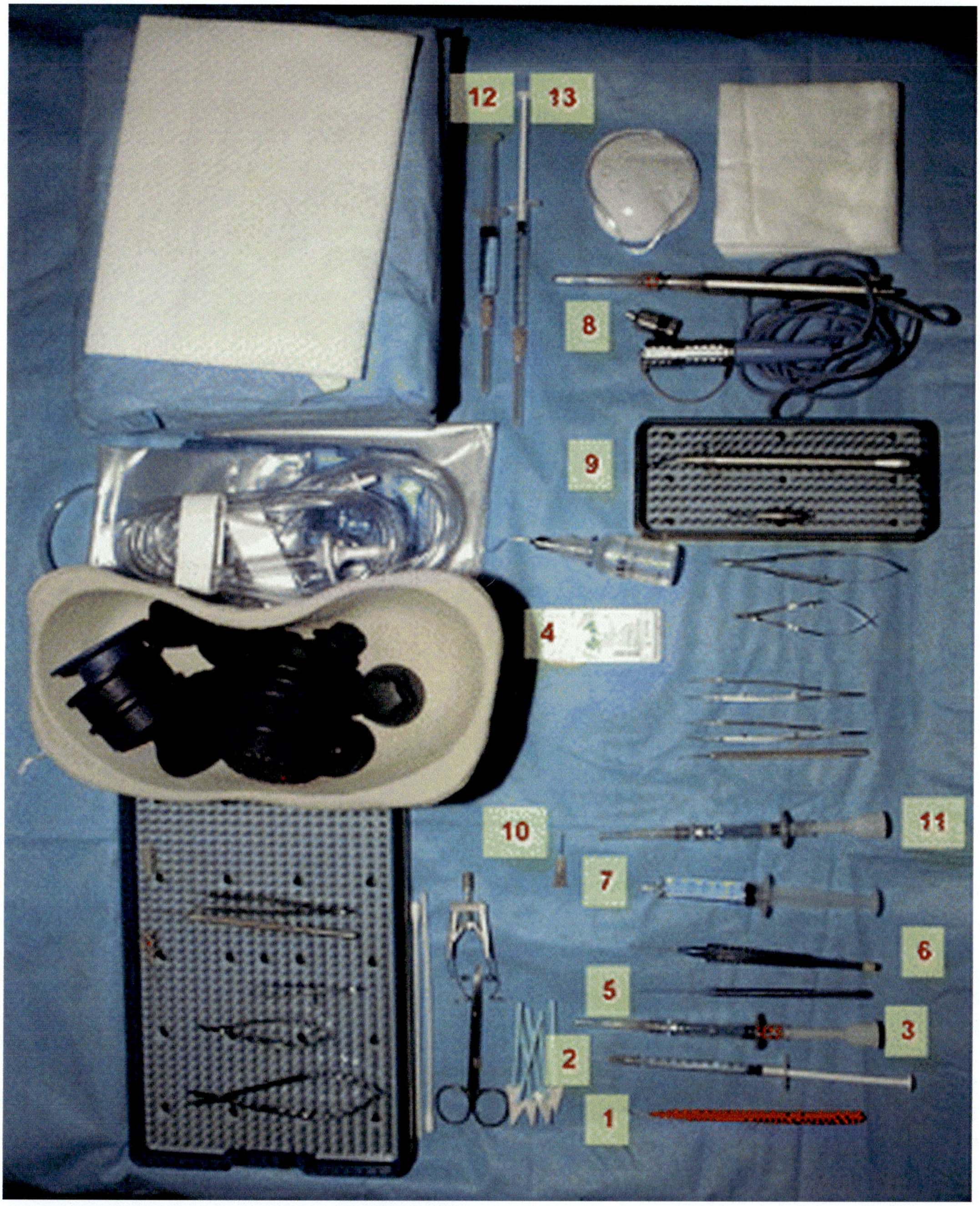

Fig. 10.5 Surgical tray for congenital cataract (Photocourtesy Morcher)

P.S. In pediatric cataracts the procedure is slightly different

- Ring caliper 4.5 mm is used
- Two sight ports of 1.0 mm are used for lens removal
- Injection of Healon into the space of Berger by means of a 41 G needle (Dorc 1270.0.100).

Instrumentation list [2]

No	Description	Comments	Ref. no	Manufacturer
1	"Bag-in-the-lens" foldable IOL	28% hydrophylic acrylic	89 A–D-E–F	MORCHER®
2	Ring caliper (4.5 – 5.0 – 6.0)	To caliper the position of the anterior capsulorhexis	Type 4 L Type 5 NO	MORCHER®
3	Tassignon caliper ring positioner	To position the ring caliper in the eye	sh-7017	EyeTech
4	Lkeda angled 30° capsulorhexis 23.0 g forceps	To perform anterior and posterior capsulorhexis	Fr 2268	EyeTech
5	Straight scissors in curved shaft	To adjust the capsulorhexis if needed	Fr 2295c	EyeTech
6	Naviject injector atraumatic/naviglide cartridge 2.5-IP injector set foldable cartridge 2.8-IP injector set foldable	Up to + 20.0 diopters For all diopters	Lp 604,420 Lp 604,410	Medicel
7	Rycroft/ Helsinki hydrodissection needle 27G	To inject dispersive viscoelastic behind the posterior capsule	1273E	Steriseal Oasis
8	41G needle (same type from two different manufacturers)	Idem than 7 but to be used in babies and children	E7370 1270.0.100	Bausch & Lomb Dorc
9	Corydon cannula	Curved hydrodissection cannula		Beaver Visitec Moria

Surgical protocol in detail according to the University of Gothenburg, Sweden

Video 10.3: 4 weeks old newborn
Video 10.4: 2 1/2 years child
Video 10.5: IOL implantation

Paracentesis and Tunnel (Fig. 10.6)
The superior rectus muscle is clamped with a surgical forceps and a holding suture (silk 4.0) is fixated to the muscle. Continue with a small peritomy at 1:30 and then a 20 g paracentesis with Alcon V-lance. Inject Healon GV in the anterior chamber. You can stain the anterior capsule with Vision Blue but the lens capsule stains

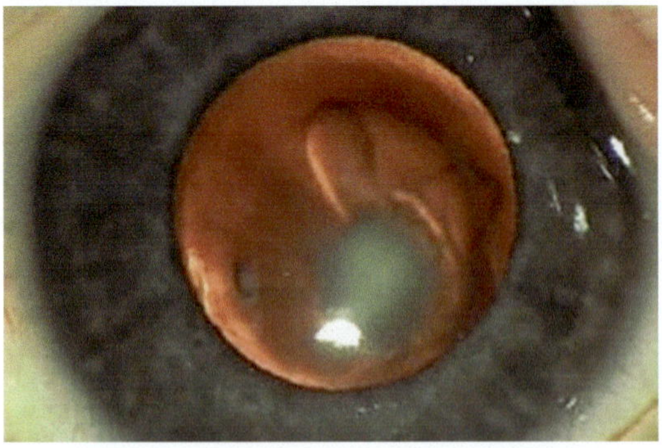

Fig. 10.6 A congenital cataract with posterior pole opacification

much less compared to adults. The next step is a peritomy at 12 o'clock, dissect a 3 mm wide sclerocorneal tunnel first with the crescent knife then enter the anterior chamber with an ordinary tunnel knife. Place a 5.0 mm caliper ring (Morcher) with a ring caliper inserter (Eye tech) or a Sinskey hook onto the anterior lens capsule.

Anterior capsular rhexis (Fig. 10.7)

Puncture the anterior capsule with a cystotome. If the lens capsule is too fibrotic puncture it with a 20G lance (Alcon). Puncture the lens capsule in an area without disturbing reflections so that the capsular rhexis can begin in a controlled fashion. The capsular rhexis is performed with the Ikeda forceps (Eye Tech), always make short strokes/movements with the forceps and observe the whole time how the rhexis behaves. In the inferior periphery the rhexis often has a tendency to move outwards; just the opposite to the superior periphery where the rhexis has the tendency to move inwards. If necessary recenter the caliper ring. If the lens capsule is too fibrotic and the rhexis cannot be continued then use the curved 20G scissors (Eye Tech). Finally, remove the caliper ring.

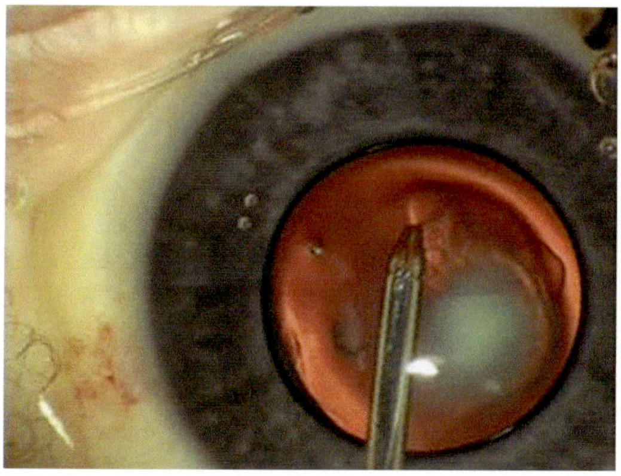

Fig. 10.7 Anterior capsular rhexis with the Ikeda forceps

Lens removal (Fig. 10.8)

First move the straight Helsinki cannula (Steriseal) and then the curved Corydon cannula gently behind the anterior rhexis edge to loosen the lens capsule from the lens; do not perform hydrodissection during this step. Then make a focal hydrodissection at 12 o'clock with Corydon cannula. The wave shall not reach the posterior pole of the lens as the capsule is often defective there. Aspirate the lens with the phaco handpiece or with I/A, then mobilize it and finally disintegrate with light ultrasound. Don't encroach on the periphery too much in the beginning, as the superior part at 12 o'clock can be removed in this way. This part was loosened in the beginning by slight hydrodissection. Then aspirate the cortex with the Corydon and Helsinki cannula. Remark: A stable anterior chamber is important during lens removal. If the anterior chamber collapses a few times then the pupil will become small.

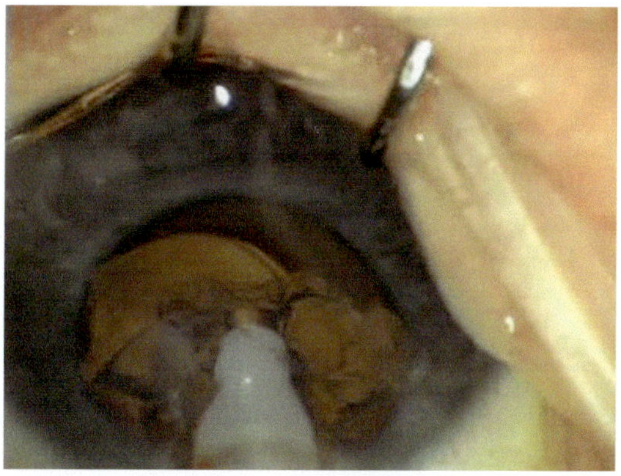

Fig. 10.8 Lens removal with phacoemulsification handpiece (Accurus machine)

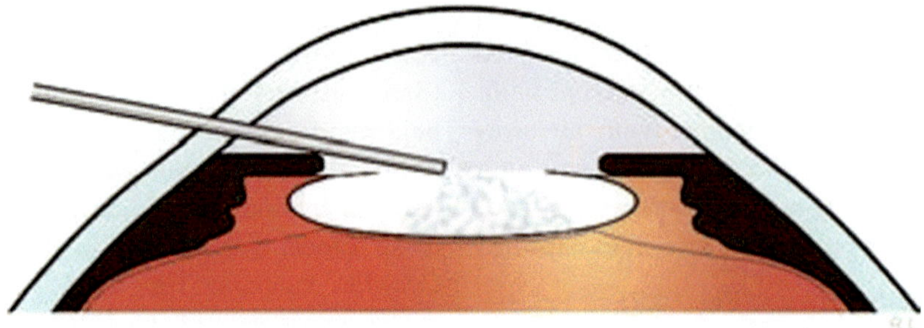

Fig. 10.9 After having emptied the capsular bag of all material (Photocourtesy Morcher)

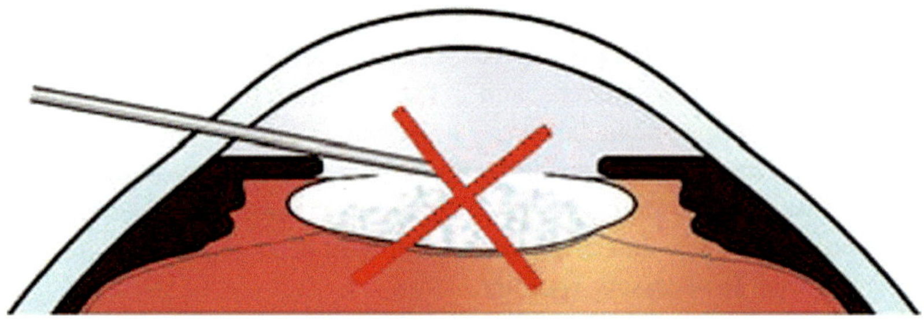

Fig. 10.10 NEVER refill the capsular bag with OVD!! (Photocourtesy Morcher)

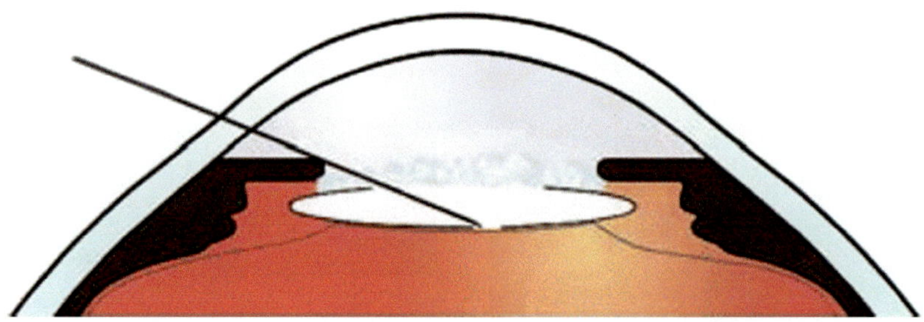

Fig. 10.11 On the contrary ONLY fill the capsular bag on top of the anterior lens capsule and bring the capsule in a horizontal plane (Photocourtesy Morcher)

Posterior capsular rhexis (Figs. 10.9, 10.10, 10.11, 10.12, 10.13, **and** 10.14)

Fill the anterior chamber with Healon GV. Do not inflate the capsular bag, make it only plane, otherwise the rhexis will not function. Puncture the posterior capsule with a 27 g needle in an area without disturbing reflections. Inject normal Healon with a thin Polytip cannula through that hole into the Berger space; be cautious that no air bubbles are present. The entire area behind the planned posterior rhexis should be filled with Healon. Then make a slow capsular rhexis with the Ikeda forceps. Make short movements as the posterior capsule is very elastic. In the lower half the rhexis often becomes substantially greater than expected. If necessary

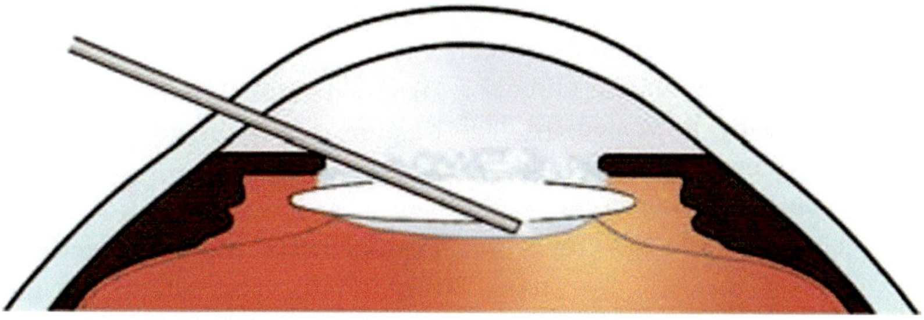

Fig. 10.12 After puncturing the posterior capsule inject the OVD through the hole until the blister is slightly larger than the anterior capsular rhexis (Photocourtesy Morcher)

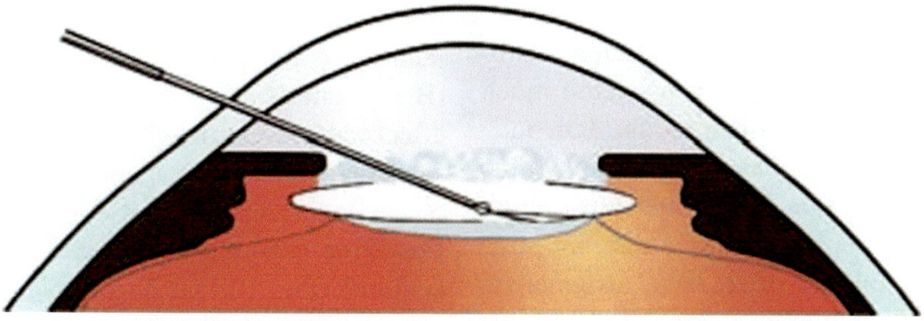

Fig. 10.13 Perform then the posterior capsular rhexis of the same size as the anterior capsular rhexis (Photocourtesy Morcher)

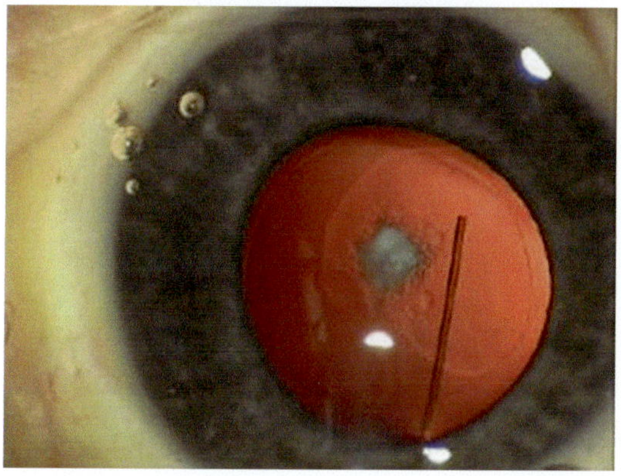

Fig. 10.14 Inject Healon with a thin Polytip cannula behind the posterior capsule inside the Berger space

inject Healon with the Corydon cannula behind the anterior capsule region. The posterior rhexis should have the same size as the anterior rhexis. If it is too small then the enclavation of both rhexis sheets into the Tassignon IOL will be difficult; the rhexis may even tear. Aspirate an excess of Healon from anterior vitreous before continuing to the next step. In case of a vitreous or embryonic tissue prolapse perform an anterior dry vitrectomy. If the eye becomes soft then inject BSS into the vitreous. Repeat this procedure several times.

IOL implantation

Load the Mediject (Navicel) cartridge with the Morcher IOL and inject the IOL in direction of the corneal endothelium because the IOL drops down more than expected. Centrate the IOL with the IOL rotator before the rhexis. Note that the posterior haptic is located at 12 and 6 o'clock. First clamp the posterior haptic at 6 o'clock behind both rhexis sheets. In the next step press on the left and right sides of the anterior haptic until at least 50% of both rhexis sheets is clamped inside the groove. In the final and most difficult step the 12 o'clock part of the posterior haptic is clamped inside both rhexis sheets by pushing the IOL towards 6 o'clock and posterior. If you push too much to the posterior then the IOL will luxate into the vitreous cavity. This event is usually prevented by the two lateral haptics which are located in front of the rhexis sheets. Double check again that both rhexis sheets are clamped inside the groove of the optic.

Suture of paracentesis and tunnel (Fig. 10.15) Place a 10-0 Ethilon cross suture with three throws on the main incision. Do not make a knot yet! Close the paracentesis with a single 10-0 Ethilon suture and rotate the knot inside. Remove the Healon from the anterior chamber with BSS irrigation. Don't inject too much BSS into the anterior chamber, as the IOL may be pressed into the vitreous cavity. Remove the Healon completely. Now tighten the cross suture with a knot. The knot is sunk. On the first postoperative day children often have astigmatism of 5–6 dpt but this minimizes quickly. Close the conjunctiva with 10-0 Vicryl. Inject Miochol to avoid an iris capture and finally 0.1 ml Zinacef (Cephalosporin). Remove the holding suture on the rectus muscle, inject Betapred subconjunctivally and place an antibiotic ointment on the cornea.

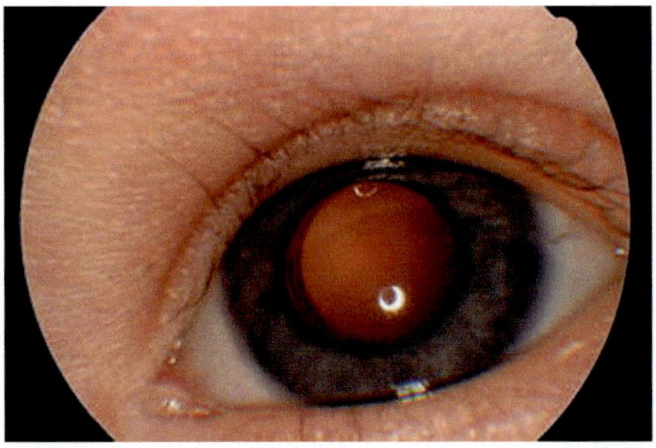

Fig. 10.15 A postoperative photograph. The Tassignon IOL's cause no inflammation compared to 3-piece IOL's and the view to fundus is excellent

Complications

Dropped IOL (happens intraoperatively): Requires a VR surgery to lift the IOL into the anterior chamber.

Postoperative iris capture (happens seldom) (Fig. 10.16): The parents are informed that if they observe an oval pupil in the child's eye to come immediately into the hospital. In the most cases a pupillary dilatation (e.g. tropicamide) is sufficient to remove the iris capture. If this is not successful, the IOL is pressed behind the iris under general anesthesia. To prevent a recurrence the eye must be treated with Azopt (Brinzolamid) drop × 2. The pathophysiologic effect may be that less aqueous is produced thus reducing the pressure against the IOL.

Posterior capsular opacification (occurs very seldom) (Fig. 10.17): A pars plana anterior vitrectomy is required.

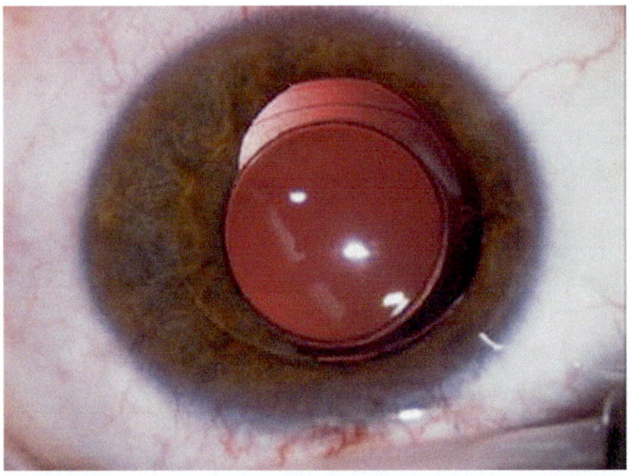

Fig. 10.16 A postoperative complication: Iris capture

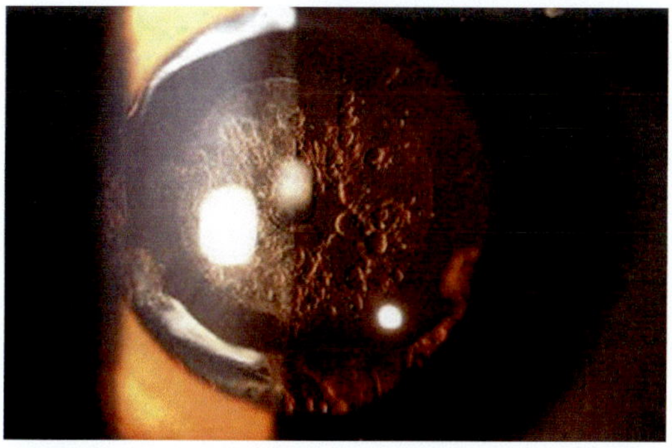

Fig. 10.17 A postoperative complication which occurs very seldom: Posterior capsular opacification

Postoperative Care with Contact Lenses

After surgery, even pseudophakic eyes are always corrected with contact lenses because the target refraction is often strongly hyperopic to prevent grave myopia when the child gets older.

If the child is aphakic the medium refraction postoperatively is about 38D (corneal plane) at 1 month of age and diminishes to about 10 diopters after the first year (28D).

Myopia above the normal and increased corneal diameter above the normal are both strong indicators for glaucoma. The child's refraction often changes 5 diopters towards myopia in less than a month.

Regarding unilateral cataracts amblyopia training is very important. To be sure that the child exercises during waking hours you can occlude the healthy eye every second day. Otherwise training 1 h daily in the waking hours is a very good as the child sleeps more in the beginning.

Materials and Companies

MORCHER® GmbH
Kapuzinerweg 12
70374 Stuttgart
Germany

References

1. Sampaolesi R, Caruso R. Ocular echometry in the diagnosis of congenital glaucoma. Arch Ophthalmol. 1982;100(4):574–7.
2. http://www.morcher.com/fileadmin/content/Broschueren_Kataloge/CATALOG-89A-TASSIGNON_2012-05-02.pdf.

Part VI
Premium IOL: Macula IOL, Add-On IOL

The amount of implanted special lenses has augmented dramatically in recent years. In this book, we will present two special lenses, the macula lens for improved reading ability and the add-on IOL. Prof. Scharioth from Recklinghausen, Germany, designed a novel macula lens which is implanted as a piggy-back IOL and allows near vision for patients with AMD. Prof. Sauder from Stuttgart, Germany, will present the use and implantation of add-on IOL's for spherical, astigmatic and presbyopic correction in pseudophakic eyes.

Scharioth Macula Lens

11

Gabor B. Scharioth

Abstract

Age-related macular degeneration has a high prevalence in industrialized societies and is the most common cause for loss of reading vision among patients older then 55 years of age (Martin et al. in Ophthalmology 119:1388–1398, 2012; Congdon et al. in Arch Ophthalmol 122:477–485, 2004). In recent years major advances have been made in the therapy of the neovascular form of age-related macular degeneration (Martin et al. in Ophthalmology 119:1388–1398, 2012; Rosenfeld et al. in N Engl J Med 355:1419–1431, 2006; Heier et al. in Ophthalmology 119:2537–2548, 2012), but reduced near visual acuity is still a major problem for all forms of age-related macular degeneration. External magnifying low visual aids are known for decades, but uncomfortable use and stigmatization in public limited their acceptance. They might affect the visual field and cannot be worn continuously. Furthermore they might be forgotten at home, lost or damaged.

Keywords

Cataract surgery · Reading distance · Ciliary sulcus · Secondary cataract · Neovascular form

Age-related macular degeneration has a high prevalence in industrialized societies and is the most common cause for loss of reading vision among patients older then 55 years of age [1, 2]. In recent years major advances have been made in the therapy of the neovascular form of age-related macular degeneration [1, 3, 4], but reduced near visual acuity is still a major problem for all forms of age-related macular degeneration. External magnifying low visual aids are known for decades, but uncomfortable use and stigmatization in public limited their acceptance. They might affect the visual field and cannot be worn continuously. Furthermore they might be forgotten at home, lost or damaged.

The amount of implanted *special lenses* has augmented dramatically in recent years. In this book, we will present two special lenses, the macula lens for improved reading ability and the add-on IOL. Prof. Scharioth from Recklinghausen, Germany, designed a novel macula lens which is implanted as a piggyback IOL and allows near vision for patients with AMD.

Supplementary Information The online version contains supplementary material available at https://doi.org/10.1007/978-3-031-84204-7_11.

G. B. Scharioth (✉)
Aurelios Augenzentrum, Recklinghausen, Germany
e-mail: Gabor.Scharioth@augenzentrum.org

U. Spandau and G. B. Scharioth (eds.), *Cutting Edge of Ophthalmic Surgery*,
https://doi.org/10.1007/978-3-031-84204-7_11

Evolution of Intraocular Low Vison Aids

Different intraocular lenses or telescopic systems were suggested for intraocular implantation. In 2006 the Italian company Lensspecial introduced the IOL VIP System. One high + power PMMA IOL was implanted in the anterior chamber angle and one high − power PMMA IOL was implanted in-the-bag. This created an intraocular Galilean telescope. The system could be implanted only during cataract surgery. Anterior chamber IOL have been shown to increase the risk of corneal decompensation and secondary glaucoma. Later this system was modified and both lenses were implanted within the capsular bag (IOL VIP revolution, Lenspecial, Italy). The two IOL are stabilized with an additional modified capsular tension ring (SALring). Magnification of this system is limited. In 2010 the Lipshitz Implantable Miniature Telescope (Vision Care Inc.) received FDA approval [5, 6]. This miniature Galilean telescope was implanted during cataract surgery and required a very large main incision of about 11–12 mm. The implant affects the visual field and is very sensible to tilt and decentration. Also diagnostics like funduscopy, fluorescein angiography and OCT might be affected. More recently Lipshitz introduced the OriLens (OptoLight, Israel) [7]. This implant uses reflection within the lens to magnify the image. It is made by PMMA and requires a main incision of about 6 mm. Patients frequently suffer from optical side effects and retina diagnostics are affected. In 2013 London Eye Hospital introduced the iolAMD [8]. This system consists of two hydrophylic acrylic IOL. First lens (−49 D) is implanted intracapsular. Second lens (+63 D and slightly decentered on haptic) is implanted into the ciliary sulcus. This creates a Galilean telescope with magnification of about 1.3 and slightly parafoveal focus. Implantation is only possible during cataract surgery and seems to be very sensible to decentration. It seems that magnification of implantable Galilean systems is limited to a maximum of 1.6 × and that this might be not sufficient for patients with advanced maculopathy. Furthermore more then 50% of patients with advanced age related maculopathy are already pseudophakic and could not benefit from such implants.

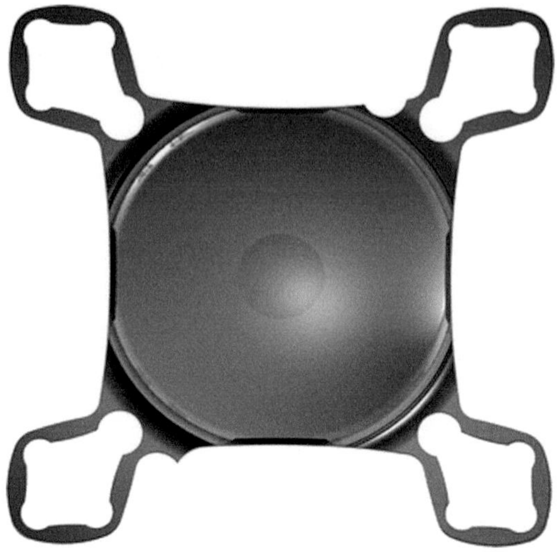

Fig. 11.1 Image of Scharioth Macula Lens (Medicontur Hungary Ltd. Hungary), lens design is based on A4 W add-on IOL (1stQ, Germany), note central optical portion of 1.5 mm diameter with + 10.0 diopters, residual optic is optically neutral and has a diameter of 6.0 mm, overall diameter is 13 mm, lens is made from hydrophilic acrylic material and requires a minimum incision size of 2.2 mm if implanted with injector

We therefore developed an implant specially designed for ciliary sulcus implantation in pseudophakic eyes (add-on technology) with sufficient magnification in near (Scharioth Macula Lens A45SML, Medicontur, Hungary) (Fig. 11.1) [9]. The add-on IOL (A4 W from 1stQ, Germany) is in clinical use for several years and has proven ease of implantation technique and low complication rate [10]. We have used a + 6.0 D version of this add-on IOL to treat hyperopic shift in vitrectomized eyes with silicone tamponade [11]. It is made from hydrophilic acrylic material and can be implanted through a minimal incision size of 2.2 mm. This lens has an overall diameter of 13 mm and an optical zone of 6.0 mm. The patented design and round polished edges prevent complication (e.g. Uveitis-Glaucoma-Hemorrhage -Syndrome, iris capture syndrome, IOL decentration, interlenticular secondary cataract "red rock syndrome" etc.) known from the previous so called piggy back IOL technique. It was developed to treat residual spherical or astigmatic errors after cataract surgery or perforating keratoplasty. Later a multifocal version became available. We modified this platform and added to a special central optic of 1.5 mm diameter and a power of + 10 D. This results in a reduced reading distance of about 15 cm and a magnification of 2 × compared to normal reading distance of 35–40 cm. Residual main part of the IOL optic is neutral (0 D). To treat residual spherical error after previous cataract surgery the SML could be ordered with additional power (up to ± 6 D). Visual field and distance vision are not affected. Retinal imaging, incl. SD-OCT is not diminished. First Scharioth Macula Lens was successfully implanted in September 2013 in a single eyed patient with advanced age related maculopathy. The eye was already treated 13 times with intravitreal antiVEGF and BCDVA was 0.12. Near vision improved from Radner 10 preoperative to Radner 4 postoperative. Four weeks postoperative patient was able to read newspaper.

Surgical Technique (Video 11.1)

Routine major incision of a minimum of 2.2 mm is required. Anterior chamber is filled with viscosurgical device. The Scharioth Macula Lens is placed in the cartridge. Special care is taken that during the folding of the winglets of the cartridge the optic of the lens is folding upwards. This will result in a controlled intraocular unfolding during implantation. While the plunger of the injector is pushed a second instrument is used through the side port incision to guide the leading haptic into the ciliary sulcus (Fig. 11.2). Usually the trailing haptics are placed into the ciliary sulcus in a second step. Proper position of the haptics and IOL centration is checked. Finally ophthalmic viscosurgical device is removed. Special care is taken to remove residual OVD between the lenses. We prefer hydroxypropylmethylcellulose to reduce

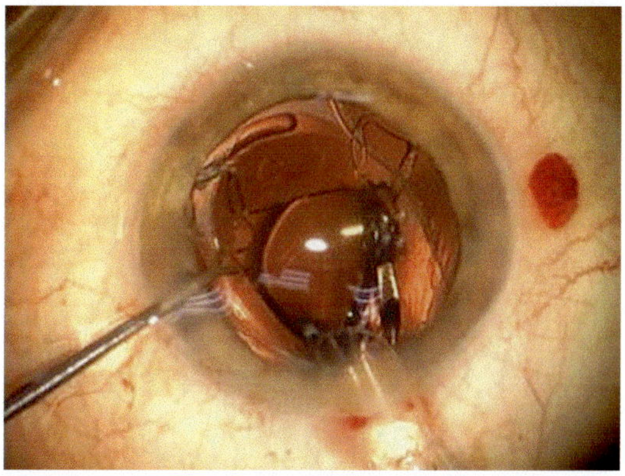

Fig. 11.2 Intraoperative situation during implantation of Scharioth Macula Lens, IOL is unfolding while second instrument is used through side port incision to guide leading haptics into ciliary sulcus

the risk for postoperative intraocular pressure spikes. Additionally one might prescribe acetazolamide per os. Finally incisions are hydrated to prevent leakage (Fig. 11.3).

The implantation can be performed during an uncomplicated cataract surgery after the standard IOL is placed in-the-bag or any time after a previous cataract surgery. If relevant cataract is present we prefer to perform first phacoemulsification and in-the-bag PCIOL implantation. SML implantation can be performed any time after if the patient is unsatisfied with the outcome of cataract surgery alone. In case of a near clear lens we perform a simultaneous surgery with immediate implantation of the Scharioth Macula Lens. In contrast to a secondary implantation years after in-the-bag implantation in this situation the SML has tendency to unfold with the leading haptics into the capsular bag. As the haptics are very soft it should not be difficult to lift the haptic and position it into the ciliary sulcus. In our experience a moderate secondary cataract does affect safeness and visual outcome. But in case of excessive secondary cataract (thick Soemmering) one should consider to remove the material to prevent decentration or tilt. All manipulations should be performed very carefully to prevent zonular damage as this could result in unstable SML positioning.

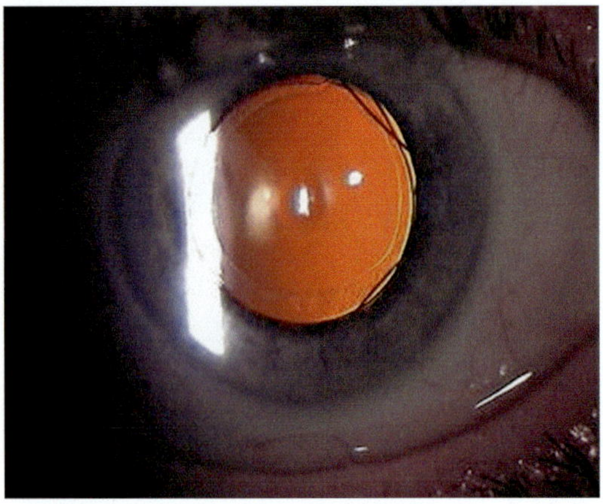

Fig. 11.3 Postoperative photo in retroillumination, well centered in-the-bag PCIOL and SML, note central portion of add-on Scharioth Macula Lens ("rain drop")

Preoperative Evaluation and Patient Selection

Patients with advanced maculopathy (e.g. AMD, diabetic maculopathy, myopic maculopathy etc.) and distance visual acuity between 0.3 (0.4) and 0.1 are good candidates. If BCDVA is better then 0.4 patients do not require low vision aid to read. In our experience preoperative testing of BCNVA at 40 cm with + 2.5 D vs. 15 cm with + 6.0 D gives a valid information about the potential of SML and if BCNVA is better at 15 cm and the patient is motivated he might be a good candidate. Patients with BCDVA worse then 0.1 or no improvement in near test (+2.5 D vs + 6.0D) might be also candidates for SML implantation but should be informed that reading vision will not be achieved. In this case a slight improvement might be helpful for daily activities (e.g. looking for coins in a wallet) if the patient is motivated and compliant.

Patients with advanced zonulopathy (e.g. pseudophakodonesis, excessive pseudoexfoliation, large zonular dialysis) are contraindicated. Patients with active maculopathy (e.g. choroidal neovascularisation, intra/subretinal fluid) should first be treated. We suggest SML implantation during a "quiet" phase of the disease. Control of visual acuity and retinal imaging shall be performed as usual. There is no contraindication to intravitreal injections. The add-on IOL implantation is reversible if IOL exchange is needed or improved technologies become available in the future.

Material and Companies Address

1stQ Deutschland GmbH

Harrlachweg 1
68163 Mannheim
Germany
http://www.1stq.de/home.

Medicontur

Herceghalmi Road 1
2072 Zsámbék
Hungary
http://www.medicontur.com.

References

1. Martin DF, Maguire MG, Fine SL, et al. Ranibizumab and bevacizumab for treatment of neovascular age-related macular degeneration: two-year results. Ophthalmology. 2012;119(7):1388–98.
2. Congdon N, O'Colmain B, Klaver CC, et al. Causes and prevalence of visual impairment among adults in the United States. Arch Ophthalmol. 2004;122(4):477–85.
3. Rosenfeld PJ, Brown DM, Heier JS, et al. Ranibizumab for neovascular age-related macular degeneration. N Engl J Med. 2006;355(14):1419–31.
4. Heier JS, Brown DM, Chong V, et al. Intravitreal aflibercept (VEGF trap-eye) in wet age-related macular degeneration. Ophthalmology. 2012;119(12):2537–48.

5. Lipshitz I, Loewenstein A, Reingewiirtz M, et al. An intraocular telescopic lens for macular degeneration. Ophthalmic Surg Lasers. 1997;28(6):513–7.
6. Lane SS, Kuppermann BD, Fine IH, et al. A prospective multicenter clinical trail to evaluate safety and effectiveness of the implantable miniature telescope. Am J Ophthalmol. 2004;137(6):993–1001.
7. Agarwal AI, Lipshitz I, Jacob S, et al. Mirror telescopic intraocular lens for age-related macular degeneration: design and prelimanary clinical results of the Lipshitz macular implant. J Cataract Refract Surg. 2008;34(I):87–94.
8. Qureshi MA, Robbie SJ, Tabernero J, Artal P. Injectable intraocular telescope: pilot study. J Cataract Refract Surg. 2015;41(10):2125–35.
9. Scharioth GB. New add-on intraocular lens for patients with age-related macular degeneration. J Cataract Refract Surg. 2015;41(8):1559–63.
10. Sauder G, Cordes A. Scope of applications and experience record with a new generation of add-on IOLs: the A4 W lens. Ophthalmo-Chirurgie. 2012;24(Suppl. 2):1–6.
11. Scharioth GB. Add-on IOLs for vitrectomized silicone oil-filled eyes. Retinal Physicians. 2014;11:31–3

AddOn® Intraocular Lenses

12

Gangolf Sauder and S. Mödl

Abstract

An add-on intraocular lens is designed to be implanted in the ciliary sulcus. In the most cases an add-on IOL is implanted secondary in the sulcus of an already pseudophakic eye. It can also be implanted simultaneously with an endocapsulary implanted lens in the ciliary sulcus.

Keywords

Intraocular lens · Corneal astigmatism · Pigment dispersion · Endothelial cell loss · Ciliary sulcus

Introduction

An add-on intraocular lens is designed to be implanted in the ciliary sulcus. In the most cases an add-on IOL is implanted secondary in the sulcus of an already pseudophakic eye. It can also be implanted simultaneously with an endocapsulary implanted lens in the ciliary sulcus.

Supplementary Information The online version contains supplementary material available at https://doi.org/10.1007/978-3-031-84204-7_12.

G. Sauder · S. Mödl (✉)
Charlottenklinik in Stuttgart, Stuttgart, Germany
e-mail: sarah.moedl@charlottenklinik.de

Although add-on IOLs no longer belong to the very latest developments in ophthalmic surgery, it is worth to look at the developments in recent years. The first add-on IOLs that are available for about 10 years were derived in their design of primary endocapsular implanted intraocular lenses, i.e. usually three-piece design with silicone or PMMA haptics and acrylat optic.

The following patient case shows, which therapeutic options add-on IOL's have:

- 76 y/o engineer with Fuchs corneal disease. The cornea decompensated after phacoemulsification of the right eye. A perforating corneal transplant was performed and resulted in a high astigmatism:
- Refraction:
  RE: – 2.0–7.0/42° = 0.9
  LE: + 2.5–0.5/90° = 0.9
- Surgery: Implantation of a toric add-on IOL in the sulcus.
- Result: Third postoperative month:
  RE: – 1.0–0.75/170 = 0.9–1.0p
  LE: + 2.5–0.5/90 = 0.9

Possible indications of add-on IOL's are:

- Astigmatic situations with unstable corneal radii e.g. keratoconus

U. Spandau and G. B. Scharioth (eds.), *Cutting Edge of Ophthalmic Surgery*,
https://doi.org/10.1007/978-3-031-84204-7_12

- ametropia after cataract surgery (instead of IOL exchange)
- lack of near vision in pseudophakic eyes
- ametropia secondary to silicone oil-filled eyes
- ametropia secondary to episcleral cerclage.

To use an add-on IOL for the possible indications, the following requirements to the design should be met:

- Highest rotational stability
- High precision of refraction in biometrics
- Stable positioning in ciliary sulcus
- Stable distance to endocapsular IOL
- No induction of pigment dispersion
- Minimal induction of positive or negative dysphotopsia.

The most recent AddOn® development by the company 1stQ (Mannheim, Germany) for the first time has adapted the design of the add-on IOL to the requirements of an implantation in the ciliary sulcus Fig. (12.1). In order to avoid contact of the optics of the add-on IOL in the ciliary sulcus with the basis IOL in the lens capsule, the overall diameter was created with a convex-concave optic design.

The IOL of AddOn® 1stQ Fig. (12.1) consists of a square basic geometry and a 6.0 mm optics. The square geometry prevents an iris capture. The hydrophilic acrylic IOL has a convex-concave optical design, which has an edge in all four quadrants of the optic rear surface, which ensures a steady distance to the base lens. The distance from the base lens is on average 0.64 mm [1]. This important design feature prevents a touch of both intraocular lenses, which might change the refraction such as diminishing the toric effect Figs. (12.2, 12.3, and12.4). On the other hand a stable refraction and refractive predictability is guaranteed Fig. (12.5).

The main feature of AddOn® IOL's is the four diamond-shaped haptics on the four corners of the square basic shape Fig. (12.1). They provide a neutral adaptation of the IOL to the anatomical conditions of the ciliary sulcus by absorbing forces acting from the outside on the haptics without transferring these to a decentering or rotational component. This feature ensures a high stability in the ciliary sulcus and is especially important for toric and multifocal AddOn® intraocular lenses.

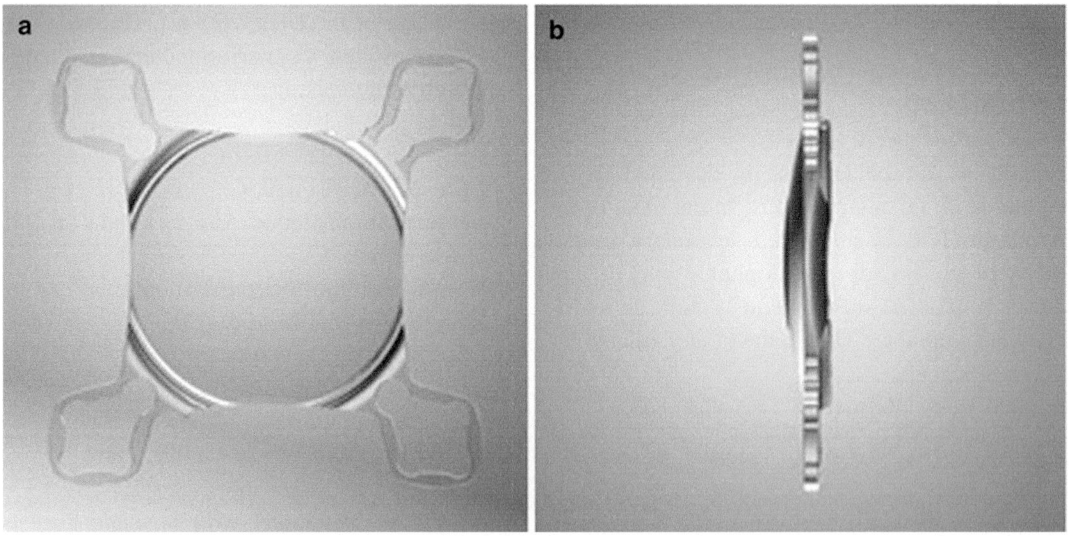

Fig. 12.1 Front-(**a**) and backview (**b**) of the AddOn® IOL (1stQ, Mannheim, Germany)

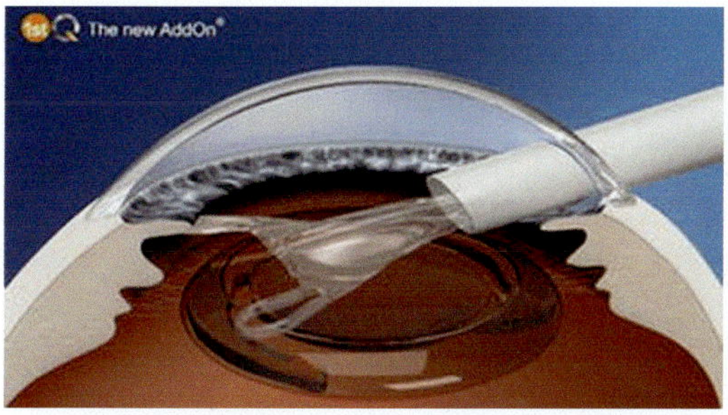

Fig. 12.2 The addON IOL is implanted into a pseudophakic eye. Fotocourtesy 1stQ (Germany)

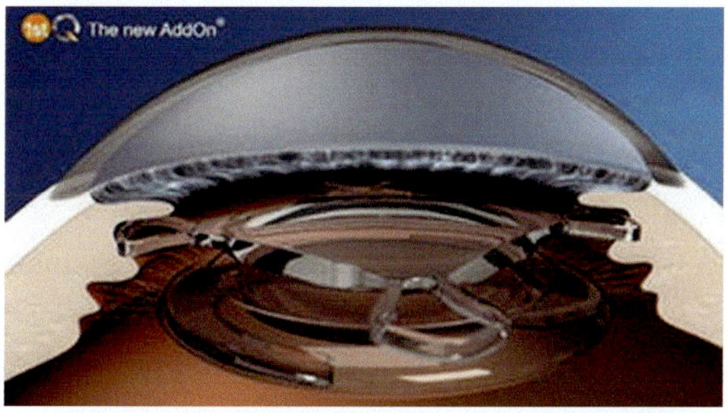

Fig. 12.3 The addON IOL is located in the ciliary sulcus. Fotocourtesy 1stQ (Germany)

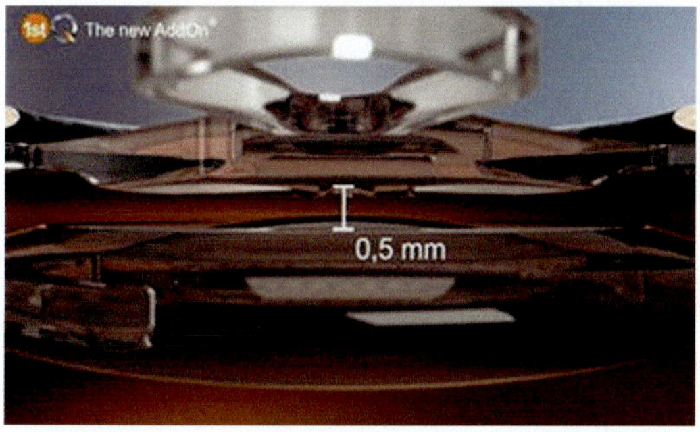

Fig. 12.4 There is a secure distance of 0.5 mm between the addON IOL and the endocapsular IOL. Fotocourtesy 1stQ (Germany)

<u>The main indications of AddOn® IOL are:</u>

1. Spheric intraocular lens AddOn®

Already pseudophakic eyes can be effectively "retrofitted" even years after the cataract operation with an AddOn® IOL. Postoperative ametropia can be corrected with a possibly complicated lens exchange or more elegant with an AddOn® IOL. In addition, an ametropia in eye with permanent silicone oil tamponade or with a cerclage can be easily corrected with an AddOn® IOL. This applies in principle all under one to three mentioned variants. Toric and spherical post-corrections are not critical, easy to perform and have a high refractive accuracy.

2. Toric intraocular lens AddOn®

An excellent indication for a toric addOn IOL is the correction of corneal astigmatism after penetrating keratoplasty or stable keratoconus in eyes with pseudophakia. The toric AddOn® IOK is implanted into the ciliary sulcus. Even if changes in the corneal geometry occur to a later time point then a repositioning (rotation) of the toric AddOn IOL is simple and feasible. If necessary, the AddOn IOL can be explanted so that the implantation of an AddOn IOL is always reversible.

If future prospective studies prove that toric AddOn® IOL are as rotationally stable or even better than a endocapsulary IOL then an AddOn IOL approach for corneal astigmatism should be considered.

3. Multifocal intraocular AddOn®

Within a prospective study it could be demonstrated that a multifocal AddOn® IOL is equal to an endocapsular toric IOL in regard to contrast sensitivity, halos and glare and even superior in subjective patient satisfaction [2]. The multifocal Array of AddOn® IOL is being investigated as part of a multicenter study. The main advantage of the addON IOL approach is of course its reversibility.

4. A more recent approach is the implantation of add-on IOL's lenses to correct undesirable dysphotopsias [3]. With an additional IOL implantation in the ciliary sulcus visual phenomenon like a shadow, or halos disappear. Larger and more extensive studies are required to investigate the precise nature of negative and positive dysphotopsias and their correction.

The calculation of the required AddOn® IOL power is essentially based on the subjective refraction. The situation is different in pseudophakic patients who wish a multifocal IOL

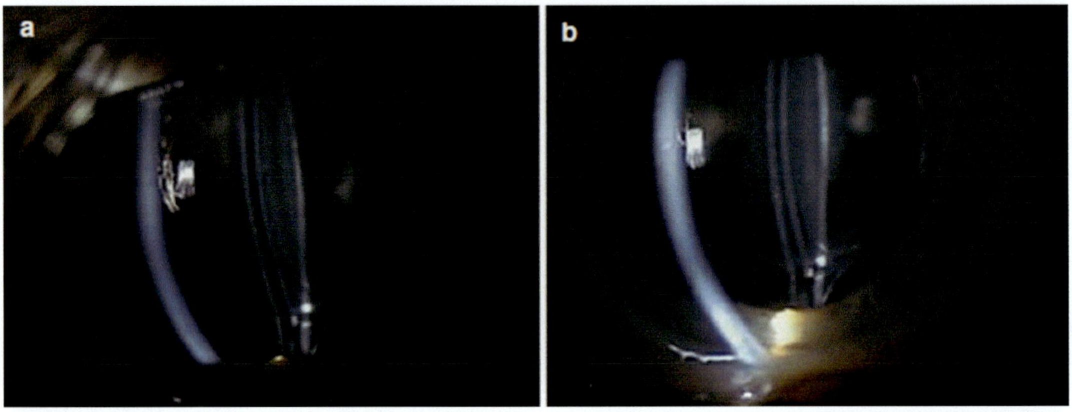

Fig. 12.5 Slit lamp view of an AddOn® IOL in the ciliary sulcus with a constant distance between the add-on IOL and the endocapsular IOL

AddOn® to improve reading vision. Here the preoperative information is paramount that a higher spectacle independence and better near vision is achieved for the price of a subjective and often also objective loss of distance vision.

The Surgical Technique (Videos 11.1 and 11.2)

Important points **before** implantation:

- Identification of the front and back surface of the IOL
- use blunt forceps for manipulation
- note orientation teeth on the IOL
- Exact positioning in shooter:
  - Complete filling with viscoelastics in the cartridge
  - Exact positioning of haptics in cartridge channel
  - note that the haptics are not jammed inside the cartridge channel
  - No temporary advancing of the IOL in the shooter

Important points **during** implantation:

- Clear cornea incision of 2.2 mm
- Inject highly viscous viscoelastic into the anterior chamber
- inject visco under the iris to simplify the implantation
- advance the IOL slowly inside shooter
- when the IOL unfolds in the anterior chamber, make a short stop with advancing of the IOL to allow the two front haptics unfold fully
- rotate the IOL 90° to ensure the haptics to unfold safely in the sulcus
- in case of simultaneous implantation of a regular IOL check that the add-on IOL does not sit endocapsulary
- inject Miochol ™ to induce miosis
- No iridectomy

Adverse Effects of AddON IOL's [2]

- No IOP elevation
- No pigment dispersion
- Minimal endothelial cell loss

In conclusion AddOn® IOL's represent a useful addition to the operational spectrum of refractive cataract surgery, be it as a primary implantation of two lenses for presbyopia or to correct corneal astigmatism. Easy atraumatic implantation and easy reversibility or post-rotation are certain advantages of the AddOn® system. The high rotational stability of the toric IOL AddOn® could also bring advantages over endocapsulary implanted toric IOLs.

Material and Companies Address

1stQ Deutschland GmbH

- Harrlachweg 1
- 68,163 Mannheim
- Germany
- http://www.1stq.de/home

Medicontur

- Herceghalmi Road 1
- 2072 Zsámbék
- Hungary
- http://www.medicontur.com

References

1. K. Mayer, G. Sauder. “Ultraschallbiomikroskopische Untersuchungen von AddOn® Intraoklarlinsen”, Masterthesis im Studiengang Augenoptik und Psychophysik der Hochschule Aalen (zur Beurteilung eingereicht)
2. S. Brandtner, G.Sauder. “AddOn MIOL versus endokapsuläre MIOL: Eine randomisierte Studie” DOC Nürnberg 2012
3. M Ny B Tt B Hj N Rm 2015 Treatment of negative dysphotopsia with supplementary implantation of a sulcus-fixated intraocular lens Graefes Arch Clin Exp Ophthalmol 253 6 973 7

Part VII Secondary IOL Implantation: Carlevale IOL, IOL Exchange

The Carlevale IOL, however, is the first foldable IOL specially designed to be used for scleral fixation. The Carlevale IOL is currently one of the most popular techniques for secondary IOL implantations. The inventor will describe the surgical technique step-by-step.

An *IOL exchange* may be necessary due to IOL opacity or wrong IOL choice. The surgery is however tricky especially for a re-implantation into the lens capsule. Dr. Spandau from Stockholm, Sweden, will show tips and tricks for IOL extraction and implantation into the lens capsule.

Carlevale IOL for Scleral Fixation

13

Carlo Carlevale

Abstract

The Carlevale IOL is the first foldable IOL specially designed to be used for scleral fixation.

Keyword

Carlevale—Scleral fixation IOL

Features of the Carlevale IOL Design

The Carlevale IOL is equipped with T shaped plugs on the top of the two close loops. Once the T shaped plugs are pulled through the scleral thickness from the ciliary sulcus to the bed of a scleral flap or scleral pocket, they open like harpoons and the IOL is stabilized to the ciliary sulcus without need of stitches (Fig. 13.1).

The loops have special design (Fig. 13.2), four arms connect the optic disc of the IOL with the loops, these arms have small nicks creating weak point, so all the haptic system is flexible and adapts to different diameter of ciliary sulcus without modification of the Effective Lens Position of the optic part of the IOL resulting in good refractive predictability (Figs. 13.2, 13.3 and 13.4).

The loops are not like a C loops or G loops, they touch the ciliary sulcus only in one point with more risk of tilting, the Carlevale IOL loops look like "wings", so they stabilize the IOL placing the two bumps in the ciliary sulcus and in the middle with the vertical part of the T shaped plug, because of these three points of contact for each side to the ciliary sulcus this IOL has very good three-dimensional stability and self-centering properties (Fig. 13.5).

The optic of the Carlevale IOL has a diameter of 6.5 mm that minimizes the risk of decreased visual acuity in case of mild decentration and creates an efficient compartmentalization between anterior and posterior segment (good separating effect in case of gas in A.C. for corneal surgery or silicone oil and gas in VR surgery).

The 10-degree vaulting between the optic disc and the loops reduces the risk of chronic iris root chaffing with pigment epithelium dispersion syndrome.

The Carlevale IOL is nowadays one of the most popular IOL for scleral fixation. In contrast to standard 3-piece IOLs, the Carlevale IOL is specifically designed for scleral fixation through a special design of the haptics. Dr. Carlevale will personally introduce his IOL and explain the surgery.

Supplementary Information The online version contains supplementary material available at https://doi.org/10.1007/978-3-031-84204-7_13.

C. Carlevale (✉)
Karol Wojtyla Hospital, Rome, Italy
e-mail: c.carlevale@tiscali.it

U. Spandau and G. B. Scharioth (eds.), *Cutting Edge of Ophthalmic Surgery*,
https://doi.org/10.1007/978-3-031-84204-7_13

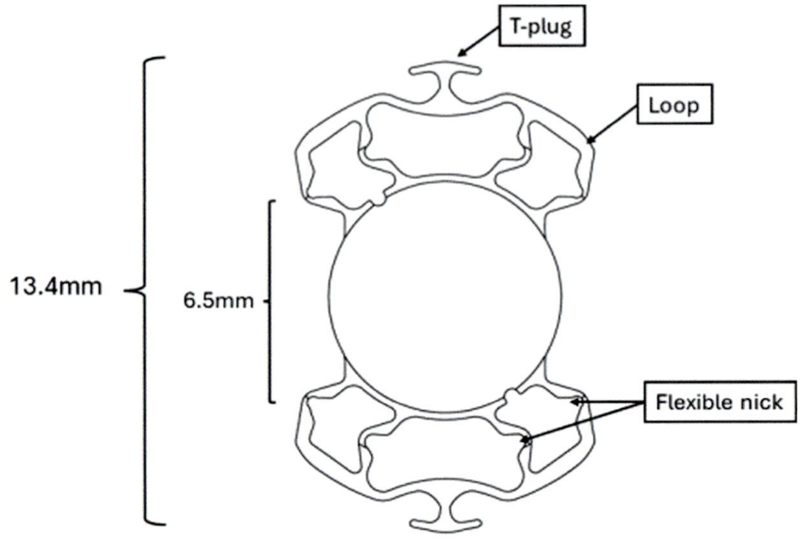

Fig. 13.1 The IOL is equiped with two T shaped plugs, they open like harpoons and stabilize the IOL to the ciliary sulcus

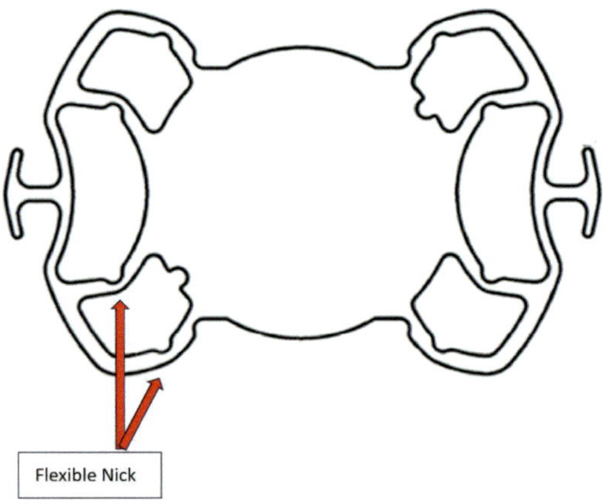

Fig. 13.2 The small nicks in the arms that are connecting the optic disk and loops creates weak points and IOL adapts to different diameter of ciliary sulcus

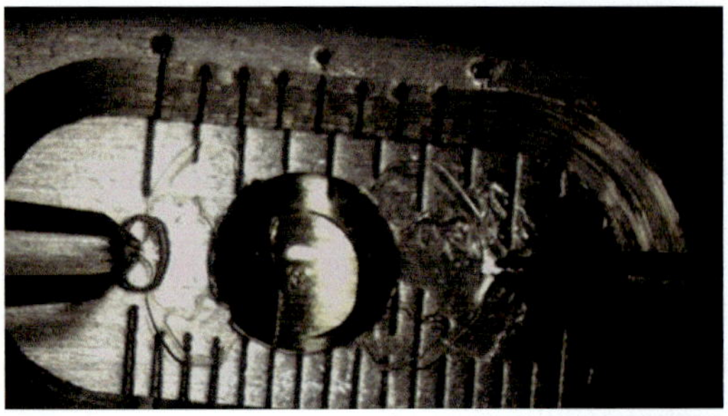

Fig. 13.3 The IOL loops stretched in a big diameter ciliary sulcus

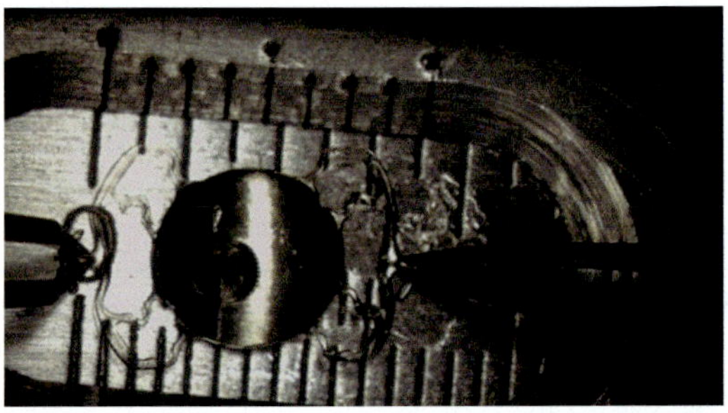

Fig. 13.4 The IOL loops constricted in a small diameter ciliary sulcus

Actually, there are two kinds of material available in the manufacture of the Carlevale IOL: acrylic hydrophilic and a co-polymer hydrophobically coated, the second one has much less chances of late opacification but is slightly less elastic than the hydrophilic one. In the co-polymer hydrophobically coated model the flat end of the harpoons allows them to adapt better inside the scleral flaps or pockets reducing the risk of erosion.

The Carlevale IOL behaves as in the bag IOL, A Constant U/S 118,0.

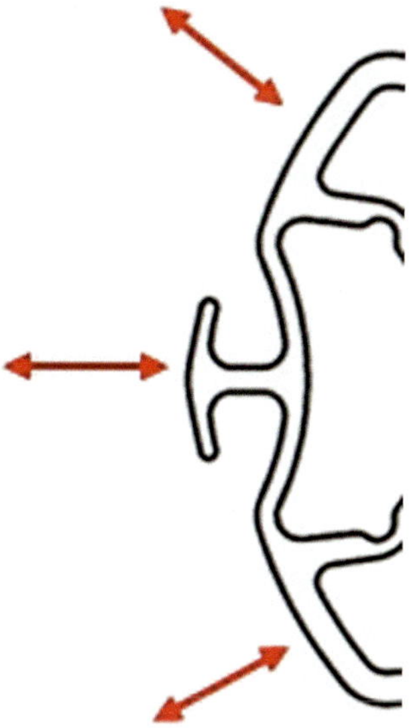

Fig. 13.5 Good three-dimensional stability due to the special loops design, they have three points of contact for each side to the ciliary sulcus

Constant with Ulib System

SRK/T = 118,5; SRKII = 118,7; Holladay1 sf = 1,42; Holladay 2 = 5.257; Barrett = 1.62 HofferQ pACD = 5,20; Haigis a0 = 1,589; a1 = 0,400; a2 = 0,100

The surgery:

Instruments

1. Anterior chamber maintainer or pars plana infusion
2. Vitrector
3. 23 G Curved Intraocular forceps (e.g. Scharioth IOL fixation forceps, DORC)
4. 22/23 G needle
5. 22/23 G side port blade
6. 2.4 - 2.75 mm main incision knife
7. Cautery or diathermy.

The surgical procedure step by step

There are several variations to implant the Carlevale IOL, here the standard variation is described that at the moment looks to be the safest procedure (Watch surgical video on Springer platform).

1. Insertion of pars plana infusion or anterior chamber maintainer.
2. Prepare two opposite 4 by 4 mm scleral flaps 180° one from each other possibly without making any initial perforation of the eye globe (hypotony will start). The ideal point to position the flaps are on the oblique meridians (to avoid the 3:00 and 9:00 clock position because of the long posterior ciliary artery). Try to cauterize as little as possible in order to maintain a healthy sclera, the ideal scleral flaps dissection to avoid late plug surface extrusion, should be as deep as 1/2 or 2/3 of the sclera's thickness.
3. Perforate each bed of the scleral flaps at 2 mm behind the limbus, using a sclerotome or better a 22/23 G needle (that will create a round hole in the sclera) (Fig. 13.6). Test that the 22/23G micro coaxial forceps fits smoothly in the scleral hole before starting to deliver the IOL in the A. C. (Anterior Chamber)(Fig. 13.7).
4. The clear cornea main incision (2.4 - 2.75 mm) is possibly positioned opposite to the

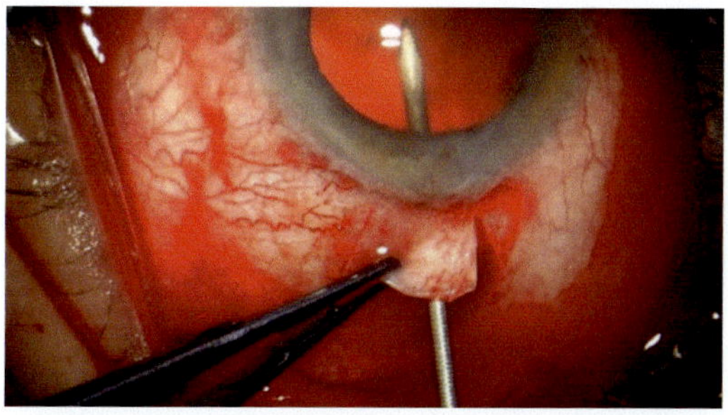

Fig. 13.6 The bed of the scleral flap is perforated at 2 mm from the limbus using a needle or sclerotome

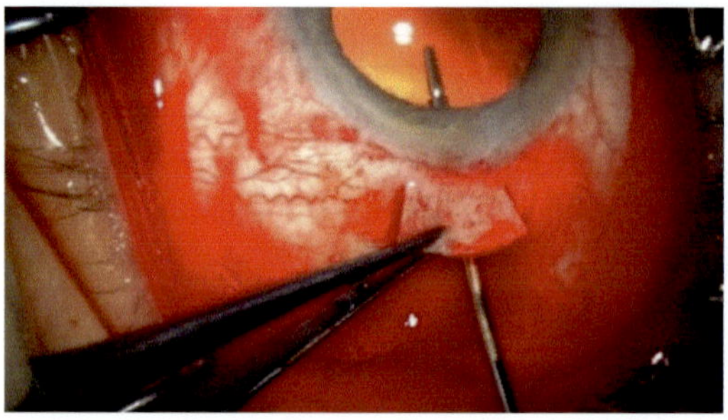

Fig. 13.7 The micro coaxial forceps should be tested in the scleral hole

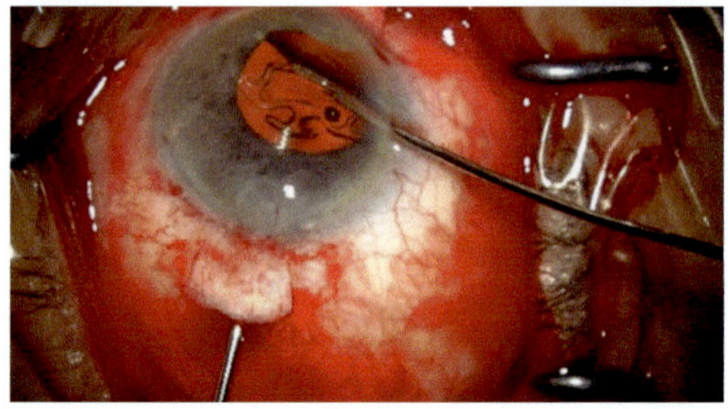

Fig. 13.9 The micro coaxial forceps grasps the trailing T shaped plug

scleral flap used to grab and externalise the leading plug.

5. Viscoelastic injection in A.C.
6. Careful loading of the IOL in the cartridge (Fig. 13.8).
7. IOL delivery in A.C.
8. The plug of the leading haptic is then grasped with intraocular micro coaxial forceps, then the forceps is carefully withdrawn till the plug appears from the hole on the bed of the scleral flap. The same maneuver is performed with the plug of the trailing haptic in the 180° scleral hole bed of the other flap. The two plugs open and stabilize the IOL to the ciliary sulcus without any need of stitches (Figs. 13.9 and 13.10).
9. Suture of the scleral flaps and conjunctiva with self-resorbing suture (Fig. 13.11).
10. Viscoelastic removal.

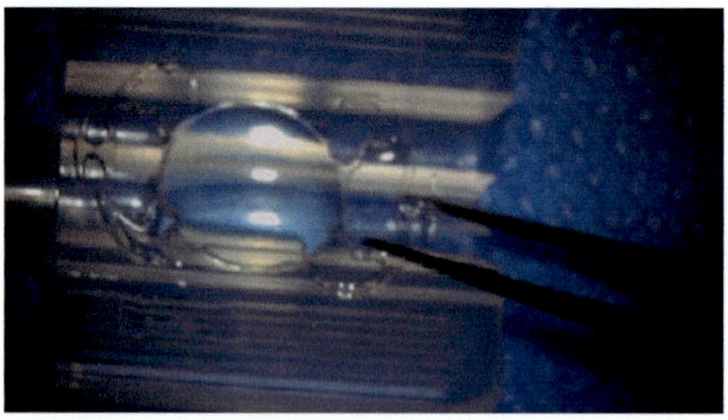

Fig. 13.8 The IOL should be carefully loaded in the cartridge to avoid any damage

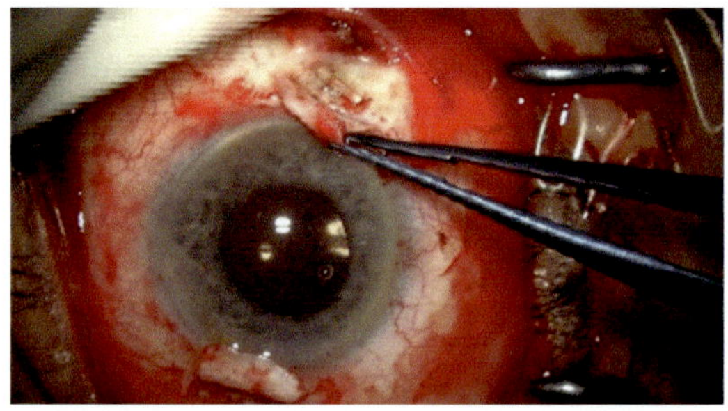

Fig. 13.10 Once the T shaped plug is externalized, it opens on the bed of the scleral flap

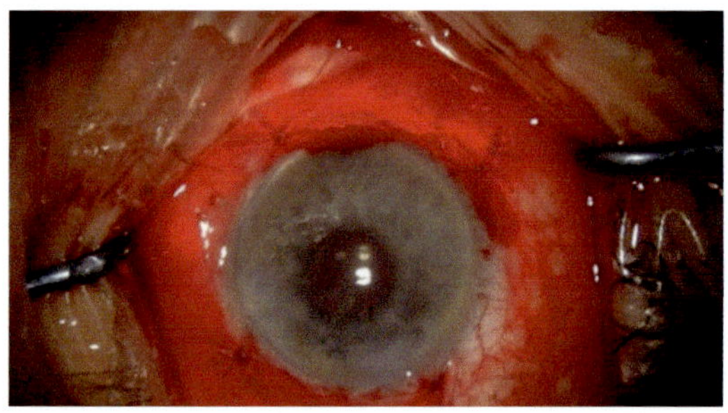

Fig. 13.11 Scleral flaps and conjunctiva are sutured with self-resorbing suture

Special Recommendations

(A) Remember always to have two curved micro coaxial forceps (if you have a deep-set eye, a big nose or prominent frontal bone will be impossible to tilt the forceps in a way to be able to grasp the "T" shaped plug at the level of the iris plane or just below it).

(B) Avoid using 25G micro coaxial forceps because during externalization there is more risk to damage the T shaped plug.
(C) Always sculpt large (4 by 4 mm) opposite thick scleral flaps to protect all around the plug to avoid late surface extrusion.
(D) Always load the IOL in cartridge of the single-use injector under microscope to avoid snatching some part of the IOL between the cartridge and the rubber piston and consequently deliver in A.C. the IOL already damaged (Fig. 13.8).
(E) Accurate vitrectomy of the anterior and vitreous base will prevent late retinal detachment.
(F) Better to suture scleral flaps and conjunctiva with 7-0 or 9-0 Vicryl, hypotony should always be avoided.

IOL Exchange

14

Ulrich Spandau

Abstract

An IOL exchange is sometimes necessary. The surgery is easy shortly after cataract surgery but difficult after several months. This chapter describes a late IOL exchange. The IOL explantation and an IOL re-implantation into the lens capsule is shown step-by-step. With the described technique a posterior capsule rupture can be avoided.

Keywords

IOL exchange · Opacified IOL · Anisometropia

An intraocular lens exchange is easier shortly after surgery because the anterior and posterior capsule can be easily separated. This separation becomes more difficult with time but even after several years an IOL extraction is possible. The most crucial point is the opening of the lens capsule and the mobilisation of the haptics. After one year it may be surgically easier to cut the haptics with scissors and leave them in the lens capsule.

The surgical trick is to open the anterior rhexis with a 27G cannula and inject viscoelastics into the capsular bag. A surgical video can be seen on my youtube website with the following link: https://youtu.be/72XjD_svdJ4?si=Gnz5xCLS0iCDs_5h

<u>Instruments</u>

1. 15° paracentesis knife
2. 2.4 mm tunnel incision knife
3. Maybe: Iris spatula
4. Push–pull instrument or Sinskey hook (Fig. 14.1)
5. Capsulotomy scissors (Fig. 14.2)
6. 27G needle cannula

<u>Individual steps</u>

(1) Paracentesis
(2) Injection of viscoelastics in capsular bag
(3) Opening of capsular bag
(4) Mobilisation of IOL
(5) Rotation of IOL on iris
(6) Cutting of IOL
(7) Extraction of IOL
(8) Implantation of IOL

U. Spandau (✉)
Department of Ophthalmology, University of Stockholm, Stockholm, Sweden
e-mail: ulrich_spandau@yahoo.de

U. Spandau and G. B. Scharioth (eds.), *Cutting Edge of Ophthalmic Surgery*,
https://doi.org/10.1007/978-3-031-84204-7_14

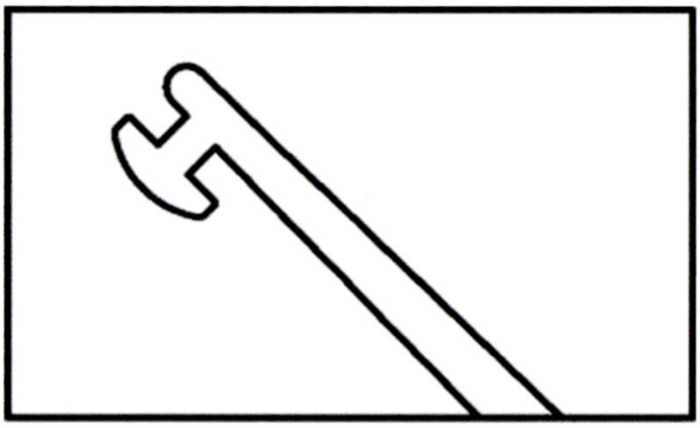

Fig. 14.1 A push–pull instrument, alternative Sinskey hook. Indication: Manipulator of nucleus, iris and IOL (Geuder 16,175)

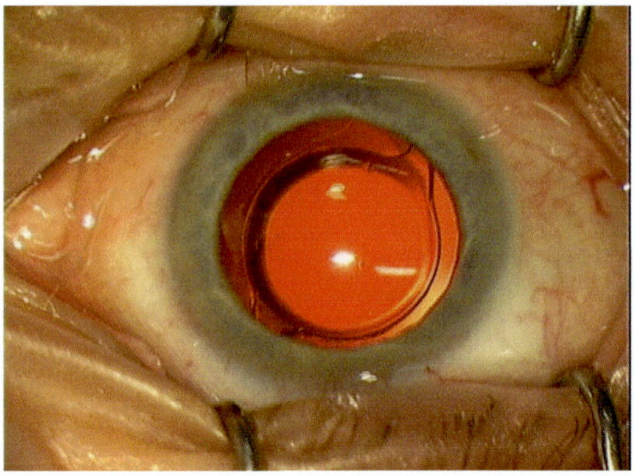

Fig. 14.3 Preoperative status. A highly myopic patient, who was dissatisfied with his postoperative refraction of + 1.0Y D

The surgery step-by-step:

(1) Paracentesis
(2) Injection of viscoelastics in capsular bag
(3) Opening of capsular bag

Begin with a paracentesis at 10 o'clock and 2 o'clock and a main incision at 9 o'clock. Inject viscoelastics into the anterior chamber (Fig. 14.3). Now comes the difficult part of surgery. Attach a 27G needle cannula on the viscoelastics cannula and bend the needle. Then inject viscoelastic between the anterior capsule and the IOL. Try to start at the haptics. Be cautious with the needle cannula: You can easily pierce the posterior capsule. As soon as you could inject a small bleb of viscoelastics switch the needle cannula to the regular cannula and open the capsular bag. This has to be done 360° (Figs. 14.4, 14.5 and 14.6).

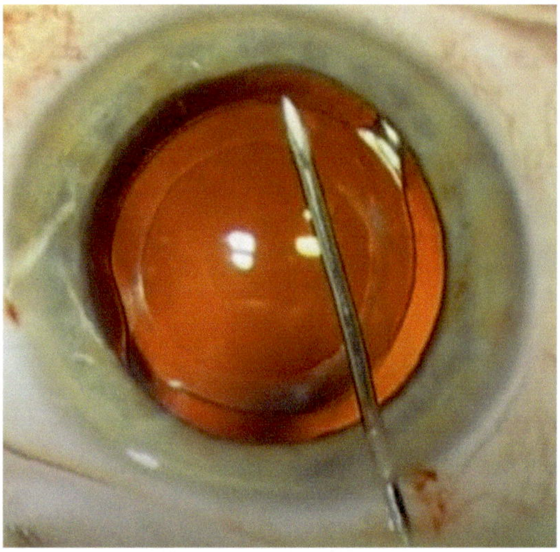

Fig. 14.4 A 27G cannula is attached to a viscoelastics syringe and opens the anterior lens capsule

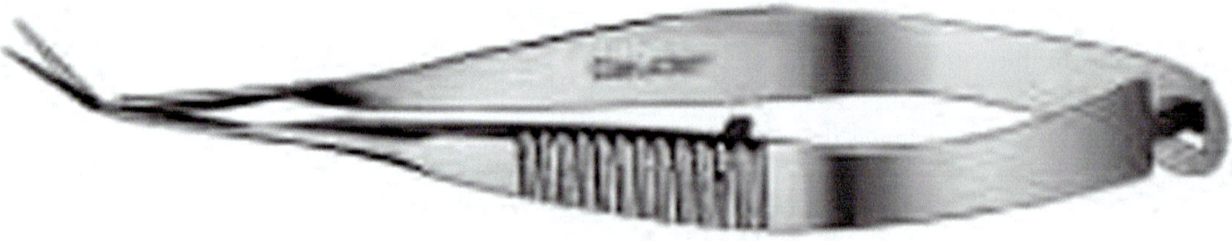

Fig. 14.2 Capsulotomy scissors. Indication: Cutting of an IOL (Geuder 19,776)

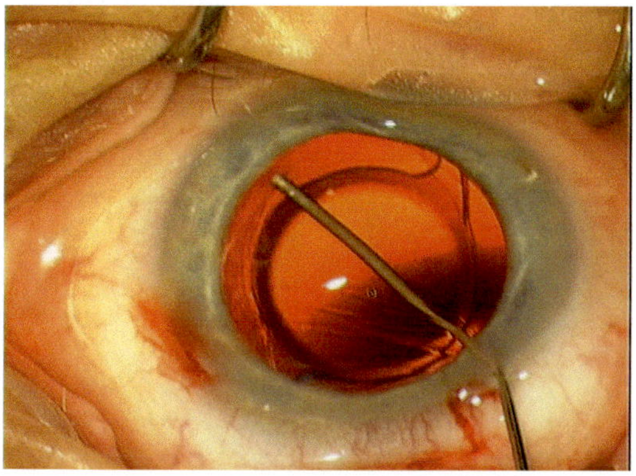

Fig. 14.5 Place the tip of the viscoelastic cannula between the anterior lens capsule and the IOL and inject viscoelastics in order to inflate the lens capsule

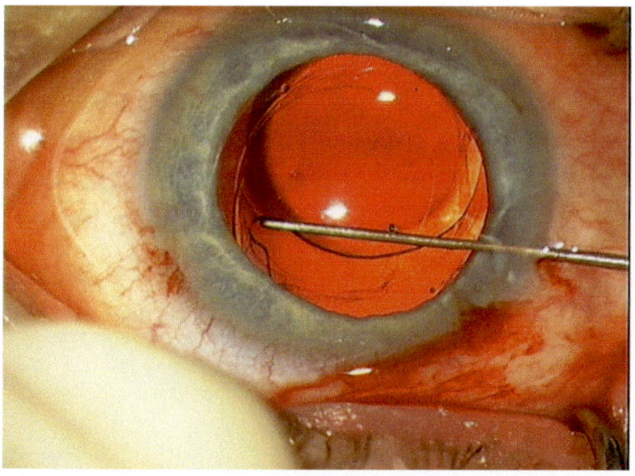

Fig. 14.6 Separate also the haptic from the lens capsule

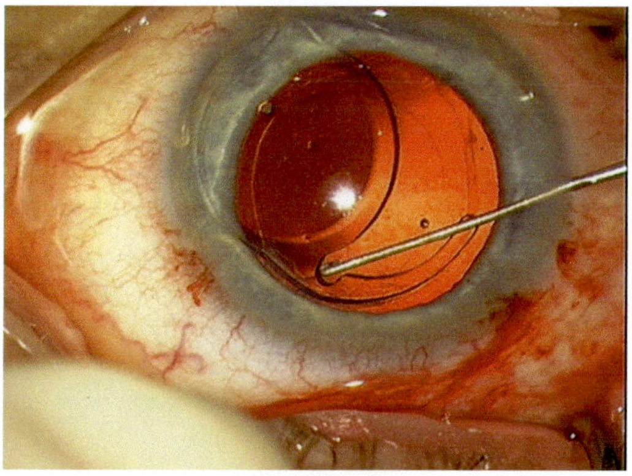

Fig. 14.7 Rotate the IOL out of the capsular bag with help of a push–pull or Sinskey hook. Inject viscoelastics behind the IOL to avoid a posterior capsular defect

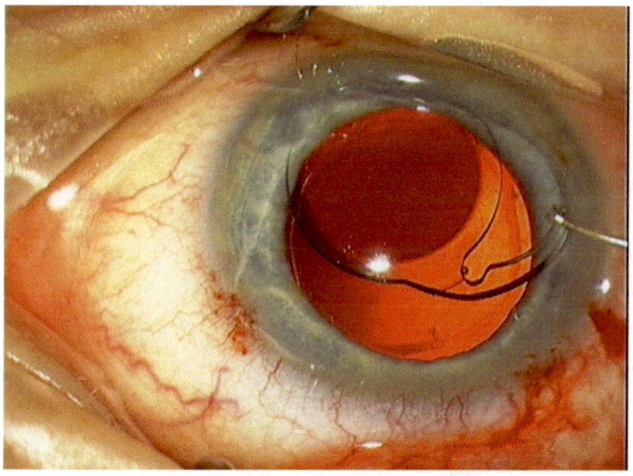

Fig. 14.8 Rotate a haptic towards the main incision

(4) Mobilisation of IOL
(5) Rotation of IOL on iris
(6) Cutting of IOL

Try cautiously to loosen the haptic with a push–pull manipulator or an iris spatula (Fig. 14.6). This manoeuvre is difficult at the haptics. If the IOL is mobilised, then rotate it outside the capsular bag (Fig. 14.7). Then luxate it with a rotational movement onto the iris (Fig. 14.8). The next step is the cutting of the IOL (Figs. 14.9, 14.11). Do not cut the IOL completely; leave 1–2 mm at the edge. Important regarding the cutting is that you begin to cut LEFT to the haptic (not right) (Fig. 14.12). From there you cut the optic into 2 halves but leave 1–2 mm at the end (Fig. 14.10).

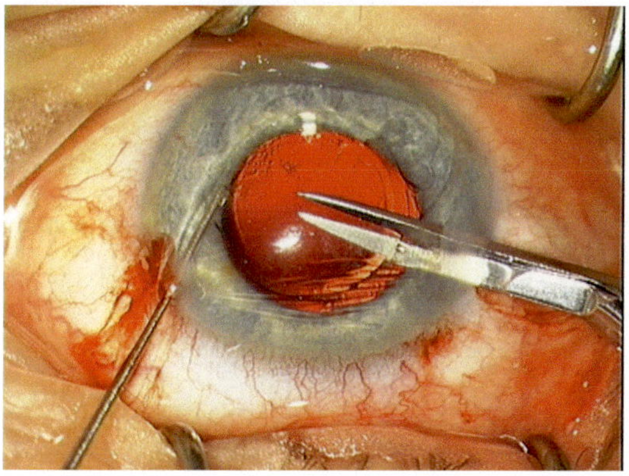

Fig. 14.9 Cut the IOL with the capsulotomy scissors

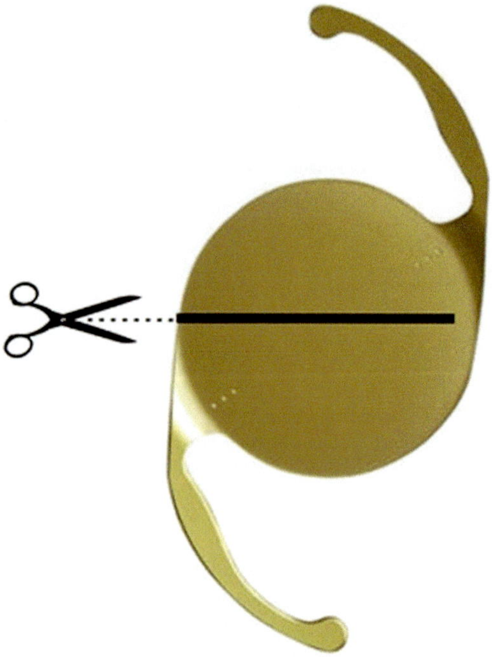

Fig. 14.10 Drawing how the IOL has to be cut. It is important to start the cutting on the left side (and not the right side) of the haptic

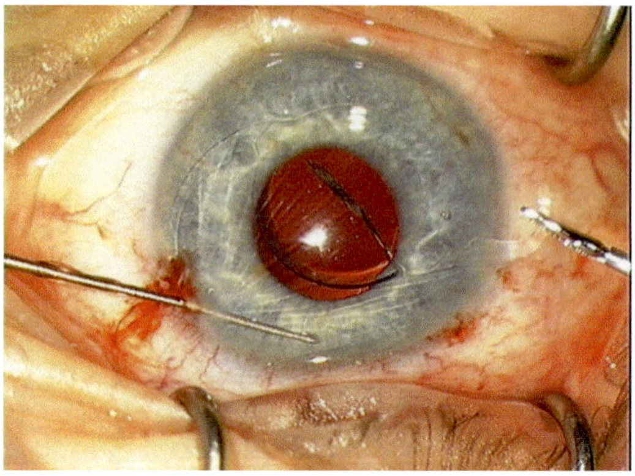

Fig. 14.12 Cut only 95% of the IOL. Then grasp the haptic with a surgical forceps

(7) Extraction of IOL
(8) Implantation of IOL

Pull the haptic through the main incision and then extract the first half of the optic, the second half of the optic follows automatically (Figs. 14.13 and 14.14). Implant finally the IOL

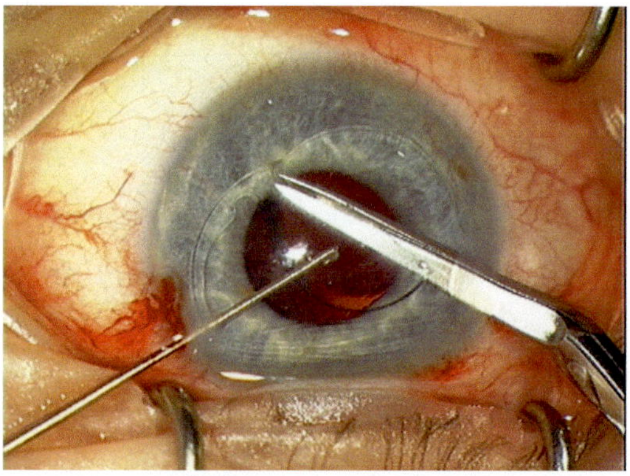

Fig. 14.11 If necessary, stabilize the IOL to avoid a damage of the endothelium

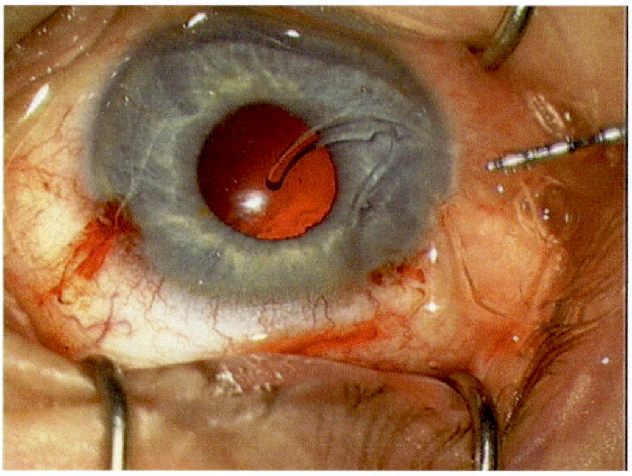

Fig. 14.13 Extract the first half of the IOL

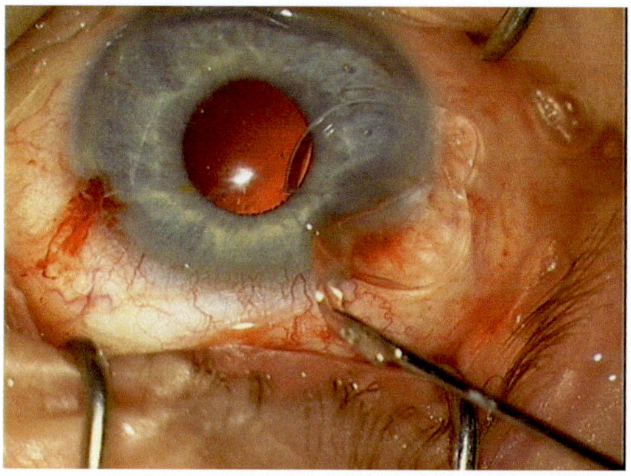

Fig. 14.14 Then extract the second half of the IOL

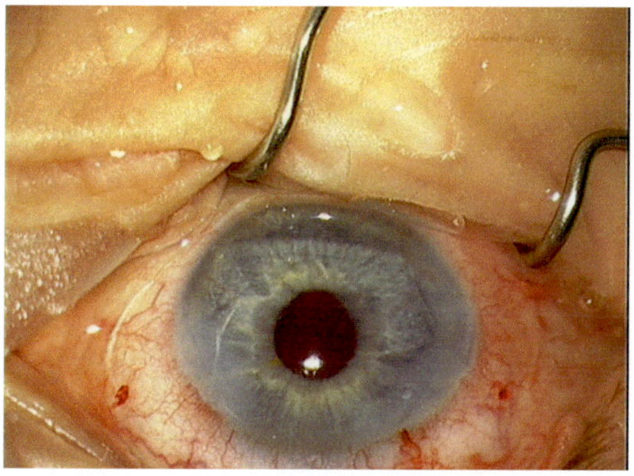

Fig. 14.15 Implant the new IOL into the bag

and inject cefuroxime as endophthalmitis prophylaxis (Fig. 14.15).

***Remark*:** The IOL extraction is easier if you cut the IOL in 4 quadrants.

Part VIII
Retina: Amniotic Membrane, Robotic Surgery

Vitreoretinal surgery has undergone dramatic changes in the last 10 years through the introduction of trocars. The most recent development the usage of amniotic membranes for indications such as macular hole, PVR perforations, optic disc pit and morning glory syndrome. Dr. Spandau from Stockholm, Sweden, will demonstrate a vitrectomy with usage amnion membrane in a patient with retinal detachment.

Will robotic surgery be the future in ocular surgery and replace the surgeon? Dr. Charles Mango from New York, USA, will report about the latest state of robotic technology for eye surgery.

Gene Therapy with Voretigene Neparvovec (Luxturna®) 15

Maximilian Gerhardt and Siegfried Priglinger

Abstract

Over the last decades, significant progress has been made in ocular gene therapy, culminating in the approval of Voretigene neparvovec, the first gene therapy for retinal dystrophies caused by biallelic mutations in the RPE65 gene, such as Leber congenital amaurosis type 2. This chapter provides an overview of the gene therapy Voretigene neparvovec explaining the therapy's structure, mechanism of action, and the surgical procedure involved. Furthermore, it highlights important considerations for planning, executing, and following up on the therapy.

Keywords

Luxturna · Leber congenital amaurosis · Voretigene neparvovec

M. Gerhardt (✉)
Department of Ophthalmology, LMU University Hospital, Ludwig-Maximilians Universität, München, Germany
e-mail: maximilian.gerhardt@med.uni-muenchen.de

S. Priglinger
Ludwig-Maximilians Universität, München, Germany

The Dawn of a New Era—Ocular Gene Therapy in Clinical Practice

Molecular biology has made remarkable strides in medicine over the past decades. Key technologies such as modern sequencing methods, gene manipulation, and gene transfer have paved the way for the development of gene therapy approaches. Advances in molecular genetic diagnostics have significantly expanded our understanding of hereditary eye diseases. Today, we are aware of more than 280 genes linked to inherited retinal conditions (https://sph.uth.edu/retnet). The eye's accessibility, the ability to administer low-dose drugs locally, and its partial immune privilege contribute to a reduced risk of toxic and immunogenic reactions compared to systemic treatments [1].These factors, along with the fact that many hereditary eye diseases are monogenic, have positioned ocular gene therapy at the forefront of the entire gene therapy field [2].

Molecular genetic analysis is an indispensable prerequisite for accurately diagnosing retinal dystrophies, as the various forms can only be properly classified at the molecular genetic level. Historically, classification was based on morphological appearance, autofluorescence, and functional characteristics, with many conditions named after their first describers. It is now understood that defects in different genes can produce a nearly identical clinical phenotype. Conversely, different mutations within the same

U. Spandau and G. B. Scharioth (eds.), *Cutting Edge of Ophthalmic Surgery*,
https://doi.org/10.1007/978-3-031-84204-7_15

gene can result in highly variable clinical presentations, often with significantly different disease progressions.

RPE65-Associated Inherited Retinal Diseases

In 1869, Theodor von Leber described a form of congenital blindness, marked by severely reduced vision before the age of one, nystagmus, reduced pupillary responses, and tapetoretinal degeneration [3]. Today, we know that Leber congenital amaurosis (LCA) encompasses a genetically diverse group of retinal diseases with varying forms and degrees of severity, all characterized by progressive loss of retinal function. More than 20 genes have been linked to this type of retinal dystrophy. The subtype of LCA (LCA2) that can be treated with the first and only approved ocular gene therapy, Voretigene neparvovec, is associated with mutations in the RPE65 (retinal pigment epithelium-specific 65kDa) gene, first reported by Marlhens et al. in 1997 [4]. This condition is typically inherited in an autosomal recessive manner. Affected individuals suffer from retinal degeneration, which typically involves early night blindness and visual field loss with vision progressively worsening over time, leading to legal blindness. Significant visual impairment may be present at birth, occur slightly later—as seen in severe early childhood-onset retinal dystrophy (SECORD)—or develop in early adulthood, as with the subtype of retinitis pigmentosa (RP20), leading to progressive and severe vision loss. Mutations in the RPE65 gene are found in an estimated 6% of LCA patients and approximately 2% of autosomal recessive retinitis pigmentosa cases [5–10].

Mechanism of Action and Molecular Structure of Voretigene Neparvovec

Voretigene neparvovec adresses mutations in the RPE65 (retinal pigment epithelium-specific) gene, which encodes the enzyme retinoid isomerohydrolase. Depending on the type of mutation in the RPE65 gene, varying degrees of functionally impaired proteins are being translated. The varying levels of residual enzyme activity are believed to account for the different clinical courses and symptoms observed in affected individuals. Retinoid isomerohydrolase, produced by the RPE65 gene, is a crucial enzyme in the visual cycle, playing a key role in regenerating 11-cis-retinal [11]. As a chromophore, 11-cis-retinal is an essential component of light-sensitive visual pigments (opsins), which function as light receptors critical for the visual process. If the enzyme's function is impaired or absent, the regeneration of 11-cis-retinal is disrupted, preventing light stimuli from being processed into a normal visual response. This continuous regeneration is necessary for the initiation and maintenance of phototransduction. Rods are particularly vulnerable since they are entirely dependent on the metabolic processes occurring in the retinoid cycle in order to regenerate 11-cis-retinal. As a result, rod dysfunction typically manifests as early night blindness and visual field loss. In contrast, cones can partially compensate by utilizing 11-cis-retinol from other sources like Müller cells, which, after being oxidized to 11-cis-retinal in the outer segments of photoreceptors, supports the visual cycle to some extent [12–15].

Voretigene neparvovec is a recombinant gene transfer vector that uses the capsid of an adeno-associated viral vector of serotype 2 (AAV2) as a transport vehicle for the coding sequence (cDNA) of human RPE65 and other regulatory elements including the chicken beta-actin (CBA) promoter combined with a cytomegalovirus (CMV) enhancer element (Fig. 15.2). This therapeutic principle is referred to as gene supplementation or gene augmentation therapy. Voretigene neparvovec is administered via subretinal injection and is taken up by RPE cells through receptor-mediated processes. Once taken up by the nucleus, the single-stranded cDNA is first converted into double-stranded DNA, which is transcribed into messenger RNA (mRNA) in a further step. The mRNA is subsequently translated in the cytosol, leading to the production of the corresponding protein, the enzyme retinoid isomerohydrolase (RPE65 protein) (Fig. 15.1).

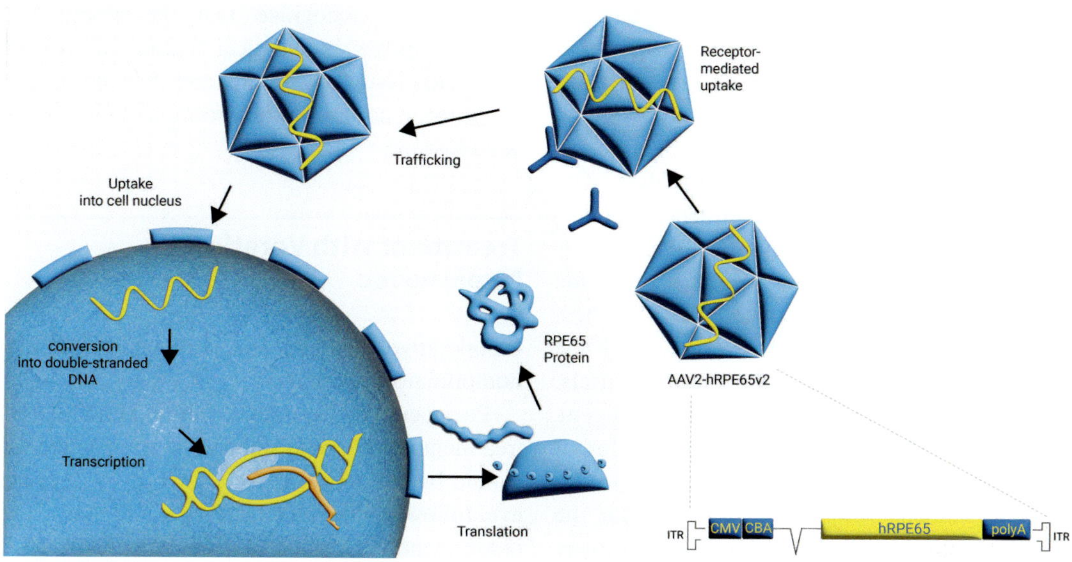

Fig. 15.1 Mechanism of action and molecular structure of Voretigene neparvovec (©LMU)

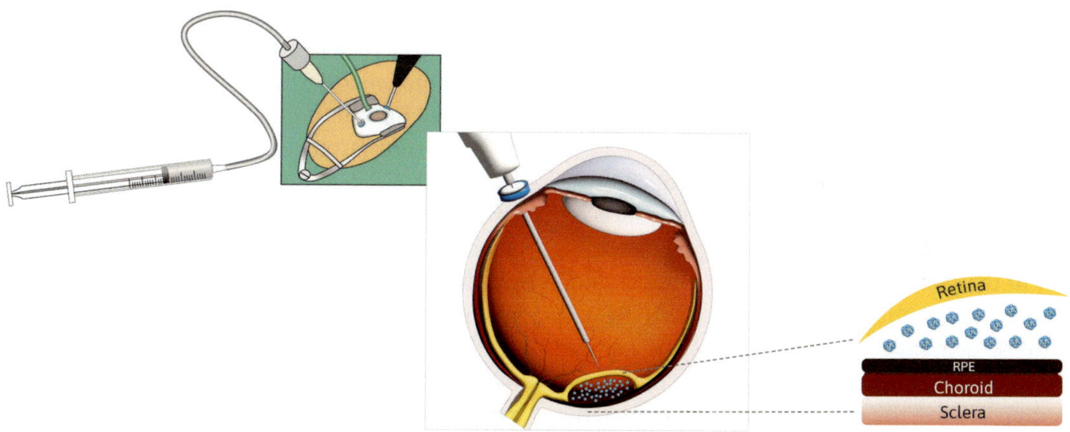

Fig. 15.2 Schematic Illustration of Voretigene neparvovec administration (©LMU)

The Pivotal Study of Voretigene Neparvovec

In the phase 3 study conducted between 2012 and 2015 in Philadelphia and Iowa, 20 patients were treated with Voretigene neparvovec at intervals of 6 to 18 days, while 9 additional patients completed the study as controls [16]. The primary endpoint was defined as the change in performance on the 'Multi-luminance Mobility Testing' (MLMT) course after one year. This test assessed the ability to navigate a course, partially equipped with obstacles, under varying standardized lighting conditions (ranging from 1 to 400 lx, across 7 possible lighting levels). The secondary endpoint measured changes in light sensitivity using the full-field light sensitivity threshold (FST) test, which employed white light in the pivotal study. Results indicated improvements in both functional vision and light sensitivity. For instance, 13 (65%) of the treated patients—but none from the control group—were able to complete the course at the lowest light level (1 lx) [16].

The treatment with Voretigene neparvovec is designed to provide long-term improvement in vision, but its exact duration of effect is still unknown due to lack of long-term data. The clinical trial outcomes of Voretigene neparvovec align with preclinical findings, demonstrating sustained results for up to 7.5 years in the full-field light sensitivity threshold (FST) test and 5 years in the multi-luminance mobility test (MLMT) from the Phase I and Phase III trials, respectively [16–19]. In conclusion, Voretigene neparvovec's therapeutic effect endures for at least a decade in animal models and up to 7.5 years in humans [20]. It is expected that the treatment may provide lasting benefits for many years, but it is unclear if all patients will maintain improvements indefinitely or if some might require additional interventions later in life.

Who Is Eligible for Treatment with Voretigene Neparvovec?

A fundamental requirement for treatment with Voretigene neparvovec is the identification of biallelic mutations in the RPE65 gene. In addition to the genetic finding and the clinical diagnosis of an inherited retinal dystrophy (IRD), it must be demonstrated that a sufficient number of functional retinal cells are still preserved. Comprehensive diagnostics, including imaging techniques such as optical coherence tomography (OCT) and fundus autofluorescence, along with functional assessments including best-corrected visual acuity (BCVA), perimetry, retinal sensitivity and electrophysiological assessments, play a crucial role in this evaluation. It is important to recognize that the absence of ERG responses is a typical feature of RPE65-associated retinal dystrophy and does not necessarily mean complete photoreceptor function has been lost [5].

Treatment with Voretigene Neparvovec

Preoperative planning and perioperative immunomodulatory therapy.

Perioperative systemic immunomodulatory treatment with prednisolone (or an equivalent) should be administered for a total of 17 days per eye, following the manufacturer's guidelines. The recommended regimen is detailed in Table 15.1. The purpose of perioperative immunosuppression is to minimize the risk of an immune response to the AAV2 vector capsid or the transgenic product, the retinal pigment epithelium-specific 65 kDa protein (RPE65). Prior to initiating immunomodulatory therapy and gene therapy, any active infectious disease in the patient should be ruled out. Conducting a differential blood count with CRP, hepatitis serology, and serology for toxoplasmosis, Lyme disease, and Syphilis is recommended. Additionally, an HIV test and a quantiferon test should be performed to rule out HIV infection and tuberculosis, respectively.

Surgical Administration of Voretigene Neparvovec

Gene therapy with Voretigene neparvovec requires special training and should only be performed by experienced retinal surgeons. Ideally, the surgeon should have expertise in

Table 15.1 Perioperative immunomodulatory regimen

Pre-operative	3 days prior to administration of Voretigene Neparvovec	Prednisone (or aequivalent) 1mg/kg bw/day (maximum daily dose: 40 mg)
Post-operative	4 days (including the day of administration)	Prednisone (or aequivalent) 1mg/kg bw/day (maximum daily dose: 40 mg)
	Followed by 5 days (on postoperative days 5–9)	Prednisone (or aequivalent) 0, 5 mg/kg bw/day (maximum daily dose: 20 mg)
	followed by 5 days with one dose given every two days	Prednisone (or aequivalent) 0, 5 mg/kg bw/day (maximum daily dose: 20 mg)

vitreoretinal surgery for children and adolescents, be proficient in subretinal injections, and be familiar with the intraoperative conditions and potential complications associated with dystrophic retinas. On the day of surgery, a strict schedule must be adhered to from the production and transport of the gene therapy drug to its intraoperative administration in the operating room. The preparation provided by the distributing pharmaceutical company consists of a concentrate and a solvent used to prepare the injection solution. It is delivered in a frozen state and must be stored at temperatures below −65 °C until it is ready for use. Typically, the hospital pharmacy (or alternatively, a trained laboratory) prepares the solution, ideally with prior experience in handling viral vectors. To be authorised to prepare and obtain Voretigene neparvovec, training provided by the manufacturer or distributing pharmaceutical company is mandatory.

Once thawed and prepared, Voretigene neparvovec must be surgically administered within 4 h. To achieve this, successful coordination and clear, timely communication between all parties involved—hospital pharmacy staff, transport service, anesthesiologists, operating room personnel, and surgeons—is essential. The gene therapy drug is supplied in two 1 ml syringes, each containing 0.8 ml of the prepared injection solution.

To administer Voretigene neparvovec, a pars plana vitrectomy is performed according to standard surgical practice, followed by a subretinal injection of the vector solution to deliver the gene therapy directly to the target cells, the retinal pigment epithelium (Fig. 15.2).

Particular attention should be paid to complete removal of the vitreous body at the posterior pole. This may involve the use of triamcinolone acetonide to enhance visualization of the vitreous. A circumscribed peeling of the internal limiting membrane (ILM) at the site of injection may be performed to reduce resistance during subretinal injection [21]. Prior to injection, the syringe containing the vector solution is connected to an injection cannula. It is then inserted into the eye through a vitrectomy trocar and placed onto the retina at least 2 mm away from the fovea, applying gentle pressure in the region of the superior vascular arch, the preferred site of injection. As per the manufacturer's guidelines, the same volume as used in the pivotal study, 0.3 ml of the injection solution (containing 1.5×10^{11} vector genomes) should be administered into the subretinal space. A small amount of the vector solution is slowly injected until the formation of a subretinal bleb becomes evident. The remaining volume is then gradually administered until the full 0.3 ml dose is delivered. This can be achieved manually with the aid of an assisting surgeon or using an electronically controlled injecting device. Before proceeding with the injection, the intraocular pressure must be reduced to 10 mmHg to decrease intraocular resistance and ensure that the subretinal injection is successful. It is crucial that the retina is not punctured by the subretinal injection needle during the initial injection attempt, but rather gently indented with light pressure. The retinotomy should be created solely by the pressure of the injection and should not be induced mechanically to minimize the risk of iatrogenic damage. When choosing the injection site, it is essential to avoid markedly atrophic areas or other retinal abnormalities such as scars or pigment epithelial clumping near the injection site, as these increase the risk of iatrogenic damage and injection failure. In general, the location and success of the injection can be assessed clinically. However, intraoperative optical coherence tomography (iOCT) offers high-resolution visualization, aiding in the safe administration of the vector solution by providing a detailed assessment of injection site, subretinal bleb, and any epiretinal changes that may be present [22, 23] (Fig. 15.3).

Following the administration of Voretigene neparvovec, a fluid-air exchange is obligatory. The purpose of this is twofold: first, to remove any injection solution that may have leaked into the vitreous cavity and to temporarily protect it from the anterior uveal structures using an air endotamponade; second, the air bubble may help further seal the retinotomy. At the end of surgery, sclerotomies should be sutured to prevent

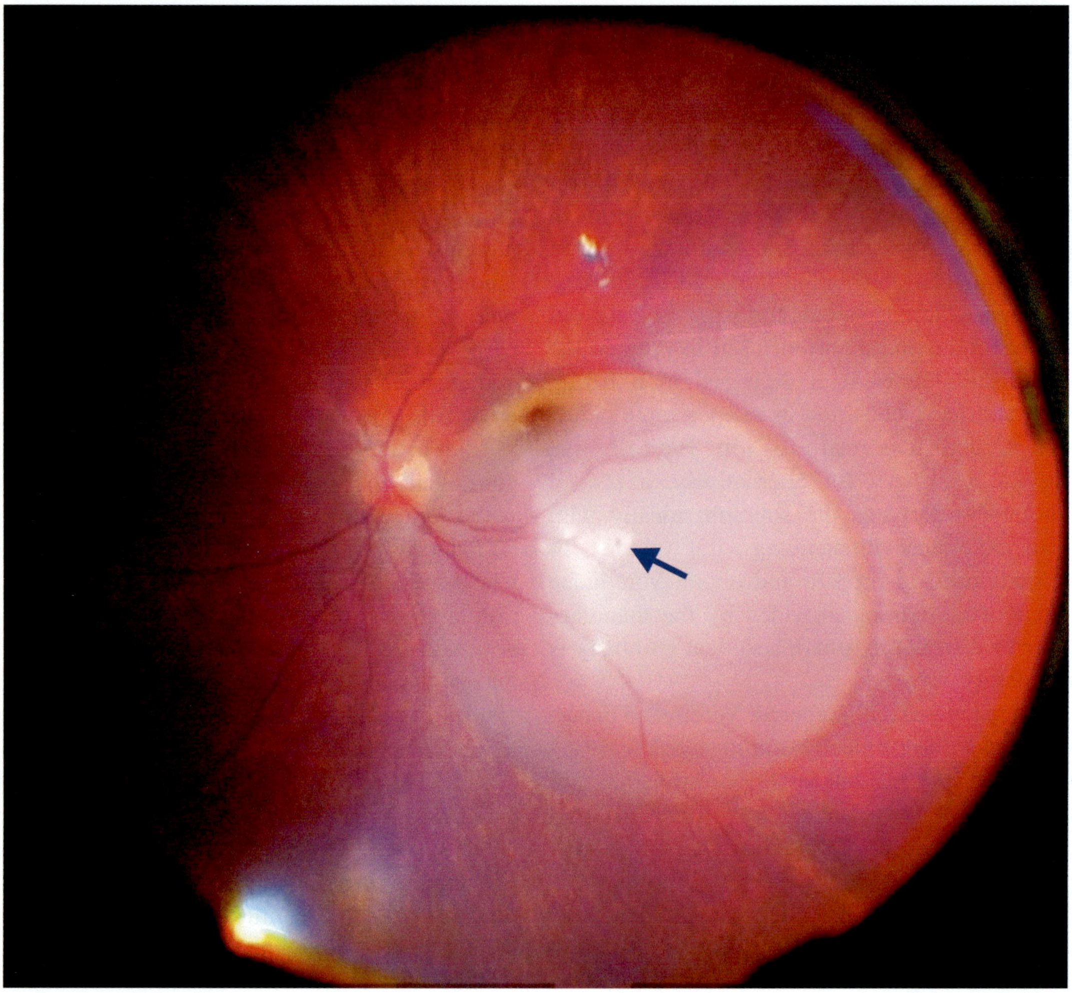

Fig. 15.3 Intraoperative view after subretinal injection of Voretigene neparvovec. Arrow indicates the injection site (surgeon's view. Image is inverted and laterally reversed, surgeon S. Priglinger ©LMU)

leakage of vitreous fluid. During the immediate postoperative course, the patient should remain in a flat, supine position, ideally until the following day.

Postoperative Care and Follow-Up

Postoperative treatment includes the administration of antibiotic and steroid eye drops as well as the continuation of systemic immunomodulatory therapy (Table 15.1). As generally recommended after vitreoretinal surgery, patients are advised to avoid strenuous activities, water exposure and air travel for the duration of the endotamponade to ensure proper healing and to reduce the risk of complications. Patients should monitor for any unusual symptoms such as increased pain, vision changes, or redness, and attend all follow-up appointments for proper recovery. Recommended follow-up appointments should be scheduled for days 1, 7, 14, and 30 after the operation, and then every three months in the first year. Treatment of the second eye should be dependent on the recovery process of the first eye and the patient's preference. In clinical practice, an interval of about 4 weeks from the first operation has proven to be useful and well tolerated by patients. The time between the two treatments should be no less than 6 days, as this was the shortest interval used in the pivotal study. Possible complications that may require treatment in the immediate postoperative period include increased intraocular inflammation (vitritis), increased intraocular pressure, and retinal detachment [21, 24]. These should be recognised and treated in a timely manner to ensure a favourable treatment outcome.

References

1. Willett K, Bennett J. Immunology of AAV-mediated gene transfer in the eye. Front Immunol. 2013;4:261.
2. Auricchio A, Smith AJ, Ali RR. The future looks brighter after 25 years of retinal gene therapy. Hum Gene Ther. 2017;28:982–7.
3. Leber T. Uber retinitis pigmentosa und angeborene amaurose. Graefes Arch Clin Exp Ophthalmol. 1869;15:1–25.
4. Marlhens FB, Griffoin C, Zrenner JM, Amalric E, Eliaou P, Liu C, Harris SY, Redmond E, Arnaud TM, Claustres B, Hamel MCP. Mutations in RPE65 cause Leber's congenital amaurosis. Nat Genet. 1997;17:139–41.
5. Gu S, Thompson DA, Srikumari CRS, Lorenz B, Finckh U, Nicoletti A, Murthy KR, Rathmann M, Kumaramanickavel G, Denton MJ, Gal A. Mutations in RPE65 cause autosomal recessive childhood-onset severe retinal dystrophy. Nature Genet. 1997;17:194–7.
6. Morimura H, Fishman GA, Grover SA, Fulton AB, Berson EL, Dryja TP. Mutations in the RPE65 gene in patients with autosomal recessive retinitis pigmentosa or Leber congenital amaurosis. Proc Nat Acad Sci. 1998;95:3088–93.
7. Chung DC, Traboulsi EI. Leber congenital amaurosis: clinical correlations with genotypes, gene therapy trials update, and future directions. J AAPOS. 2009;13:587–92.
8. den Hollander AI, Roepman R, Koenekoop RK, Cremers FP. Leber congenital amaurosis: genes, proteins and disease mechanisms. Prog Retin Eye Res. 2008;27:391–419.
9. Weleber RG, Michaelides M, Trzupek KM, Stover NB, Stone EM. The phenotype of Severe Early Childhood Onset Retinal Dystrophy (SECORD) from mutation of RPE65 and differentiation from Leber congenital amaurosis. Invest Ophthalmol Vis Sci. 2011;52(1):292–302.
10. O'Neill MJF, Stumpf AM. Retinitis Pigmentosa 20; RP20. Online Mendelian Inheritance in Man 2017. https://www.omim.org/entry/613794. Accessed 20 Aug 2019.
11. Redmond TM, et al. Rpe65 is necessary for production of 11-cis-vitamin A in the retinal visual cycle. Nat Genet. 1998;20(4):344–51.
12. Travis GH, Golczak M, Moise AR, Palczewski K. Diseases caused by defects in the visual cycle: retinoids as potential therapeutic agents. Annu Rev Pharmacol Toxicol. 2007;47:469–512.
13. Wang JS, Kefalov VJ. An alternative pathway mediates the mouse and human cone visual cycle. Curr Biol. 2009;19:1665–9.
14. Sato S, Kefalov VJ. Sis retinol oxidation regulates photoreceptor access to the retina visual cycle and cone pigment regeneration. J Physiol. 2016;594:6753–65.
15. Sato S, Frederiksen R, Cornwall MC, Kefalov VJ. The retina visual cycle is driven by cis retinol oxidation in the outer segments of cones. Vis Neurosci. 2017;34:E004.
16. Russell S, Bennett J, Wellman JA, Chung DC, Yu ZF, Tillman A, Wittes J, Pappas J, Elci O, McCague S, Cross D, Marshall KA, Walshire J, Kehoe TL, Reichert H, Davis M, Raffini L, George LA, Hudson FP, Dingfield L, Zhu X, Haller JA, Sohn EH, Mahajan VB, Pfeifer W, Weckmann M, Johnson C, Gewaily D, Drack A, Stone E, Wachtel K, Simonelli F, Leroy BP, Wright JF, High KA, Maguire AM. Efficacy and safety of voretigene neparvovec (AAV2-hRPE65v2) in patients with RPE65-mediated inherited retinal dystrophy: a randomised, controlled, open-label, phase 3 trial. Lancet. 2017;390:849–60.
17. Maguire AM, Simonelli F, Pierce EA, Pugh EN Jr, Mingozzi F, Bennicelli J, Banfi S, Marshall KA, Testa F, Surace EM, Rossi S, Lyubarsky A, Arruda VR, et al. Safety and efficacy of gene transfer for Leber's congenital amaurosis. N Engl J Med. 2008;358:2240–8. https://doi.org/10.1056/NEJMoa0802315.
18. Maguire AM, High KA, Auricchio A, Wright JF, Pierce EA, Testa F, Mingozzi F, Bennicelli JL, Ying GS, Rossi S, Fulton A, Marshall KA, Banfi S, et al. Age-dependent effects of RPE65 gene therapy for Leber's congenital amaurosis: a phase 1 dose-escalation trial. Lancet. 2009;374:1597–605. https://doi.org/10.1016/S0140-6736(09)61836-5.
19. Maguire AM, Russell S, Chung DC, Yu ZF, Tillman A, Drack AV, Simonelli F, Leroy BP, Reape KZ, High KA, Bennett J. Durability of Voretigene Neparvovec for Biallelic RPE65-mediated inherited retinal disease: phase 3 results at 3 and 4 years. Ophthalmology. 2021;128(10):1460–8. https://doi.org/10.1016/j.ophtha.2021.03.031.
20. Leroy BP, Fischer MD, Flannery JG, MacLaren RE, Dalkara D, Scholl HPN, Chung DC, Spera C, Viriato D, Banhazi J. Gene therapy for inherited retinal disease: long-term durability of effect. Ophthalmic Res. 2023;66(1):179–96. https://doi.org/10.1159/000526317.
21. Gerhardt MJ, Priglinger CS, Rudolph G, Hufendiek K, Framme C, Jägle H, Salchow DJ, Anschütz

A, Michalakis S, Priglinger SG. Gene therapy with Voretigene Neparvovec improves vision and partially restores electrophysiological function in pre-school children with Leber congenital Amaurosis. Biomedicines. 2022;11(1):103. https://doi.org/10.3390/biomedicines11010103. PMID: 36672611; PMCID: PMC9855623.

22. Xue K, Groppe M, Salvetti AP, MacLaren RE. Technique of retinal gene therapy: delivery of viral vector into the subretinal space. Eye (Lond). 2017;31(9):1308–16.

23. Vasconcelos HM Jr, Lujan BJ, Pennesi ME, Yang P, Lauer AK. Intraoperative optical coherence tomographic findings in patients undergoing subretinal gene therapy surgery. Int J Retina Vitreous. 2020;6(1):13. https://doi.org/10.1186/s40942-020-00216-1. PMID: 32377379; PMCID: PMC7193395.

24. Kessel L, Christensen UC, Klemp K. Inflammation after Voretigene Neparvovec administration in patients with RPE65-related retinal dystrophy. Ophthalmology. 2022;129(11):1287–93. https://doi.org/10.1016/j.ophtha.2022.06.018.

16 Amniotic Membrane in Retinal Surgery

Ulrich Spandau

Abstract

The usage of amniotic membranes is currently a hot topic in vitreoretinal surgery. The indications are a large macular hole, PVR perforations, optic disc pit and morning glory syndrome. We used an Optos photograph of the retina to determine the size of the amniotic membrane. The amniotic membrane consists of three layers; the epithelium, the stroma and the chorion. The latter has adhesive properties. Place the amniotic membrane with the sticky side (chorionic side) on the retina. The amniotic membrane is best fixated under the retina in order to prevent future dislocation. An epiretinal placement is necessary in pathologies such as optic disc pit or morning glory syndrome (Figs. 16.1, 16.2, 16.3, and 16.4). For epiretinal amniotic membranes a silicone oil tamponade is advisable because gas tamponades result often in dislocations.

Keywords

Amniotic membrane · Morning glory syndrome · Vitreoretinal surgery · Retinal surgery

Instruments

1. 25G trocars
2. Chandelier light
3. 25G endgripping forceps (Ultra Peel forceps, DORC)
4. PFCL
5. 23G MVR blade
6. Silicone oil (Figs. 16.1, 16.2, 16.3, and 16.4).

Individual Steps

(1) Insertion of trocars and chandelier light
(2) Vitrectomy
(3) External drainage of subretinal fluid
(4) Preparation of amniotic membrane
(5) Insertion of Amniotic membrane in vitreous cavity
(6) Correct placement of amniotic membrane
(7) Injection of PLCL or direct FAX to fixate the membrane
(8) Silicone oil tamponade.

U. Spandau (✉)
Stockholm University Hospital, Stockholm, Sweden
e-mail: ulrich_spandau@yahoo.de

U. Spandau and G. B. Scharioth (eds.), *Cutting Edge of Ophthalmic Surgery*,
https://doi.org/10.1007/978-3-031-84204-7_16

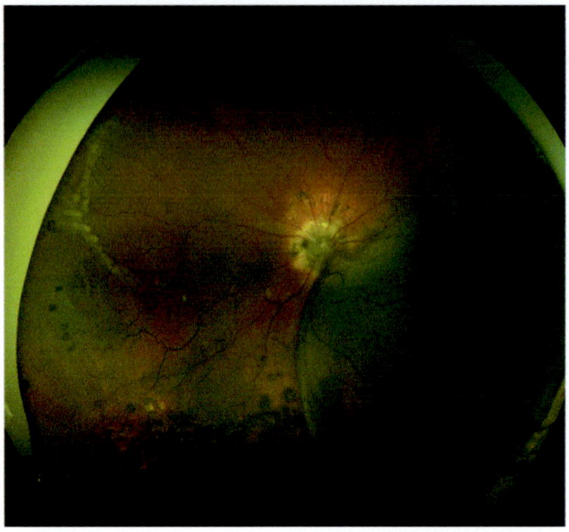

Fig. 16.1 Preoperative status of a retinal detachment with morning glory syndrome

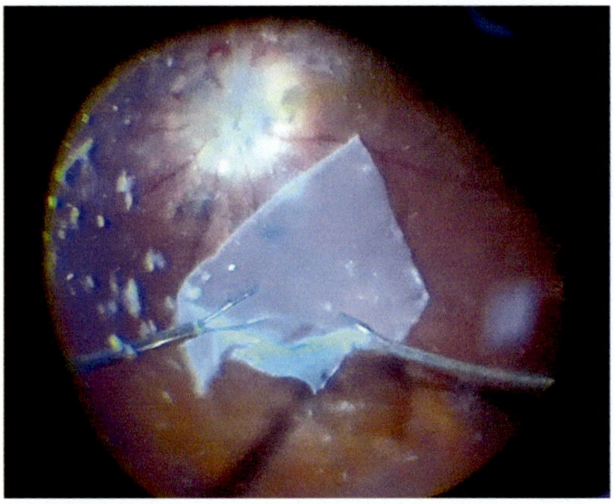

Fig. 16.2 Peroperative photograph of the amniotic membrane

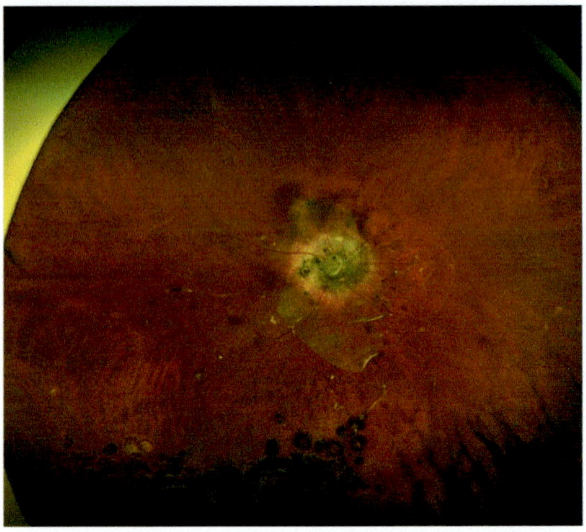

Fig. 16.3 7-months postoperative status

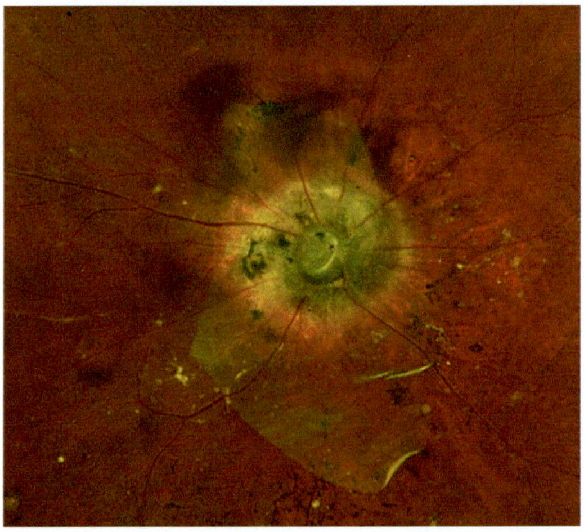

Fig. 16.4 7-months postoperative status. Note the amniotic membrane. The silicone oil was removed after ten months and the retina remains attached

The Surgery Step-by-Step

(1) Insertion of trocars and chandelier light

(2) Vitrectomy

Insert three 25G trocar cannulas and a chandelier light. A chandelier light is required for bimanual surgery. Proceed with a central vitrectomy. Induce a PVD, if necessary, stain the vitreous gel with triamcinolone. Continue with a peripheral vitrectomy.

(3) External drainage of subretinal fluid

The normal procedure would be the drainage of subretinal fluid from the retinal tear. In this case the break is located in the morning glory optic disc anomaly. In order to prevent an iatrogenic retinotomy I decided to perform an external drainage. Attach a 27G needle cannula onto a 3 cc syringe and pierce the sclera behind a bullous detachment. The subretinal fluid flows out the sclerotomy and the retina attaches.

(4) Preparation of amniotic membrane. Cut the amniotic membrane together with the paper and remove then the amniotic membrane from the paper with an endgripping forceps.
(5) Insertion of amniotic membrane in vitreous cavity
Mark the amniotic membrane at one corner with a "P" and mark the size with a caliper according to the Optos photograph. Then remove one 25G trocar, insert an endgripping forceps through the contralateral trocar cannula and externalise it through the sclerotomy (with removed trocar cannula). Feed the forceps with the amniotic membrane and internalise it into the vitreous cavity.
(6) Correct placement of amniotic membrane
(7) Injection of PLCL or direct FAX to fixate the membrane
Place the amniotic membrane with a forceps on the optic disc and inject cautiously a PFCL bubble onto the amniotic membrane. Observe that the "P" is correct. Remark: If you are not sure which side of the membrane is chorion you can find this out with a forceps (Fig. 16.2). The chorion side will attach to the forceps. Alternatively, perform a fluid against air exchange and position the amniotic membrane above the optic disc. Remark: The manipulation of the amniotic membrane is much easier under air than under PFCL.
(8) Silicone oil tamponade
Continue with a fluid against air exchange. Finalize surgery with 5000 cSt silicone oil tamponade.

Robotic Eye Surgery

17

Charles W. Mango, Angelo Tsirbas, and Jean-Pierre Hubschman

Abstract

Ophthalmology is a field at the forefront of innovation. Improvements in surgical instrumentation and refinements in surgical techniques have resulted in improved outcomes while decreasing operating time. Digital ultrahigh definition microscope utilization, real-time overlays of intraoperative OCT data, and automated laser assisted cataract surgery have been recent major contributions to our field. We believe the next revolution in ophthalmology will be the further development and acceptance of robotics.

Keywords

Robotic surgery · Surgical system · Vitreous cavity · Ocular surgery · Vinci surgical system

Introduction

Ophthalmology is a field at the forefront of innovation. Improvements in surgical instrumentation and refinements in surgical techniques have resulted in improved outcomes while decreasing operating time. Digital ultrahigh definition microscope utilization, real-time overlays of intraoperative OCT data, and automated laser assisted cataract surgery have been recent major contributions to our field. We believe the next revolution in ophthalmology will be the further development and acceptance of robotics.

Robotic Surgery History

A robot is a machine that can do the work of a person and that works automatically or is controlled by a computer [1]. Robotic surgery, or more precisely Robotic-assisted surgery had its beginnings 40 years ago with the development of the Arthrobot [2]. The robot, strapped to a

Will robotic surgery be the future in ocular surgery? Dr. Charles Mango from New York, USA, Jean-Pierre Hubschman from Los Angeles, USA, and Angelo Tsirbas from Sidney, Australia, will report on the latest state of robotic technology for eye surgery.

Supplementary Information The online version contains supplementary material available at https://doi.org/10.1007/978-3-031-84204-7_17.

C. W. Mango (✉)
Department of Ophthalmology, Weill Cornell Medical College Angelo, New York, NY, USA
e-mail: cmango@hotmail.com

A. Tsirbas · J.-P. Hubschman
Department of Ophthalmology at the David Geffen School of Medicine, University of California Los Angeles (UCLA), Los Angeles, CA, USA

U. Spandau and G. B. Scharioth (eds.), *Cutting Edge of Ophthalmic Surgery*,
https://doi.org/10.1007/978-3-031-84204-7_17

patient's leg, positioned the leg via voice commands from the surgeon. This allowed the surgeon to operate without the need of an assistant for this task. In 1985, the Puma Robot was used to assist in guiding a needle for a brain biopsy [3]. In 1992 the PROBOT was designed and utilized in the first robotic prostatic surgery. Also in 1992, ROBODOC, a robotic system designed to assist in hip replacement surgeries was developed [4]. ROBODOC was tasked with precisely carving out the femur during a hip replacement [5], improving the fitting process as compared to the prior method of carving the femur by hand.

Further development of medical robotic systems yielded the AESOP in 1994. It was a voice activated robot that was used to hold and position an endoscope. The surgeon would say: "AESOP move left" and the positioning arm would move until the "Stop" command was given. Building on this, the next generation ZEUS Robotic Surgical System was developed for microsurgery procedures such as suturing a beating heart [6].

In 2000, the Da Vinci Surgical System was approved for use by the US FDA [7]. The Da Vinci Surgical system incorporates a three-dimensional surgical monitor, a surgeon control area, and three robotic slave arms (Fig. 17.1). The robotic arms have seven degrees of movement that allow for the surgeon's wrist and finger motions to be precisely mimicked. Each of the robotic arms can be equipped with a variety of instrumentation to allow for specialized surgical procedures. The monitor and surgeon control area can be separated from the robotic slave arm portion of the machine allowing for remote surgery. This remains the current and most widely used system to our present day. Mainstream use of robotics using this surgical platform have overtaken the fields of Urology [8–11], Gynecology [12, 13], and Cardiovascular surgery [14–16].

Robotic Eye Surgery History

Robotic eye surgery has a relatively short history compared to robotic surgery in general. Whereas other surgical fields have accumulated a significant clinical experience using robotic surgery on patients, the focus of Ophthalmic surgeons has been on demonstrating the feasibility of specific ocular procedures using a robot in a laboratory setting. There are several reasons for this cautious approach to robotic acceptance in the field of Ophthalmology. Ocular surgery already employs minimally invasive techniques providing rapid recovery and excellent outcomes. Eye surgeons have good control and excellent views with the current standard of optical microscopes. Lastly, maneuverability of ophthalmic instruments poses little problem for experienced surgeons with trained hands.

Robotic surgery has addressed the limitations of traditional surgery in other surgical disciplines. Benefits of this system, compared to traditional surgery have demonstrated increased precision, improved range of motion, tremor elimination, increased surgeon safety, and ability to maneuver in confined anatomic spaces [17–21]. These are all central facets to advancement in any surgical field and by extension to ocular surgery. In other words, there is always room for improvement for surgeon control, safety, and patient outcomes in any surgical field.

In 1989, Guerrouad and Vidal described and developed the first robot dedicated to eye surgery, the Stereotaxical Microtelemanipulator (SMOS). The SMOS included a spherical micromanipulator that provided for 6 degrees of freedom. It demonstrated improved accuracy of specific tasks compared to manual surgery, but was slower [22].

The Robot Assisted MicroSurgery (RAMS) workstation developed by Steve Charles and collaborators with NASA's Jet Propulsion Laboratory was first described in 1997 [23].

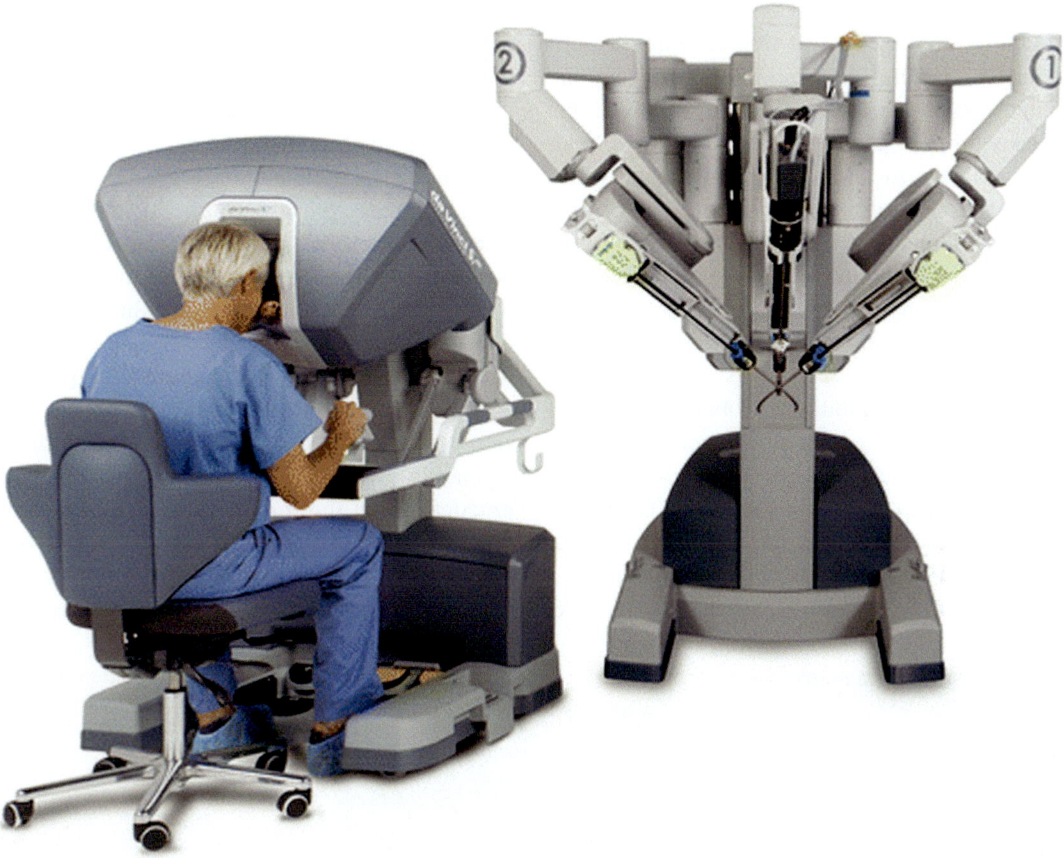

Fig. 17.1 Da Vinci Surgical System showing surgeon looking into console viewer, robot with arms separated physically from surgeon's console (Image courtesy of Intuitive Surgical)

The RAMS workstation is a compact robot that allowed for extensive precision of movement down to 15 microns along with motion scaling, that is where large movements in the surgeon's hand are translated to micro-movements by the robot.

At the same time, Northwestern University developed a robot that allowed for retinal vessel cannulation inside a cat's eye. The retinal vessels ranged in internal diameter from 20 to 130 microns [24].

In 1998, Yu et al. developed a patented spherical manipulator, similar to the SMOS, specifically to demonstrate feasibility off intraretinal vascular drug delivery, implantation of ocular microdrainage devices and the intraretinal manipulation of microelectrodes. These tasks were successfully carried out with minimal tissue damage in a laboratory setting [25].

Japanese collaborators created a prototype robotic system based on the SMOS platform that was designed to aid in multiple specific tasks of vitreoretinal surgery [26]. This robot facilitated successful surgical induction of a posterior vitreous detachment, retinal vessel sheathotomy using 25-gauge microscissors, and microcannulation of retinal vessels with a diameter of 100 microns in porcine eyes.

Investigators at Johns Hopkins University developed a steady hand manipulator (SHM) for retinal microsurgery [27]. The design places the pivot point of the articulating probe at the sclera (as it would be in traditional vitreoretinal surgery), Placing the remote center of motion (RCM) at this location minimizes undesirable tension on the eye wall. The SHM provided filtration of tremor that was demonstrated experimentally. Further innovations by this group include intra-operative retina registration that syncs with pre-operative imaging to guide treatment delivery to a specific point on the retina [28]. The Micron, a microsurgical tool that reduces unintentional tremor while preserving eye-hand coordination was also developed and tested. Surgeons experienced up to 52% reduction in error in validation experiments using the Micron [29].

In 2006 the feasibility of robotic ocular surgery and robotic ocular telesurgery using the Da Vinci Surgical System was demonstrated through a series of studies [30, 31]. The experiments were performed on harvested porcine eyes placed in an anatomical position using a foam head on a standard operating room table. Visualization of the eye was achieved with a 3D endoscope camera directly above the globe, thus mimicking a view through a standard operating microscope. The 2 robotic arms were placed on either side of the globe at a 45-degree angle, resembling the same approach used by a surgeon to maximize exposure to the ocular surface. The surgeons performed the procedures while positioned at the surgeon control area that was located across the operating room suite. External ocular surgery (cornea suture laceration repair) was performed and deemed feasible (Fig. 17.2). Anterior segment procedures (clear cornea incision creation and anterior capsule capsulorhexis formation) were performed and felt not to be practical given the impossibility to position the remote center of motion at the fulcrum, which caused undue tissue strain. Posterior segment procedures (core vitrectomy and trocar insertion

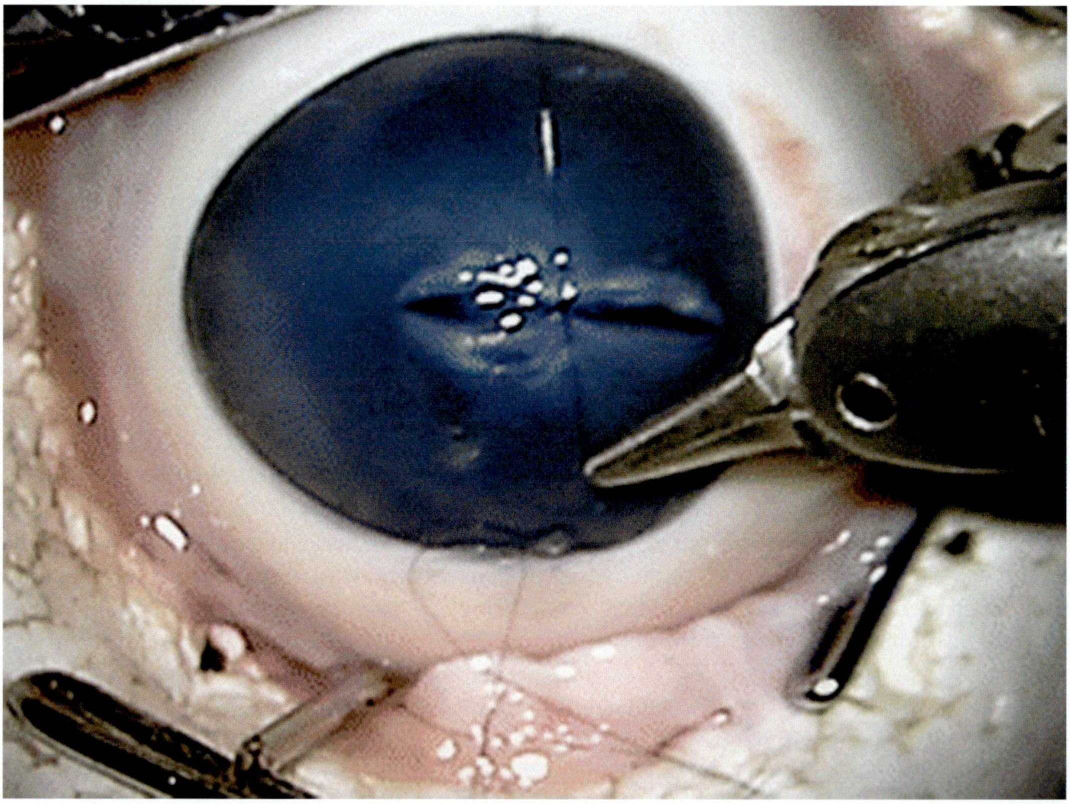

Fig. 17.2 Surgeon's view through the Da Vinci Surgical System showing suture closing of a corneal laceration. A black diamond robotic micro-forcep (controlled by robotic arm) is shown holding one end of the suture. The other robotic micro-forcep is out of the picture frame holding the other end of the suture (Image courtesy of A Tsirbas)

/ removal) proved possible, although limitations were noted secondary visualization (difficult view of posterior chamber) and robotic arm issues that did not allow for refined movements within the vitreous cavity.

We have learned over these past several decades that robotics lends itself to ocular surgery in unique ways compared with other surgical disciplines. Tactile feedback mechanisms are advantageous for other surgical fields but are not a necessity for eye surgery. Ocular surgeons rely primarily on visualization as their main tool for performing delicate intraocular tasks. Tremor elimination and motion scaling mechanisms are very important in a microsurgical field involving the eye [21, 32]. Within the confines of the orbit and eyeball, each movement needs to be precise and tremor free. Tremor reduction and motion scaling components of some of these robotic systems has demonstrated this advantage be employed in eye surgery.

Robotic Eye Surgery Today (Video 14.1)

Recent advancements have been made to overcome some of the cumbersome limitations of using the Da Vinci Surgical System.

In order to allow for a more natural vitrector motion by placing the remote center of motion at the fulcrum, a smaller micro robot, the Hexapod Surgical System (HSS) was created [33]. The HSS is mounted to an arm of the Da Vinci Surgical System. The precision and dexterity of this approach was validated by successful insertion of a vitreous cutter through a sclerotomy in porcine eyes.

A robotic forceps advancement, the "Micro hand," was developed to allow for a membrane peeling function necessary in many types of vitreoretinal surgeries [34]. This device was designed to mimic a human hand and is pneumatically controlled, allowing titration of grasping force. Four fingers, with a length of 4 mm each, were used to manipulate fresh retinal tissue of porcine cadaver eyes.

Steerable micro-robots with an outer diameter of less than 500 μm were created and injected through a 23 g needle into the vitreous cavity of cadaver porcine eyes. Using a wireless electromagnetic control headset, researchers were able to achieve coordinated movement of the robots and targeted placement along the retina surface [35]. These micro-robots may act as a future drug delivery system that can be moved to a specific place in the eye (once injected into the eye) using robot steering technology.

Retinal vascular cannulation robots that allow for telemanipulation have been developed [36, 37]. Preliminary feasibility testing shows that this outperforms standard vascular cannulation. An integrated robotic intraocular snake, a submillimeter intraocular dexterous robot prototype has been built [38]. It can eventually be utilized as a steerable needle, steerable forceps, or steerable cannula.

The Intraocular Robotic Interventional Surgical System (IRISS) is a dedicated microsurgical platform capable of performing complete ophthalmic procedures [39]. The design features a remote console which could facilitate telesurgery. The IRISS design includes a head-mounted stereoscopic visualization system, two joystick controls with tremor filtration and scaled motion, custom designed arms appropriately sized to accommodate commercially available instrumentation, and two closely approximated remote centers of motion (pivot points) to reduce tissue stress at the point of ocular entry (Figs. 17.3 and 17.4). Recent trials have focused on three complex ocular procedures: lens capsulorhexis in cataract surgery, 23-gauge core vitrectomy, and retinal vein cannulation. The team is currently developing automated capabilities of the IRISS platform for cataract surgery.

The PRECEYES Surgical System is a prototype robotic system that is being developed primarily for vitreoretinal surgery [40]. It is mounted at the side of the head during vitrectomy surgery and can be brought into place and used as needed (Fig. 17.5). It functions to scale down movements for better precision, filters out tremors, and allows the instrument to freeze in place if the surgeon's hand relaxes. This robotic system is going to be tested for its ability to deliver gene therapy into the subretinal space for a variety of inherited disorders [41].

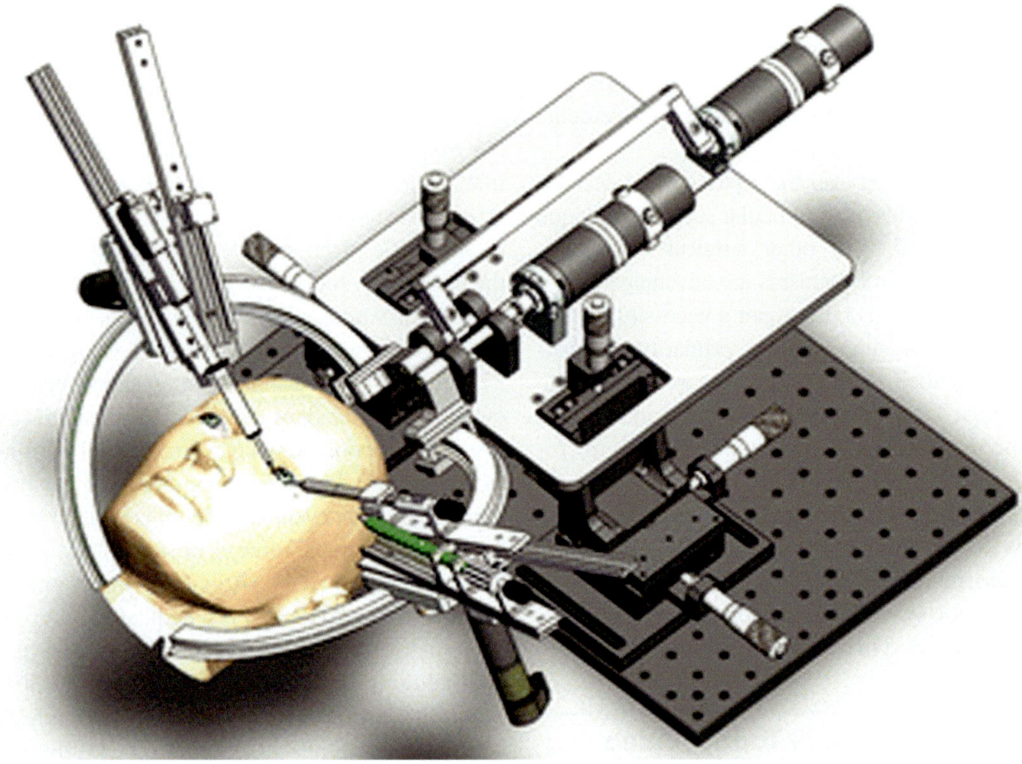

Fig. 17.3 Intraocular Robotic Interventional Surgical System (IRISS) schematic view: custom designed arms appropriately sized to accommodate commercially available instrumentation, and two closely approximated remote centers of motion (pivot points) to reduce tissue stress at the point of ocular entry (Image courtesy of JP Hubschman)

In 2015, the first human case of robot assisted eye surgery, a pterygium removal, was performed on a 73-year-old patient using the DaVinci robotic surgical system [42].

Today we realize ocular surgery is a field that continues to benefit from incremental advances in robotic technology. Improved instrument engineering, precision scaled movements, integrated tremor reduction, and improved maneuverability are all key advancements that robotic integration currently provides.

Robotic Eye Surgery of the Future

The feasibility of telesurgery was demonstrated in 2001 when Marescaux and colleagues performed the first transatlantic robotically assisted surgery on an animal model [43]. This was followed by the first transatlantic robotically assisted laparoscopic cholecystectomy in a human being [44]. Since then, telesurgery has been demonstrated successfully on multiple occasions [45]. Ocular robotic telesurgery may also be feasible, bringing emergency eye care to distant and hard-to-reach locales, such as an isolated island or war torn nation.

In 2016, the Smart Tissue Autonomous Robot (STAR) demonstrated for the first time the ability of a fully autonomous robot to suture up intestine on a live pig [46]. Autonomy would be a logical next step in robotic eye surgery. Performing routine and replicative tasks such as trocar insertions, infusion connection, and trocar removal could save the surgeon valuable time and energy on each case. Future advancements

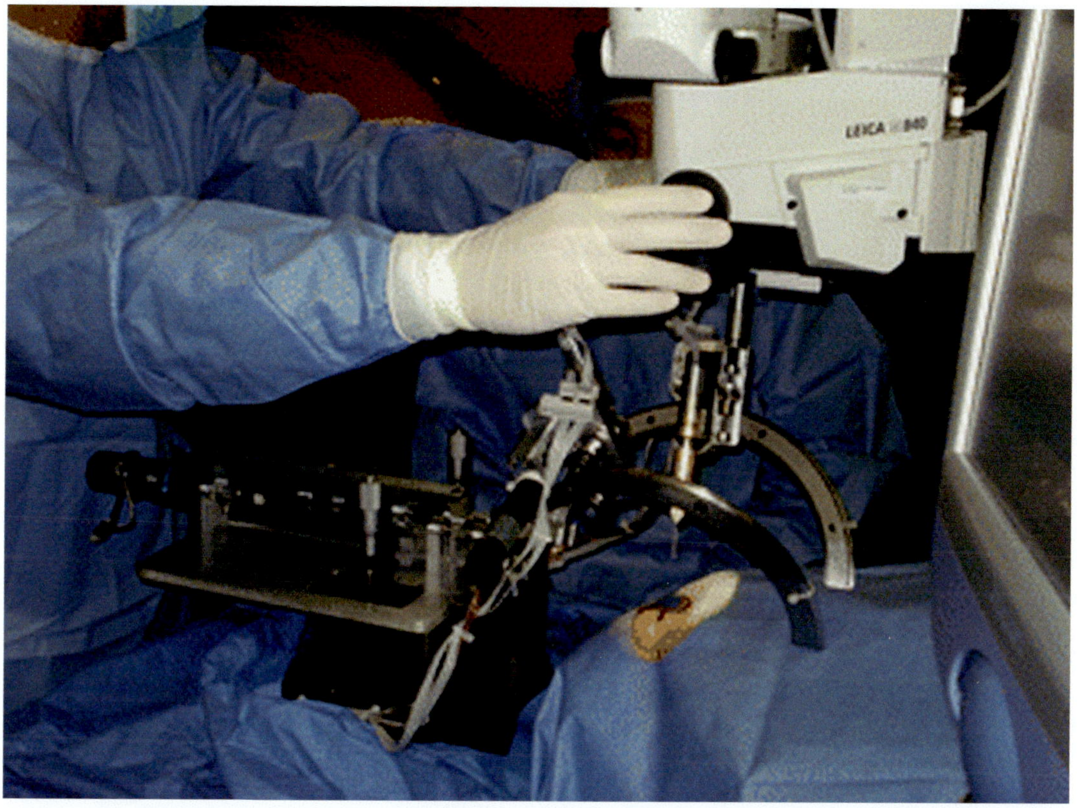

Fig. 17.4 Intraocular Robotic Interventional Surgical System (IRISS) working prototype (Image courtesy of JP Hubschman)

in sensor technology that prevents the vitreous cutter from hitting the retina would allow for a core vitrectomy to be an automated task. Perhaps 1 day, even the most delicate vitreoretinal surgical tasks such as internal limiting membrane peeling will be an automated experience.

Visualization improvements may be the next forefront that dovetails with robotic advancements. 3D ultra-high definition displays with overlayed intraoperative OCT data are already present. Perhaps a full immersion with virtual reality headsets will be the next frontier providing the ability to look around from inside the vitreous cavity. A miniature robotic controlled camera mounted on the end of a vitrector probe would allow for this experience. The surgeon would be able to virtually stand in the vitreous cavity and look up at the underside of the iris simply by looking upwards with virtual reality goggles on. Every structure of the eye would be within potential view and accessible to surgical intervention.

Tele-mentoring is the creation of a virtual classroom, and current robotic and audio/visual infrastructure allows for this to exist. In the first demonstration of tele-mentoring, a laparoscopic colectomy was performed by a novice surgeon taking instructions from an expert surgeon located across a medical campus [47]. Since then, tele-mentoring has been implanted across continents with improving success [48–53]. Ocular surgery lends itself well to the mentoring process as one-on-one training has been the standard over time. It is easy to envision a senior ocular surgeon lending real-time advice (via audio/visual connection) and providing control assistance (via robotic connection) to a novice surgeon located at a remote site.

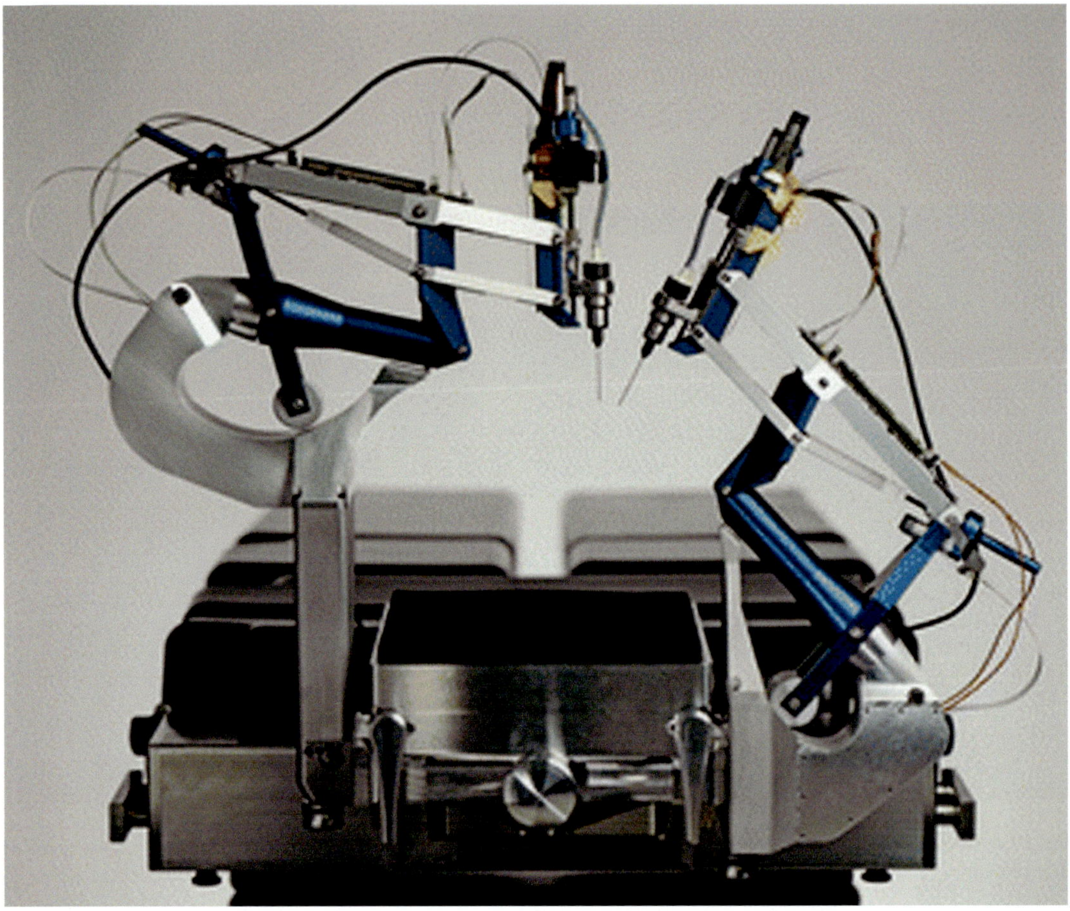

Fig. 17.5 PRECEYES Surgical System prototype showing how it is mounted on the side of the patient's head rest (Image courtesy of PRECEYES)

Conclusion

There are many benefits to the integration of robotics into the field of Ophthalmic surgery. The first advantage is improved precision. Tremor reduction and motion scaling components of current robotic systems allow for this. Whether cannulating a retinal vein or grasping an epiretinal membrane, robotic assistance improves upon traditional manual methods at these tasks. Safety is another benefit that is enhanced with robotic surgery. By means of operating at a distance, the surgeon should rarely come into direct contact with any sharps. This reduces the risk of a surgeon injury considerably and is especially relevant when operating on patients with communicable disease. Lastly, the ability to enhance already excellent visualization platforms by augmenting additional data is a tremendous benefit.

While recognized engineering challenges persist, advancements in ocular robotic surgical systems are forthcoming. Future advances such as autonomic surgical tasks will allow for surgeons to save their energy to focus on the most critical aspects of the procedure while the robot performs the routine portions. Expansion of telesurgery and tele-mentoring capabilities beyond what we have now will enable teaching and assisting others throughout the world.

Ophthalmology has always been an innovative field. With current robotic technology and forward thinking ideas, the potential for the future is unlimited.

References

1. [Robot]. In Merriam Webster Online, Retrieved May 9, 2016, from http://www.merriam-webster.com/dictionary/citation
2. Medical Post 23: 1985 (PDF)
3. YS Kwoh J Hou EA Jonckheere S Hayall 1988 A robot with improved absolute positioning accuracy for CT guided stereotactic brain surgery IEEE Trans Biomed Eng 35 2 153 61
4. AR Lanfranco AE Castellanos JP Desai WC Meyers 2004 Robotic surgery Ann Surg 239 1 14 21
5. J Pransky 1997 ROBODOC—a surgical robot success story Indust Robot Int J. 24 3 231 3
6. Meadows, Michelle. Computer-assisted surgery: an update. FDA Consumer magazine. Food and Drug Administration. Archived from the original on 9 May 2016
7. A Labontiu 2001 The da Vinci surgical system performing computer-enhanced surgery Osp Ital Chir. 7 367 72
8. JP Ruurda IAMJ Broeders RPM Simmermacher 2002 Feasibility of robot-assisted laparoscopic surgery Surg Laparosc Endosc Percutan Tech. 2002 12 41 5
9. R Kumar AK Hemal 2005 Emerging role of robotics in urology J Min Access Surg. 1 202 10
10. P Dasgupta B Challacombe D Murphy 2006 (2006) Coming full circle in robotic urology BJU Int 98 4 5
11. S Kaul R Laungani R Sarle 2007 Da Vinci-assisted robotic partial nephrectomy: technique and results at a mean of 15 months of follow-up Eur Urol 51 186 91
12. C Diaz-Arrastia C Jurnalov G Gomez C Townsend Jr 2002 Laparoscopic hysterectomy using a computer-enhanced surgical robot Surg Endosc 2002 16 1271 3
13. Beste TM, Nelson KH, JA D. Total laparoscopic hysterectomy utilizing a robotic surgical system. J Soc Laparoendosc Surg. 2005;9:13–5
14. MR Katz F Praet Van D Canniere de 2006 Integrated coronary revascularization: percutaneous coronary intervention plus robotic totally endoscopic coronary artery bypass Circulation 114 473 6
15. RS McClure B Kiaii RJ Novick 2006 Computer-enhanced telemanipulation in mitral valve repair: preliminary experience in Canada with the da Vinci robotic system Can J Surg 49 193 6
16. AP Kypson WR Chitwood 2006 Robotic cardiovascular surgery Expert Rev Med Devices 3 335 43
17. M Hashizume K Konishi N Tsutsumi 2002 A new era of robotic surgery assisted by a computer-enhanced surgical system Surgery 2002 131 S330 3
18. SM Prasad SM Prasad HS Maniar 2004 Surgical robotics: impact of motion scaling on task performance J Am Coll Surg 199 863 8
19. JD Hernandez SD Bann Y Munz 2004 Qualitative and quantitative analysis of the learning curve of a simulated surgical task on the da Vinci system Surg Endosc 18 372 8
20. K Moorthy Y Munz A Dosis 2004 Dexterity enhancement with robotic surgery Surg Endosc 18 790 5
21. M Gomez-Blanco CN Riviere PK Khosla 2000 Intraoperative tremor monitoring for vitreoretinal microsurgery Stud Health Technol Inform. 70 99 101
22. Guerrouad A, Vidal P SMOS: stereotaxical microtelemanipulator for ocular surgery. In: Engineering in medicine and biology society, 1989. images of the twenty-first century, proceedings of the annual international conference of the IEEE engineering in 1989. IEEE; 1989. p. 879–80
23. S Charles H Das T Ohm 1997 Dexterity-enhanced telerobotic microsurgery Adv Robotics 1997 5 10
24. PS Jensen KW Grace 1997 Toward robot-assisted vascular microsurgery in the retina Graefes Arch Clin Exp Ophthalmol 235 11 696 701
25. Yu DY, Cringle SJ, IJ C. Robotic ocular ultramicrosurgery. Sust N Z J Ophthalmol. 1998;26(Suppl 1):S6–8
26. Uneri A, Balicki MA, Handa J, Gehlbach P, Taylor RH, et al. (2010) New steady-hand eye robot with micro-force sensing for vitreoretinal surgery. In: 2010 3rd IEEE RAS and EMBS international conference on biomedical robotics and biomechatronics
27. B Mitchell J Koo I Iordachita P Kazanzides A Kapoor 2007 Development and application of a new steady-hand manipulator for retinal surgery IEEE ICRA. 2007 623 9
28. Fleming IN, Voros S, Vagvolgyi B, Pezzementi Z, Handa J, et al. Intraoperative visualization of anatomical targets in retinal surgery. In: Applications of computer vision, IEEE workshop;2008:1–6
29. RA MacLachlan BC Becker JC Tabarés GW Podnar LA Lobes 2012 Micron: an actively stabilized handheld tool for microsurgery IEEE Trans Robotics 28 195 212
30. A Tsirbas C Mango E Dutson 2007 Robotic ocular surgery Br J Ophthalmol 91 18 21
31. DH Bourla JP Hubschman M Culjat A Tsirbas A Gupta 2008 Feasibility study of intraocular robotic surgery with the da Vinci Surgical System Retina 28 154 8
32. Riviere CN, Jensen PS. A study of instrument motion in retinal microsurgery. In: 21st Annual conference of IEEE engineering medicine and biology social. Chicago; 2000
33. JL Bourges JP Hubschman J Wilson S Prince TC Tsao 2011 Assessment of a Hexapod surgical system for robotic micro-macro manipulations in ocular surgery Ophthalmic Res 46 25 30

34. JP Hubschman JL Bourges W Choi A Mozayan A Tsirbas 2010 'The Microhand:' a new concept of micro-forceps for the ocular robotic surgery Eye 24 364 7
35. Bergeles C, Kummer MP, Kratochvil BE, Framme C, Nelson BJ. Steerable intravitreal inserts for drug delivery: in vitro and ex vivo mobility experiments. In: Procedings of the 14th international conference on medical image computing and computer assisted intervention; 2011
36. Gijbels A, Vander Poorten EB, Gorissen B, Devreker A, Stalmans P, Reynaerts D Experimental validation of a robotic comanipulation and telemanipulation system for retinal surgery; 2014
37. Caers P, Gijbels A, De Volder M, Gorissen B, Stalmans P, Reynaers D, Vander Poorten EB. Precision experiments on a comanipulated robotic system for use in retinal surgery. In: Proceedings of the 2011 SCATh joint workshop on new technologies for computer/robot assisted surgery; 2011 July; Graz; 2011.p. 11–13. 2011
38. X He V Geirt van P Gehlbach R Taylor 2015 Iordachita I (2015) IRIS: integrated robotic intraocular snake IEEE Int Conf Robot Autom. 2015 1764 9
39. Rahimy E, Wilson J, Tsao TC, Schwartz S, JP H. Robot-assisted intraocular surgery: development of the IRISS and feasibility studies in an animal model. Eye (Lond). 2013;27(8):972–8
40. Eye, robot, the ophthalmologist. 2015:19–25
41. Preceyes enters into collaborations with Nighstar and the University of Oxford to develop subretinal drug delivery technology. Press Release. Accessed 9 May 2016.
42. T Bourcier J Chammas PH Becmeur J Danan A Sauer D Gaucher P Liverneaux D Mutter 2015 Robotically assisted pterygium surgery: first human case Cornea 34 10 1329 30
43. J Marescaux J Leroy M Gagner 2001 Transatlantic robot-assisted telesrugery Nature 413 379 80
44. J Marescaux J Leroy F Rubino 2002 Transcontinental robot-assisted remote telesurgery: feasibility and potential applications Ann Surg 235 487 92
45. J Marescaux F Rubino 2004 Robot-assisted remote surgery: technological advances, potential complications, and solutions Surg Technol Int. 12 23 6
46. A Shademan R Decker J Opfermann S Leonard A Krieger P Kim 2016 Supervised autonomous robotic soft tissue surgery Sci Transl Med. 4 337
47. JC Rosser M Wood JH Payne TM Fullum GB Lisehorn LE Rosser PJ Barcia RS Savalgi 1997 Telementoring: a practical option in surgical training Surg Endosc 11 852 5
48. BR Lee JA Caddedu G Janetschek P Schulman SG Docimo RG Moore AW Partin LR Kavoussi 1998 International surgical telementoring: our initial experience Stud Health Technol Inform. 50 41 7
49. BR Lee DJ Png L Liew M Fabrizio MK Li JW Jarrett LR Kavoussi 2000 Laparoscopic telesurgery between the United States and Singapore Ann Acad Med Singapore 29 655 68
50. BR Lee JT Bishoff G Janetschek P Bunyaratevej W Kamolpronwijit JA Cadeddu S Ratchanon S O'Kelley LR Kavoussi 1998 A novel method of surgical instruction: international telementoring World J Urol 16 367 70
51. Micali S, Virgili G, Vannozzi E, Grassi N, Jarrett TW, Bauer JJ, Vespasiani G, JAvoussi JR. Feasibility of telementoring between Baltimore (USA) and Rome, Italy. J Endourol. 2000;14:493–6
52. E Taniguchi S Ohashi 2000 Construction of a regional telementoring network for endoscopic surgery in Japan IEEE Trans Inf Technol Biomed 4 195 9
53. M Cubano BK Poulouse MA Talamini R Stewart LE Antosek R Lentz R Nibe M Nutka M Mendoza-Sagaon 1999 Long disgtance telementoring: a novel tool for laparpscopy aboard the USS Abraham Lincoln Surg Endosc 13 673 8

Index

U. Spandau and G. B. Scharioth (eds.), *Cutting Edge of Ophthalmic Surgery*,
https://doi.org/10.1007/978-3-031-84204-7